Contemporary
Geriatric
Medicine

Volume 1

Contemporary
Geriatric Medicine

Editor-in-Chief: STEVEN R. GAMBERT • Milwaukee, Wisconsin

A Continuation Order Plan is available for this series. A continuation order will bring delivery of each new volume immediately upon publication. Volumes are billed only upon actual shipment. For further information please contact the publisher.

Contemporary
Geriatric
Medicine

Volume 1

Edited by

Steven R. Gambert, M.D.

Chief, Section of Geriatrics and Gerontology
Department of Medicine
Associate Professor of Medicine and Physiology
The Medical College of Wisconsin
Milwaukee, Wisconsin

Geriatrician-in-Chief
Long-Term Care Gerontology Center
Milwaukee, Wisconsin

Chief, Geriatrics Section
Medical Service
Wood Veterans Administration Medical Center
Wood (Milwaukee), Wisconsin

PLENUM MEDICAL BOOK COMPANY
NEW YORK AND LONDON

Library of Congress Cataloging in Publication Data

Main entry under title:

Contemporary geriatric medicine.

(Contemporary geriatrics)
Includes bibliographical references and index.
1. Geriatrics. I. Gambert, Steven R., 1949–
RC952.C594 1983   618.97   83-10978

ISBN-13: 978-1-4684-4516-9   e-ISBN-13: 978-1-4684-4514-5
DOI: 10.1007/978-1-4684-4514-5

© 1983 Plenum Publishing Corporation
233 Spring Street, New York, N.Y. 10013
Softcover reprint of the hardcover 1st edition 1983

Plenum Medical Book Company is an imprint of Plenum Publishing Corporation

Contributors

RONALD D. ADELMAN, M.D. ● Instructor in Clinical Medicine, Division of General Medicine, Department of Medicine, College of Physicians and Surgeons, Columbia University, New York, New York 10032

URIEL S. BARZEL, M.D. ● Associate Professor of Medicine, Endocrine Section, Department of Medicine, Montefiore Hospital and Medical Center, Albert Einstein College of Medicine, Bronx, New York 10467

EDWARD W. CAMPION, M.D. ● Chief, Geriatrics Unit, Massachusetts General Hospital; and Instructor in Medicine, Division on Aging, Harvard Medical School, Boston, Massachusetts 02115

EDMUND H. DUTHIE, JR., M.D. ● Assistant Professor of Medicine, Associate Chief, Section of Geriatrics and Gerontology, Department of Medicine, The Medical College of Wisconsin, Milwaukee, Wisconsin 53226; and Chief, Nursing Home Care Unit, Wood Veterans Administration Medical Center, Wood, Wisconsin 53193

CORNELIUS J. FOLEY, M.D. ● Medical Director, Jewish Institute for Geriatric Care, New Hyde Park, New York 11042; Assistant Professor, School of Medicine, State University of New York at Stony Brook, Stony Brook, New York 11794; and Chief of Geriatric Medical Education, Long Island Jewish and Hillside Medical Center, New Hyde Park, New York 11040

STEVEN R. GAMBERT, M.D. ● Chief, Section of Geriatrics and Gerontology, Department of Medicine, Associate Professor of Medicine and Physiology, The Medical College of Wisconsin, Milwaukee, Wisconsin 53226; Geriatrician-in-Chief, Milwaukee Long-Term Care Gerontology Center, Milwaukee, Wisconsin 53226; Chief, Geriatrics Section, Medical Service, Wood Veterans Administration Medical Center, Wood, Wisconsin 53193;

and Director, Geriatrics Service, Milwaukee County Medical Complex, Milwaukee, Wisconsin 53226.

MICHELE G. GREENE, M.D. ● Staff Associate, Division of General Medicine, Department of Medicine, College of Physicians and Surgeons, Columbia University, New York, New York 10032

STEPHEN C. JACOBS, M.D. ● Associate Professor of Urology, Department of Urology, The Medical College of Wisconsin, Milwaukee, Wisconsin 53226; and Chief, Urology Section, Surgery Service, Wood Veterans Administration Medical Center, Wood, Wisconsin 53193

FRED G. KANTROWITZ, M.D. ● Chief of Rheumatology Unit, Beth Israel Hospital; and Assistant Professor of Medicine, Harvard Medical School, Boston, Massachusetts 02115

MICHAEL H. KEELAN, JR., M.D. ● Professor of Medicine, Section of Cardiology, Department of Medicine, The Medical College of Wisconsin, Milwaukee, Wisconsin 53226; and Milwaukee County Medical Center, Milwaukee, Wisconsin 53226

DONALD A. MAHLER, M.D. ● Chief, Pulmonary Function Laboratory, and Assistant Professor of Medicine, Pulmonary Section, Department of Medicine, Dartmouth Medical School, Hanover, New Hampshire 03756

GABE J. MALETTA, M.D. ● Program Director, Geriatric Research, Education, and Clinical Center, Minneapolis Veterans Administration Medical Center, Minneapolis, Minnesota 55417

MARC L. MILLER, M.D. ● Rheumatology Fellow, Beth Israel Hospital; and Clinical Fellow in Medicine, Harvard Medical School, Boston, Massachusetts 02115

JOSEPH B. MURPHY, M.D. ● Assistant Professor of Urology, Department of Urology, The Medical College of Wisconsin, Milwaukee, Wisconsin 53226

THOMAS W. SHEEHY, M.D. ● Professor of Medicine, The University of Alabama in Birmingham, School of Medicine, Department of Medicine; and Chief, Medical Services, Veterans Administration Medical Center, Birmingham, Alabama 35233

MICHAEL M. STEWART, M.D. ● Associate Professor of Clinical Medicine, Division of General Medicine, Department of Medicine, College of Physicians and Surgeons, Columbia University, New York, New York 10032; and Vice President, The Rockefeller Foundation, New York, New York 10036

REIN TIDEIKSAAR, P.A., Ph.D. ● Coordinator of Geriatric Education, Department of Geriatrics and Adult Development, and Assistant Professor of Geriatrics, Mt. Sinai School of Medicine, New York, New York 10029

PANAYIOTIS D. TSITOURAS, M.D. ● Assistant Professor of Medicine, Sections of Geriatrics and Gerontology and of Endocrinology, Department of Medicine, The Medical College of Wisconsin, Milwaukee, Wisconsin 53226; and Staff Geriatrician, Geriatrics Section, Medical Service, Wood Veterans Administration Medical Center, Wood, Wisconsin 53193

Preface

This volume marks the first of a new series, *Contemporary Geriatric Medicine,* joining the ever growing "Contemporary" family. As with the other "Contemporary" volumes, our goal is to assist the reader in maintaining currency in a rapidly changing field. Perhaps no field has shown such major advances in such a short time as geriatrics. Over the last several years, the "demographic imperative" has become a source of concern for many, including clinicians, scientists, economists, and health planners.

Our geriatric knowledge base continues to grow, often making it difficult to keep abreast of advances and current therapeutic modalities. *Contemporary Geriatric Medicine* presents the state-of-the-art thinking regarding a variety of topics all of major concern to the health practitioner caring for the elderly person. The authors, for the most part serving as members of a stable editorial board, have chosen topics that should have immediate interest to the readership. By having a stable editorial board, continuity is ensured in successive volumes. Every two years, a subsequent issue will either address new thoughts on already presented topics or focus on new topics of current interest. As with the other "Contemporary" series volumes, the every other year interval is intended to allow new findings to develop and be tested. It also provides the authors with time to provide the highest quality of work.

In attempting to present the state of the art of geriatric medicine, we dedicate this book to the clinician who cares for the elderly on a continuing basis. Geriatricians, although skilled in the special needs and problems of the elderly, are few and far between and can only scratch the surface in providing comprehensive health care for the growing number of elderly. By presenting an easy-to-read group of essays, we attempt to keep the nongeriatrician abreast of the current state of the art regarding the special needs and problems of the elderly.

In this first volume, our editorial board has been given the liberty of providing whatever background information they felt necessary to place their topics into proper perspective. Material has not been confined to that which has appeared during the preceding year. As with the other "Contemporary" volumes, the emphasis has been to introduce new material within the context of earlier work and also what is likely to result in the future.

The editors are appreciative of the opportunity given to develop the *Contemporary Geriatric Medicine* series. Particular thanks go to Ms. Hilary Evans of Plenum for her steadfast confidence. Appreciation is also given to our previous mentors who have helped mold our careers, to our secretaries, and to our families who have given support and understanding to this time-consuming venture. Most of all we thank our elderly patients for providing the clinician with the impetus to develop new strategies and knowledge upon which *Contemporary Geriatric Medicine* is based.

Steven R. Gambert

Milwaukee

Contents

Chapter 1
Geriatric Cardiology and Blood Pressure

Edmund H. Duthie, Jr., and Michael H. Keelan, Jr.

Chapter 2
Pulmonary Aspects of Aging

Donald A. Mahler

Chapter 3
Gastroenterology and the Elderly

Thomas W. Sheehy

Chapter 4
Rheumatology in Geriatrics

Marc L. Miller, Fred G. Kantrowitz, and Edward W. Campion

Chapter 5
Genitourinary Problems in the Elderly

Stephen C. Jacobs and Joseph B. Murphy

Chapter 6
Endocrinology and Metabolism in the Elderly

Uriel S. Barzel, Steven R. Gambert, and Panayiotis D. Tsitouras

Chapter 7
Neuropsychiatric Problems in the Elderly

Gabe J. Maletta

Chapter 8
Nutritional Problems in the Elderly

Cornelius J. Foley and Rein Tideiksaar

Chapter 9
Preventive Medicine for the Elderly

Ronald D. Adelman, Michele G. Greene, and Michael M. Stewart

Geriatric Cardiology and Blood Pressure

Edmund H. Duthie, Jr., and Michael H. Keelan, Jr.

1.1. Cardiovascular Morbidity–Mortality

Degenerative disease of the cardiovascular system remains the leading cause of mortality and morbidity in the elderly patient. Coronary artery disease accounts for approximately 40% of all deaths beyond age 55 years.[1] An impressive reduction in fatalities due to ischemic heart disease has been seen in the United States during the past 15 years. This favorable statistic applies to both sexes, whites and nonwhites, and patients over age 65 years as well. For white males age 65 to 74 years, the death rate from ischemic heart disease has fallen from 2119 per 100,000 in 1968 to 1642 per 100,000 in 1977.[1] The decrease in mortality has not been accompanied by a comparable reduction in the incidence of coronary attacks (Framingham study).[2] Nonetheless, reduction in mortality does appear to be real and there are multifactoral explanations for it. Change in smoking habits, awareness of diet, better physical fitness, new pharmacologic agents, and coronary bypass all play a responsible role. Other therapeutic advances, particularly in the prevention and treatment of rheumatic fever and the surgical treatment of cardiac disease,

EDMUND H. DUTHIE, JR. • Section of Geriatrics and Gerontology, Department of Medicine, The Medical College of Wisconsin, Milwaukee, Wisconsin 53226; and Nursing Home Care Unit, Wood Veterans Administration Medical Center, Wood, Wisconsin 53193.   MICHAEL H. KEELAN, JR. • Section of Cardiology, Department of Medicine, The Medical College of Wisconsin, Milwaukee, Wisconsin 53226; and Milwaukee County Medical Center, Milwaukee, Wisconsin 53226.

have increased the lifespan of cardiac patients. Degenerative disease superimposed on preexisting valvular heart disease has resulted in an increasing population of elderly patients with "hybrid" heart disease. Appropriate therapy depends on early recognition of the underlying disease process and understanding its pathophysiology. This task is made more difficult because the clinical history is often atypical or the physical signs are masked by the effects of aging on the cardiovascular system. It is appropriate to review the consequences of aging on the cardiovascular system at this point.

1.2. Cardiovascular Anatomy and Physiology

1.2.1. Anatomic Changes

Anatomic changes occur in the heart and peripheral arteries with advancing age. Minor degrees of calcification of the aortic and mitral valves have been described in up to 33% of autopsies in patients over age 70 years who had no cardiac failure.[3] Progression of this process results in atrioventricular conduction block and aortic stenosis.[4,5] The large arteries develop intimal thickening and cellular proliferation. Modified smooth muscle cells enter the intima and synthesize connective tissue proteins and polysaccharides. Lipid accumulates in the media and elastin fibers are lost or become cross-linked while calcium is deposited. Arteries with the most elastin have the greatest amount of calcification (iliac > coronary > renal > hepatic > aorta). There is increased collagen in all layers of the vessel wall. Blood vessel deformation, force transmission, and elasticity are a function of these fiberous proteins. Bader has shown that increased stiffness does occur in large vessels with advancing age.[6] In smaller blood vessels (arterioles), similar changes have been reported. Basement membrane thickening has been described in the capillaries of some vascular beds. These biochemical and anatomic vascular changes contribute to the increase in peripheral resistance that occurs with aging and the resultant rise in impedance (afterload) to cardiac ejection. The same changes may explain the decline in baroreceptor sensitivity in the elderly.[7]

1.2.2. Intrinsic Cardiac Function

Peak heart rate response to maximal exercise decreases with age. There is no significant difference in the resting heart rate, however. Resting cardiac output is lower in elderly individuals and an increase in output with exercise is limited by both decreased stroke volume and limited heart rate response.[8] Maximal aerobic capacity, which defines the limits of the oxygen transport system, is necessarily reduced as well.

1.2.3. Autonomic Reflexes

The primary function of the circulatory system is to maintain blood flow and tissue perfusion over a wide variety of physiologic demands. Although certain regional vascular beds (cerebral, renal, coronary) maintain autoregulatory control mechanisms, the circulatory system as a whole depends upon a series of complex reflexes to regulate systemic blood pressure and flow. The carotid baroreceptors have been studied most extensively. There has been increasing interest in the role of cardiopulmonary receptors more recently. The integrity of these reflex arcs assures that vital organ perfusion is maintained despite abrupt change in position or level of activity. Change in heart rate, peripheral vascular resistance, or cardiac contractility reflect the activation of cardiovascular reflexes. Disturbances in autonomic function may occur as a result of alteration in the afferent limb, efferent limb, or the "gain" of the reflex itself. Chronic congestive heart failure, chronic renal failure, diabetes mellitus, many neurologic disorders, and some cases of hypertension are but a few of the disorders which have been associated with abnormal baroreceptor response. Attenuation of baroreceptor activity has also been described as a function of age.[7]

1.2.4. Pulse Wave Characteristics

Pulsatile flow of blood into the central aorta produces a characteristic pressure wave. The normal arterial pressure pulse depends on several factors including the distensibility of the central aorta, the stroke volume, the rate of peripheral runoff, and the reflection of waves from the periphery. The initial upstroke or percussion wave precedes a brief anacrotic delay which is followed by the tidal wave producing the peak pressure of the aortic pulse curve. The tidal wave presumably results from the summation of waves that are reflected from the periphery. The less distensible central aorta in the elderly patient results in a higher peak pressure for a given stroke volume. Stiffer peripheral vessels increase the velocity of the reflected waves thereby producing an earlier tidal wave with attenuation of the anacrotic notch. These changes can mask serious aortic stenosis in elderly patients.

1.3. Clinical Evaluation

Tortuosity of the great vessels can impede venous return. Unilateral cervical venous distention (usually left) is seen most commonly. The full-blown superior vena cava syndrome may be the presenting finding in a patient with ascending aortic aneurysm. Auscultation of the heart in the geriatric patient is often complicated by deformities of the chest wall or chronic obstructive lung disease. The pulmonic component of S2 is frequently indistinct and all heart tones may be difficult to hear. If the second sound is single, it may be impossible to distinguish whether it is due to aortic or pulmonary valve closure. This is particularly perplexing in the assessment of elderly patients with ejection murmurs in whom the diagnosis of aortic valvular stenosis is suspected. Auscultation over the carotid arteries is helpful since the aortic component of S2 is usually heard clearly in the great vessels and the absence of this sound strongly suggests that A2 is diminished. A soft fourth heart sound is commonly heard in patients over 40 years and is not necessarily an indication of ventricular pathology. A palpable apical A wave (the equivalent of a loud S4) does indicate left ventricular dysfunction, often a pathologic reduction in compliance. Auscultation of a third heart sound in the elderly patient almost always indicates underlying left ventricular failure, although a physiologic S3 may be heard in patients with high output states secondary to thyrotoxicosis, anemia, or A-V fistulae. A high-frequency early systolic click generally reflects pathology of the aortic valve, but it may be heard in association with dilatation of the ascending aorta alone. Nonejection clicks are most often heard in mid-systole and may be multiple. These clicks usually indicate pathology of the mitral valve. Similar sounds may accompany pleural or pericardial disease. Routine examination of elderly patients commonly discloses a cardiac murmur. Cardiac murmurs have been described in 50 to 60% of patients over 65 years.[9] The majority of the murmurs are related to ejection of blood into the aorta. They are best heard at the base of the heart and are confined to early or mid-systole, the period of peak blood flow. These murmurs are associated with dilatation of the ascending aorta and/or sclerosis of the aortic valve. The valve orifice is rarely compromised and there is no commissural fusion. Dense calcific deposits on the aortic leaflets impede valve opening even though commissural involvement is minimal. This is the characteristic finding in elderly patients with calcific aortic stenosis. The murmur associated with significant obstruction is longer in duration and most frequently the aortic component of S2 is diminished, if not absent. Conversely, A2 may be accentuated when the murmur is associated with dilatation of the aorta and hypertension. Calcification of the mitral annulus often coexists with aortic valvar calcification. This disorder, which is more prevalent in women than in men, results in a prominent musical systolic murmur in the mid-precordium or at the apex. A diastolic rumble may be present as well although hemodynamic obstruction due to mitral annular calcification alone is infrequent.[10] Diastolic blowing murmurs most often indicate disease of the aortic valve, but if the murmur is heard best at the right sternal border, disease of the aortic root should be suspected. Frequently, these murmurs are evanescent. A patient presenting with congestive heart failure and no evidence of a murmur develops an obvious murmur several days later. The question of infectious endocarditis is raised inevitably. Conversely, a prominent diastolic blowing murmur which subsequently disappears may be heard in a patient who presents with chest pain. In this setting, the diagnosis of dissection of the aorta is considered. Improvement of cardiac output accompanying cardiac compensation results in a larger stroke volume and the appearance of a murmur in the former case, although the increase in peripheral vascular resistance which accompanies ischemic chest pain will exaggerate mild preexisting valvar incompetence in the latter instance.

Bruits over the cervical and supraclavicular arteries usually indicate pathology in the underlying vessels. In the absence of any murmur in the chest, this is generally a safe conclusion. However, it is often difficult to distinguish a referred cardiac murmur from a primary bruit in the elderly patient with combined disease. Quantitative analysis of arterial bruits using phonoangiography may be a useful method for evaluating these patients.[11] Careful evaluation of peripheral pulses is mandatory in all patients. Totally inappropriate therapy may be administered to a patient in whom upper extremity blood pressure is misrepresentative because of obstructive disease in the aortic arch or its major branches.

1.4. Laboratory Investigations

1.4.1. Electrocardiogram

The laboratory assessment of the elderly patient with suspected or proven cardiovascular disease requires a basic appreciation of the validity and potential pitfalls of the multiple tests that are available. The resting electrocardiogram and standard chest X ray still comprise the baseline evaluation for most patients. Fisch studied 671 elderly patients and found a prevalence of abnormal ECGs in 46%.[12] Abnormal left axis deviation, first degree A-V block, ST-T changes, premature atrial and ventricular systole, and atrial fibrillation were found frequently. Left bundle branch block was noted in 5% of the patients, while right bundle branch block was present in 7%. This high prevalence of abnormal ECGs did not necessarily correlate with clinical heart disease, though left bundle branch block, nonspecific intraventricular conduction defects, ST-T changes, and atrial fibrillation were more likely to be so associated. In the Tecumseh study, supraventricular premature systoles were noted in 73 per 1000 standard ECGs on patients over 70.[13] Ventricular prematures were found in 128 per 1000 patients in the same population. Subsequent studies using ambulatory monitoring found an even higher prevalence of arrhythmias. Camm et al. found major ventricular arrhythmias in 30% of 106 patients over age 75 years who were monitored for 24 hr.[14] Nonetheless, the prognosis for patients with abnormal ECGs appears to relate to clinically detectable heart disease rather than the ECG finding alone.[12] The resting ECG provides limited information regarding the cardiac rhythm or latent ischemic heart disease and no information regarding myocardial function.

1.4.2. Exercise Cardiography

Judicious use of noninvasive tests in patients with suspected ischemic heart disease provides data which is not only diagnostic but prognostic as well in many cases. Despite the adverse publicity which it has received in recent years, the graded exercise ECG is still used by most physicians to detect or confirm the diagnosis of occult coronary artery disease. This test is redundant as a diagnostic procedure in patients with classic angina pectoris whose probability of having coronary artery disease approaches 90%.[15] The predictive accuracy of the stress ECG is not that high, particularly when the resting ECG is abnormal. The test may be useful, however, as a prognostic indicator since hypotension, ST segment depression greater than 2 mm, angina pectoris, or high-grade ventricular arrhythmias which appear in the first stage of an exercise test suggest more severe disease with its attendant risk of mortality and morbidity.[16] In patients with atypical angina pectoris, the incidence of coronary artery disease approaches 50%.[15]

1.4.3. Nuclear Cardiology

The addition of radionuclide scans to the exercise protocol has enhanced the predictive accuracy for patients with atypical pain as well as those whose resting ECGs are abnormal because of bundle branch block or abnormal ST segments. The diagnostic sensitivity of the thallium-201 perfusion scan and technetium-99 ventriculographic scan are similar, but the low specificity (50%) of the latter test makes it less predictive.[17] Thallium-201 is a potassium analogue which is distributed to the myocardium in proportion to blood flow. It is injected intravenously at the peak of exercise and multiview images are obtained within 10 min after the exercise has been completed. Reduction in perfusion is manifested by decreased uptake in that myocardial region. A delayed resting scan is usually performed if the exercise study is abnormal. Persistence of a perfusion defect may be related to prior myocardial infarction (MI) or severe underlying myocardial ischemia. False-positive thallium-201 perfusion scans have been described in patients with cardiomyopathies, particularly hypertrophic cardiomyopathy, and occasionally in patients with mitral valve prolapse. The test should provide 80 to 90% sensitivity with a similar specificity.[17] Its diagnostic accuracy decreases significantly if the patient is not exercised to a satisfactory level. Preferably, this would be a symptom-limited stress test, but the patient should be exercised to a minimum of 85% of his predicted maximum heart rate in the absence of symptoms.

The exercise nuclear ventriculogram assesses myocardial wall motion and ejection fraction in response to stress. The normal ventricle improves its contractile pattern with exercise. Ejection fraction increases by at least 5% and no wall motion abnormalities are noted.[17] The sensitivity of this test for detecting coronary disease is based on the observation that the ischemic ventricle increases its end-systolic volume, decreases its ejection fraction, and/or develops a regional wall motion abnormality. After the blood pool is labeled, a resting study is performed in several projections. Exercise is completed with a bicycle ergometer in either the upright or supine position. Intermediate and maximal exercise data is collected and compared to the resting data. The shortcomings of this test include the difficulty inherent in the testing mechanics—many patients develop leg fatigue before adequate cardiac stress has occurred—and the number of false-positive tests. Port et al. found no increase in ejection fraction with exercise in the majority of normal subjects over age 60, and in those over 70 years the ejection fraction fell significantly.[18] For this reason, it is not recommended as a diagnostic test in the geriatric patient. When accompanied by a fall in systolic blood pressure and an increase in end-systolic volume, a reduction in exercise ejection fraction portends a poor outcome for patients with known coronary artery disease.[19] The resting nuclear ventriculogram is used extensively to analyze ventricular function noninvasively. It is a safe, accurate method to evaluate cardiac performance and can be repeated after a variety of interventions to assess improvement or deterioration in function. Since ventricular function is the ultimate predictor of outcome for most, if not all, patients with heart disease, this information can be used by the clinician to establish optimal therapeutic regimens. Demonstration of a discrete ventricular aneurysm by this technique would dictate in favor of surgical consideration although vasodilator therapy would be preferred if the ventricle is diffusely hypokinetic.

Myocardial infarction may also be identified by nuclear techniques. The technetium-99 pyrophosphate scan is a sensitive test for identifying myocardial necrosis.[20] It is a redundant test if the diagnosis of infarction is evident by conventional means. It is most helpful for identifying infarction in the presence of preexisting ECG abnormalities, e.g., left bundle branch block, or when myocardial enzymes are elevated as a result of trauma or surgery. Since the test is usually positive for 7 or more days, it is also helpful in identifying myocardial necrosis in patients whose hospitalization may have been delayed for several days after an acute episode. The scan is not positive for 24 to 48 hr after MI and it should not be obtained before that time. It is often negative in the presence of small nontransmural infarction.[20]

1.4.4. Echocardiography

The echocardiographic examination of the heart affords a precise method for revealing all cardiac chambers, the pericardium, the valves, and the septa. Ventricular wall motion can be assessed accurately using the wide-angle sector scan commonly referred to as two-dimensional echo. The technique does have recognizable limitations which relate to unusual chest wall configurations or underlying lung pathology. These factors may limit the value of the study in some elderly patients. Both echocardiography and nuclear ventriculography offer accurate noninvasive methods for evaluating left ventricular function.

1.4.5. Ambulatory Electrocardiography

Many symptoms in elderly patients are potentially attributable to disorders of the heart rhythm. Minor arrhythmias or conduction delays which are discovered on the standard ECG can represent the "tip of the iceberg." The ambulatory Holter scan is used to detect intermittent heart block or paroxysms of atrial or ventricular tachyarrhythmia which would not be evident on the routine ECG. The 24-hr ECG often provides sufficient "clues" to the basic pathophysiology, even if there are no symptomatic episodes during the period of monitoring. Attacks which occur sporadically can also be assessed. Using a monitor which is applied at the onset of symptoms, the ECG is transmitted transtelephonically to a central recorder (often a CCU).

1.4.6. Computerized Tomography

The uses for computerized axial tomography have expanded in recent years. In our institution, it has been a valuable technique for assessing patients with potential dissection of the aorta. Sixteen of 17 dissections were identified correctly and the false-negative was also missed at the time of standard contrast aortography using invasive catheterization. The invasive study is recommended to identify the site of intimal tear more clearly once a dissection has been defined by CT scan. Current investigations are evaluating computerized tomography for visualization of the coronary arteries.

1.4.7. Invasive Procedures

1.4.7.1. Catheterization and Angiography

Any discussion of cardiologic tests would be incomplete without considering the role of invasive diagnostic procedures. Cardiac catheterization and angiography are reserved for the evaluation of patients who are potential candidates for surgical intervention. The risks involved are frequently overemphasized, particularly by individuals who are poorly informed. In a study comprising over 7500 patients who were catheterized as part of the Coronary Artery Surgery Study, the mortality rate was 0.2% and the incidence of MI was 0.25%. Systemic embolization occurred in 0.09% of the patients.[21] Hemodynamic instability rather than age is a predictor of complications. Each physician must be aware of the incidence of complications in laboratories to which he refers patients regularly.

1.4.7.2. Electrophysiology

In addition to the standard hemodynamic and angiographic procedures, invasive electrophysiologic studies are now being performed routinely in many centers. These studies are most helpful in evaluating patients with complex tachyarrhythmias or conduction abnormalities. The efficacy of antiarrhythmic agents has been established by testing patients before and after drug therapy.[22] Serious arrhythmias which have been suspected or demonstrated previously are reproduced in the laboratory. Many of these patients have symptomatic ventricular arrhythmias and are candidates for sudden death. Thorough evaluation frequently takes many hours to complete. Despite the nature of the arrhythmias and the duration of the test, the risks are remarkably low.

Aware of the potential pitfalls in the physical examination and laboratory evaluation of the elderly patient, we shall consider specific disease processes in more detail.

1.5. Coronary Artery Disease

1.5.1. Presentation and Diagnosis

Manifestations of coronary artery disease in the elderly may be quite atypical. Neurologic symptoms including confusion, weakness, and transient cerebral vascular events frequently replace the classic symptoms of anginal chest pain. Pathy reviewed the clinical presentation of MI in 387 patients over age 65 years.[23] Only 19% had the typical presentation. Dyspnea without pain was found in 20% and over 25% had neurologic presentations including confusion, stroke, or syncope. Ischemic heart disease must be suspected in patients who present with unexplained diaphoresis, dyspnea, confusion, or abdominal pain. Nonspecific ECG changes cloud the diagnosis further. In the absence of angina or electrocardiographic evidence of infarction, the diagnosis of ischemic heart disease is made by one or a combination of the tests described previously.

Recognition of ischemic heart disease invites the more perplexing question— What is the prognosis? Resting left ventricular dysfunction and multivessel coronary disease are predictors of a poor prognosis.[24] Jones et al. have found that prognosis may relate to the exercise response of the left ventricle regardless of the coronary anatomy.[25] Confirmation of these observations by other investigators would establish the exercise nuclear ventriculogram as an invaluable adjunct in the management of patients with established coronary disease.

1.5.2. Therapy

The treatment of patients with symptomatic coronary disease focuses on two clinical syndromes: (1) stable angina pectoris and (2) unstable disease including unstable angina pectoris and MI. Several factors have been responsible for a dramatic change in the medical approach to treatment. The pathophysiology of the ischemic process is better understood and potent pharmacologic agents have emerged.

Table I. Beta-Blocking Agents

	Relative beta$_1$ selective	Lipophilic	Usual dose range
Atenolol	+	+	50–200 mg 1×/day
Metoprolol	+	++	50–200 mg bid
Nadalol	0	+	40–320 mg 1×/day
Propranolol	0	+++	10–80 mg tid or qid
Timolol	0	+	10–30 mg bid

1.5.2.1. Beta-Blockers

Beta-adrenergic blocking agents form the cornerstone of therapy for patients with symptomatic coronary disease. Recent reports suggest that these drugs may be protective against future coronary events as well.[26,27] Reduction in overall mortality (39.4%) and sudden death (44.6%) following acute MI was seen in the Norwegian Multicenter Study.[27] The Beta-Blocker Heart Attack Study Group found similar results in this country.[26] Mortality was reduced by 26%, and in both studies patients over age 65 years also benefited. Propranolol was the first beta-blocker released in this country. Newly available agents include timolol, atenolol, nadolol, and metoprolol. A recent review by Frishman summarizes the activities of these newer drugs.[28] Although beta$_1$ selective blockade or hydrophilic properties may make one drug better tolerated than another, it is clear that all drugs are effective in managing cardiovascular disease when given in appropriate dosage (Table I). Severe bronchospasm (even with selective beta$_1$-blockers) and congestive heart failure are serious side effects. Fatigue, lassitude, nightmares, and gastrointestinal upset are annoying. Bradycardia is normally seen with beta-receptor blockers, but disproportionate reduction in heart rate may occur at relatively low doses. It is advised that beta-blocker therapy be initiated at low doses with titration to a level which controls symptoms. These drugs are effective because they reduce myocardial oxygen demand. While present data suggest that larger doses of propranolol reduce mortality after MI, it remains to be seen whether or not a smaller dose will accomplish the same result.

1.5.2.2. Nitrate and Calcium Channel Blockers

Nitroglycerin and other nitrates are added to the regimen to further reduce oxygen requirement by decreasing myocardial wall tension. Nitroglycerin also results in a more favorable distribution of myocardial blood flow. Documentation of vasospasm as a mechanism for myocardial ischemia and infarction has resulted in the widespread use of calcium channel blockers, such as verapamil and nifedipine, which are potent vasodilators. These drugs have been released recently in this country and an extensive review of drug mechanisms and merits has been

Table II. Calcium Channel Blocking Agents

	Vasodilation	Contractility	Conduction	Usual dosage
Verapamil	+ +	− −	− −	80–160 mg q 8 hr
Nifedipine	+ + +	0	0	10–30 mg tid or qid
Diltiazem	+ +	−	−	60–90 mg q 8 hr

reported by Stone et al.[29,30] The drugs not only relieve coronary vasospasm, but dilate peripheral vessels as well. The latter effect results in decreased myocardial wall tension by reducing afterload. Sinus node automaticity and A-V conduction are depressed and this effect is more prominent with verapamil than nifedipine.[31] Verapamil must be used with caution in patients who are being treated simultaneously with beta-blocking agents (Table II).

1.5.2.3. Antiplatelet Agents

The role of antiplatelet agents in the management of chronic ischemic heart disease remains controversial. The proposed mechanisms of potential benefit have been summarized in reviews of major clinical trials of aspirin, dipyrimadole, and sulfinpyrazone.[32] Although there are hypothetical reasons for using one or more of these drugs, the clinical proof of efficacy has not been established.

Pharmacologic management is the preferred therapeutic approach to the majority of stable symptomatic elderly patients with ischemic heart disease.

1.5.3. Unstable Angina

Progression or intractability of symptoms frequently portends a major coronary event. The patient should be hospitalized. Beta-blockers are increased to maximum levels (240 to 320 mg/day of propranolol or equivalent). Isosorbide in a dose of 10 to 40 mg every 6 hr and/or transcutaneous nitroglycerin may be of use. A calcium channel blocker is added in appropriate dosage. Many geriatric patients lead very vigorous lifestyles and are not content to reduce activities while taking large doses of multiple medications. Persistence of symptoms, intolerance of medication, or reduction in lifestyle favor a more aggressive approach to therapy. Coronary angiography is recommended to these patients anticipating coronary bypass surgery or angioplasty for qualified patients.

1.5.4. Coronary Artery Surgery

Major cardiac surgery including coronary bypass can be performed in the elderly with only a modest increase in fatality and morbidity. Multiple reports cite acceptable mortality statistics (less than 5%) in patients undergoing coronary bypass after age 65.[33-35] Chronologic age should not preclude prescription of an effective form of therapy for these patients.

1.5.5. Myocardial Infarction

Management of acute MI in the elderly does not differ significantly from therapy of younger counterparts. Nontransmural infarction, characterized by lower peak enzyme levels and absence of electrocardiographic Q wave, should be managed as a potentially incomplete infarction. Therapy should be initiated as for unstable angina. Persistence of pain in the early stages of MI should be managed with intravenous beta-blockers and nitroglycerin. Invasive monitoring of left ventricular filling pressures is recommended in these patients. Intravenous beta-blockers should not be used in patients with hypotension, severe bradycardia, or heart failure. Emergency coronary angiography and intracoronary streptokinase infusion may be indicated in select cases. Low-dose heparin (5000 units every 12 hr) is administered subcutaneously. Full anticoagulation is recommended in patients with large infarctions, congestive heart failure, or documented embolic episodes. Continuous intravenous infusion of heparin is the preferred regimen. Intravenous therapy is monitored on a daily basis with partial thromboplastin time or an equivalent test. Platelet counts should be obtained on patients who are receiving heparin, since heparin-induced thrombocytopenia has been reported with increased frequency in recent years.[36] An aggressive approach to cardiac rehabilitation will decrease the need for prolonged anticoagulant therapy. Low-level exercise tests (5 METS or heart rate 130) are advised for active patients prior to discharge. In addition to providing prognostic information regarding recurrent cardiac events, the low-level stress test provides some measure of assurance to the patient that he can accomplish activities of daily living at home without difficulty.[37]

The management of coronary disease in the elderly patient should be a highly selective and individualized effort. This approach will assure that no patient will be denied the most appropriate therapy for his condition.

1.6. Cardiomyopathy

1.6.1. Amyloidosis

The geriatric patient is subject to several forms of cardiomyopathy. Presbycardia or "senile heart" disease was a fashionable diagnosis to explain heart failure in patients with apparently normal hearts. Pomerance found structurally normal hearts in only 2.5% of 162 patients over age 75 years who died with heart failure.[38] The same author described cardiac amyloidosis in 18% of patients dying in heart failure.[38] Amyloid was found incidentally in 5% of 208 patients who did not exhibit signs of congestive failure. Seventy-one percent of patients over 90 years who had heart failure had pathologic changes of cardiac amyloidosis. When amyloid deposits are limited to the atria, heart failure is not likely to be evident. Atrial fibrillation or arrhythmias may be present. Senile cardiac amyloidosis is more common in women than in men, but marked ventricular involvement is more common in men. Amyloid heart disease is characterized by electrocardiographic conduction defects, low QRS voltage, and pseudoinfarction patterns. Amyloid deposits result in myocardial restriction and the patients manifest signs which simulate constrictive pericarditis. The diagnosis should be suspected in the patient who presents with predominantly right heart failure and the previously noted ECG abnormalities. The echocardiogram may show unusual thickening of the valves, the septum, or increased echos resulting from the amyloid deposition in the myocardium.

1.6.2. Hypertrophic Cardiomyopathy

Hypertrophic cardiomyopathy, once considered to be a disease of the young, has been described with increased frequency in patients over 60 years. The widespread use of echocardiography accounts for an appreciation of this disease in the elderly. Symptoms of angina pectoris, syncope, or heart failure combined with the characteristic bifid carotid pulse, prominent jugular A wave, and the variable systolic murmur should alert the clinician to this diagnosis. Paradoxical aggravation of symptoms with use of conventional drugs (nitrates or digitalis) provides an additional clue.

1.7. Dissection of the Aorta

1.7.1. Diagnosis

Cystic medial necrosis occurs in early or midlife as a result of connective tissue disorders such as Marfan's syndrome or Ehlers–Danlos syndrome. It is now apparent that aortic cystic medial necrosis appears as a function of advancing age.[39] This condition predisposes to dissection of the aorta particularly in the presence of arterial hypertension. The diagnosis of aortic dissection presents no problem if the triad of aortic insufficiency, unequal peripheral pulses, and neurologic defecit are found in a patient who presents with abrupt onset of severe chest pain. Such typical presentations were rarely found in our own experience of over 150 cases of aortic dissection. The key to making the diagnosis is thinking of it at all. Stroke, renal colic, acute abdominal pain, acute MI, paraplegia, or the abrupt onset of a cold extremity reflect obstruction of a major artery. The chest X ray is rarely normal in patients with aortic dissection but the ectatic aorta is often thought to be consistent with the patient's age and hypertension alone. Aortic

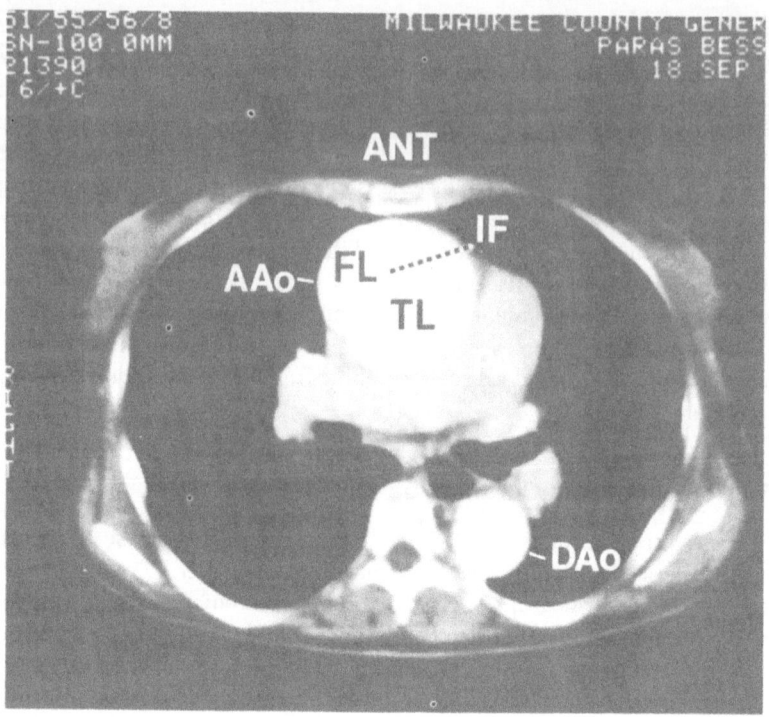

Figure 1. Thoracic CT scan with contrast. (AAo) ascending aorta; (DAo) descending aorta; (IF) intimal flap; (FL) false lumen; (TL) true lumen; (RPA) right pulmonary artery; (PA) pulmonary artery.

angiography had been the diagnostic procedure of choice, but computerized thoracic tomography has proven to be a useful screening technique (Fig. 1). Therapy should be instituted once the tentative diagnosis has been made since direct contrast angiography may precipitate rupture or extension of the dissection.

1.7.2. Therapy

Pharmacologic treatment comprises an intravenous antihypertensive (nitroprusside or trimethorphan) and beta-blockers. Surgical management must be considered on an urgent basis if the patient is hypotensive, has severe aortic regurgitation, intrapleural or intrapericardial hemorrhage, or occlusion of a major artery. Persistence of pain despite control of blood pressure is also an indication for early surgery. Surgical management is recommended for cases of dissection which involve the ascending aorta. Pharmacologic management has been successful in treating patients with dissection, but late complications are more frequent.[40] Elderly patients with complicating illnesses should be treated medically. Long-term management of all patients should include antihypertensives and beta-blockers.

1.8. Valvular Heart Disease

1.8.1. Aortic Valve Disease

Valvular heart disease is often suspected because of the high prevalence of cardiac murmurs in the elderly population. Calcific aortic stenosis is the most frequent cause of left ventricular outflow obstruction. In contrast to rheumatic or congenital aortic stenosis, both of which result in severe commissural effusion, stenosis occurs because of dense calcific deposits on the aortic side of the cusps. The mechanical impedance to outflow is often underestimated because the peripheral findings which characterize aortic stenosis in younger patients are lacking.[41] Associated arteriosclerotic disease of the aorta results in a moderate degree of systolic hypertension (160 to 180 mm Hg) in spite of a large peak systolic transvalvular gradient (50 to 120 mm Hg) (Fig. 2). The murmur is often louder at the apex due to lung disease or associated mitral annular calcification. This finding further confuses the diagnosis. Calcification is readily recognized at fluoroscopy or by echocardiography, but posterior–anterior chest X rays are misleading since the aortic valve overlies the thoracic spine. Differentiation of aortic stenosis from the commonly described aortic sclerosis (nonobstructive involvement of the annulus

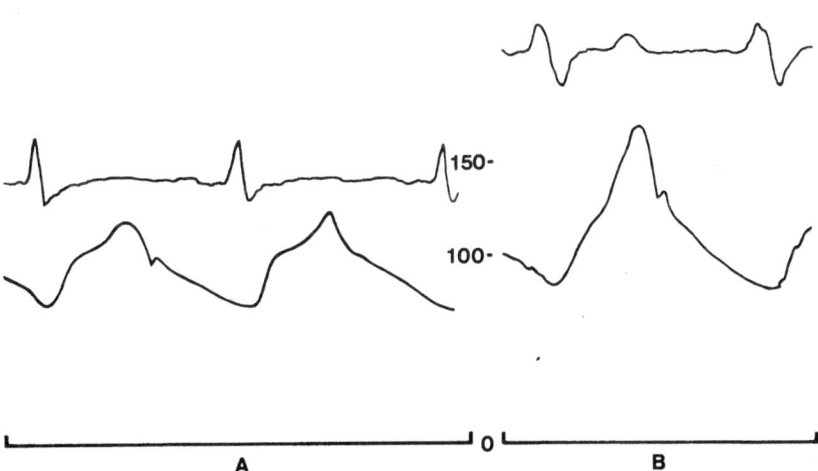

Figure 2. Aortic stenosis. Carotid pulse. Fast speed recording. Scale 0–150 mm Hg. (A) 25-year-old. Peak transvalvar gradient 60 mm Hg. (B) 76-year-old. Peak transvalvar gradient 100 mm Hg.

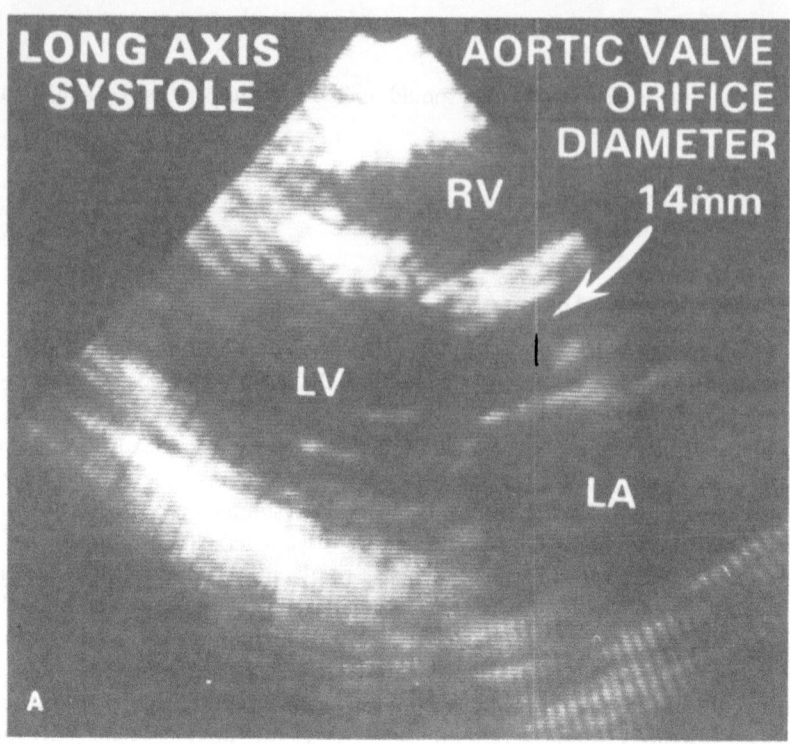

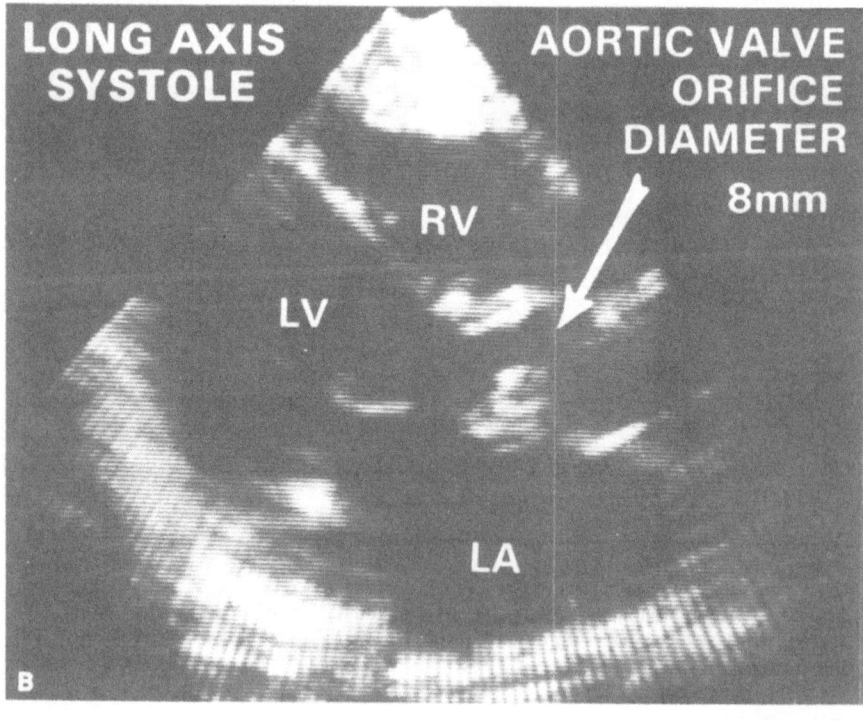

and leaflets) may be difficult in some patients. Transvalvular gradients have been correlated with the amount and pattern of calcium seen radiographically. Intensive "ring" calcification is generally associated with a significant gradient.[42] Two-dimensional echocardiography helps to distinguish the lesions in patients whose aortic valve orifice can be outlined clearly (Fig. 3).[43] Dense calcification is very echogenic and may preclude identification of the orifice. Ventricular wall thickness and motion are also useful in the differential diagnosis. Cardiac catheterization is indicated in the presence of clinical signs and symptoms of severe disease. When symptoms are questionably related to valvular obstruction and the degree of stenosis is not well delineated by noninvasive means, catheterization should be performed. Calcific aortic stenosis may progress dramatically within 2 to 3 years.[44] Thus, patients with modest gradients and minimal symptoms require careful and frequent reevaluation.

1.8.2. Mitral Valve Disease

Rheumatic mitral stenosis, most frequently a disease of middle age, may progress with such indolence that the major manifestations are delayed until the seventh or even eighth decade. In our clinic, several new cases of mitral stenosis are "discovered" each year in elderly patients, usually because of embolic complications. Moderate obstruction in the presence of a sedentary lifestyle need not result in severe dyspnea. Atrial fibrillation and hemostasis results in thrombus formation and embolization. Strokes or evidence of pseudobulbar palsy may result. Mitral stenosis should be considered in the differential diagnosis of stroke, regardless of age, particularly in the presence of atrial fibrillation. The echocardiogram is highly sensitive and the diagnostic test of choice. The mitral valve orifice can be quantitated using the sector scan.

Mitral Valve Prolapse

Mitral valve prolapse, another valvular lesion usually described in younger patients, may be responsible for major disability in elderly patients. We have shown a decided incidence of complication of prolapse including ruptured chordae tendenae and endocarditis. Of 40 patients over 60 years old with echocardiographic findings of mitral valve prolapse, congestive heart failure was noted in 25%.[45] Five patients required valve surgery and three of the five had ruptured chordae. Atypical chest pain, troublesome arrhythmias, or fleeting neurologic complaints in a patient with a variable systolic murmur or click should arouse suspicion of this diagnosis. Classical physical findings and/or the echocardiogram confirm its presence. Mitral valve prolapse is a syndrome with diverse causes and coronary artery disease should be considered in addition to myxomatous degen-

←───────────────────────────────────────

Figure 3. Aortic stenosis 2-D-echocardiogram. (A) Aortic sclerosis—no significant gradient. (B) Severe aortic stenosis—gradient 80 mm Hg.

eration. Sudden aggravation of symptoms and a murmur of increasing intensity may result from papillary muscle infarction or ischemia rather than endocarditis or chordal rupture.

1.8.3. Valve Surgery

The operative risk for valve replacement in the elderly is 2 to 3 times the average risk but is still highly acceptable.[33] Patients with symptomatic aortic valve disease should be considered for early operative intervention. Chronic mitral valve disease may be managed pharmacologically until disabling (NYHA Class II → III) symptoms dictate in favor of surgery. Acute regurgitant lesions of either the mitral or the aortic valve usually produce progressive heart failure which is refractory to medical management. Early hemodynamic assessment and surgical treatment is recommended since procrastination generally results in multisystem failure which increases the surgical risk significantly.

1.8.4. Endocarditis

The diagnosis of bacterial endocarditis in the elderly may be overlooked because of other more obvious signs or symptoms. In an autopsy study, Cooper et al. found almost half of the 68 undiagnosed cases occurred in patients over 65 years old.[46] These patients often presented with neurologic manifestations. Blood cultures should be obtained in any patient with fever and a heart murmur while the patient is being carefully evaluated for other evidence of endocarditis.

1.9. Atrial Septal Defect

Many congenital cardiac defects have been described in elderly patients. Other than aortic valve disease, atrial septal defect is the only lesion found with sufficient prevalence to be considered here. Atrial septal defect causes atrial arrhythmia, heart failure, and paradoxical arterial embolism. The murmur is frequently nonspecific and the clue to the diagnosis lies in the X ray, which demonstrates increased pulmonary blood flow, and the electrocardiogram, which usually demonstrates conduction delays in the right ventricle. Echocardiography is the diagnostic test of choice and it demonstrates large right ventricular dimensions with or without paradoxical motion of the interventricular septum.

1.10. Syncope

Neurologic signs and symptoms are common manifestations of heart disease in the elderly. Valvular disease, MI, dissection of the aorta, or endocarditis may be associated with focal or global neurologic deficits. Syncopal or presyncopal attacks may also reflect intrinsic neurologic disease or cerebral vascular disease. These symptoms are frequently elicited from patients who have abnormal ECGs. Findings of extra systoles, atrial fibrillation, mild sinus bradycardia, or bundle branch block arouse suspicion of a sustained arrhythmia as the explanation of "dizzy" spells. Pacemaker implantation is warranted for those patients whose symptoms are clearly related to documented bradyarrhythmias.

1.10.1. Heart Block

Longitudinal studies of elderly patients with bundle branch block have shown a low incidence of sudden death due to complete heart block. More often, morbidity and mortality in these patients is related to the underlying cardiac disease. Of 452 patients with chronic bifascicular block followed prospectively by Dhingra et al., 29 patients progressed to second- or third-degree heart block.[47] Twenty progressed spontaneously while 9 had an apparent cause. The cumulative incidence for spontaneous block was 7.1% at 5 years. Sudden death in 14% of these cases was most often due to ventricular fibrillation. This series was not restricted to elderly patients, although the mean age was 62 years. Rodstein et al. followed 300 patients whose average age was 82 years.[48] Ninety-seven patients had right bundle branch block and a hemiblock and 60 patients had left bundle branch block. The remainder had left anterior hemiblock. The cumulative risk for developing heart block was 1.5% per year for the first 5 years and 2.5% for each year thereafter. Risk was evenly divided between left and right bundle branch block and least for left anterior hemiblock alone. The need for invasive electrophysiologic studies and/or prophylactic pacing in asymptomatic patients with incomplete trifascicular block has been debated, but most investigators conclude that these studies and tests are not warranted.[49]

1.10.2. Sick Sinus Syndrome

Sinus node dysfunction is another cause for intermittent severe bradycardia. The sick sinus syndrome should be suspected as a cause for neurologic symptoms in patients with severe sinus bradycardia, sinoatrial block, or intermittent sinus arrest. An ectopic atrial rhythm may herald the onset of this syndrome, in which case the presenting sign may actually be a tachyarrhythmia. A ventricular pacemaker or in some cases an atrial-ventricular sequential pacemaker is the treatment of choice. Disorders of impulse formation may be due to otherwise silent MI and that diagnosis must be considered when symptoms begin abruptly.

1.10.3. Ventricular Arrythmias

The prevalence of ventricular premature beats in the elderly has already been discussed. Ventricular premature beats are often found incidentally on routine examination. The significance of this arrhythmia in a patient who presents with a syncopal or presyncopal attack must be assessed in that light. Ambulatory ECG monitoring is the most widely used means of assessing this problem. Documentation of ventricular tachycardia or finding high-grade ventricular arrhythmias in association with poor left ventricular function are indications for antiarrhythmic therapy.[50]

1.10.4. Diagnosis and Treatment

Instruction of the patient or an immediate family member in the technique of taking the pulse is an inexpensive and often productive means of identifying arrhythmogenic neurologic disorders. Invasive electrophysiologic studies are indicated in patients with recurrent unexplained episodes. DiMarco et al. established a presumptive electrophysiologic diagnosis in 17 of 25 patients with recurrent syncope of unknown cause.[51] A focal neurologic deficit is not explained on the basis of arrhythmia alone. Coexistent local vascular disease or a primary neurologic disorder must be considered. Two-dimensional echocardiography has been used as a "screening" examination for patients with neurologic deficits of unknown cause. Lovett et al. studied 138 patients with one or more episodes of focal cerebral ischemia using two-dimensional cardiac ultrasound.[52] Seventy percent of the studies provided no new information. The echo is most likely to provide helpful information if the patient has clinical evidence of heart disease with or without atrial fibrillation.

Vasodilation without arrhythmia may account for hypotension and a decrease in cerebral blood flow. Carotid sinus hypersensitivity or autonomic dysfunction may result in cerebral symptoms by this mechanism. Vasodilation may also occur as a reflex response to myocardial ischemia. In our experience, the "vagal reaction" of this type is most likely to occur in the presence of inferior myocardial ischemia or infarction. In a patient with an otherwise unexplained vasovagal reaction, occult myocardial ischemia must be considered in the differential diagnosis.

The key to proper management of the elderly patient with neurologic symptoms is a diagnostic approach which encompasses thorough neurologic and cardiologic evaluation.

1.11. Cardiovascular Pharmacology

The rational use of drugs in geriatric patients requires an awareness of the potential changes in drug sensitivity as well as a knowledge of altered pharmacokinetics. Nitrates, digitalis, diuretics, and antiarrhythmic agents comprise basic armentarium for managing the cardiac patient. As a result of recent investigations, beta-blockers and calcium channel blockers will undoubtedly be used more frequently in the future. The kinetics of several commonly used cardiovascular agents have been studied in the older population.

1.11.1. Digitalis

Digoxin is cleared from the body in a largely unaltered state via renal excretion. Digoxin dose should be modified because of the decrease in creatinine clearance which is recognized in the elderly. Digoxin levels should be monitored frequently in the setting of changing renal function and monitoring is also suggested when over- or underdosing is suspected.[53] In addition to the well-known arrhythmic and gastrointestinal symptoms associated with digitalis toxicity, confusion or psychosis may be signs of digitalis excess in the elderly. Routine monitoring of serum digoxin level in patients whose clinical status is otherwise stable is needless and unwarranted.

1.11.2. Antiarrhythmics

When antiarrhythmic therapy is indicated for the treatment of malignant ventricular extra systoles, the efficacy of treatment should be monitored with Holter scans and serum drug levels. Quinidine is metabolized in the liver, but some of the drug is cleared directly by the kidney. Excessive quinidine levels may result in a paradoxical increase in ventricular arrhythmias manifested by the "Torsade de Pointe" pattern of ventricular tachycardia (Fig. 4).[54] Haphazard administration of antiarrhythmic agents, most of which have major side effects, is potentially dangerous. Treatment should not be altered unless therapeutic failure is clearly demonstrated in the presence of adequate serum drug levels. Procainamide and disopyramide are the other currently approved antiarrhythmic agents for chronic therapy of the ambulatory patient. Disopyramide must be used with caution in patients with marginal ventricular function since its use has precipitated congestive heart failure in susceptible patients.

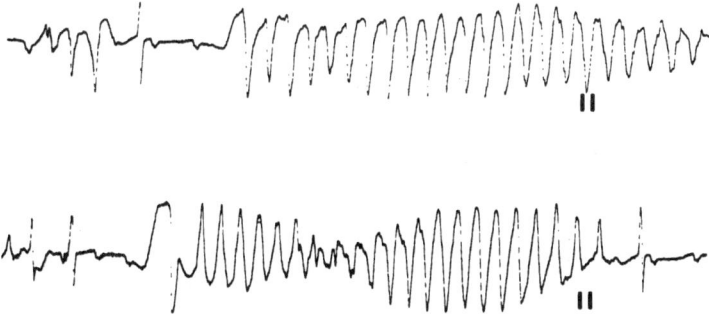

Figure 4. Torsade de Pointe—bidirectional ventricular tachycardia—continuous lead II.

1.11.3. Propranolol

Propranolol is metabolized by the liver. The first pass extraction is reduced in elderly patients. Correlation of drug levels with efficacy or side effects has not been well-established for this drug, but it is best to use it cautiously in the elderly patient in view of its negative chronotropic and negative inotropic effects.

Drug interactions are also important considerations. The effect of quinidine on serum digoxin levels is now well-recognized.[55] Cimetidene, the commonly used H2-receptor blocker, influences hepatic metabolism of propranolol and lidocaine.[56,57]

1.11.4. Vasodilators

Major advances have been made in the pharmacologic approach to refractory heart failure. Vasodilators are now used routinely.[58] Impedance to ejection (afterload) is reduced with arterial vasodilators. Forward cardiac output is enhanced and symptoms of fatigue, cold extremities, and mental obtundation are improved. Systemic venous dilatation (preload reduction) decreases pulmonary capillary pressure with a resultant reduction in dyspnea. Nitrates, hydralazine, prazosin, and captopril have been used successfully (Table III). Newer inotropic agents have been used investigationally with variable success.[59]

1.12. Preoperative Evaluation

The preoperative evaluation of elderly patients most frequently focuses on the cardiorespiratory system. In 1964, Arkins et al. reported mortality of 10.8% for surgical patients over age 70 years who did not have coronary artery disease.[60]

Table III. Vasodilators

	Usual dose	Preload	Afterload
Parenteral			
Nitroglycerin	15–100 μg/min	+++	+
Nitroprusside	10–200 μg/min	++	+++
Oral			
Isosorbide	10–40 mg q 4 hr	+++	+
Hydralazine	50–150 mg tid	0	+++
Prazosin	5–10 mg tid	++	++
Captopril	25–150 mg tid	0	+++
Cutaneous			
Nitroglycerin			
Patch	10–20 cm² daily	+++	+
Paste	½-2 inch q 4 hr		

When coronary disease was diagnosed preoperatively, the mortality doubled. Recent infarction and preoperative life-threatening disease were predictors of poor prognosis. In a more recent review, Goldman et al. evaluated 1001 patients over age 40 years.[61] Three hundred twenty-four patients were over age 70. Age alone was a moderate predictor of cardiac complications and/or death, but recent MI (within 6 months) and evidence of congestive heart failure were the strongest predictors of major complications. Emergency surgery, thoracic or abdominal operation, rhythm other than sinus, and poor general condition were additional factors. Harken cites the role of malnutrition as a surgical risk factor in the elderly cardiac patient and suggested that hyperalimentation might improve the risk.[62] Elective surgery for the patient with overt congestive heart failure should be deferred until hemodynamic stability is achieved. Complications during urgent surgery can be minimized if invasive hemodynamic monitoring is initiated preoperatively. Since recent infarction is also a consistent predictor of perioperative complications, elective surgery should be delayed for 6 months after MI. Stable angina pectoris does not appear to increase risk at the present time. Older studies indicate an 8 to 16% surgical mortality in patients with angina pectoris,[63] although in a more recent report, Goldman et al.[61] cited a 4% risk. This figure is still sufficiently high to warrant thorough preoperative evaluation whenever feasible. If a patient is unable to complete a low-level stress test without incidence (hypotension, ST depression greater than 2 mm, major arrhythmia, or severe angina), the surgery is delayed. If coronary bypass is a realistic consideration, angiography is recommended. Optimal pharmacologic management is recommended for the patient in whom revascularization is not a therapeutic option. Beta-blockers should not be abruptly withheld preoperatively and invasive monitoring is recommended intraoperatively. Judicious use of nitroglycerin intravenously will help to reduce myocardial oxygen demand and minimize the perioperative risks. Electrocardiograms and myocardial enzymes should be obtained daily for several days since MI is more likely to occur several days postoperatively than intraoperatively.[64] Patients with unstable angina should be managed in a similar fashion and every attempt should be made to stabilize the patient preoperatively. Intraoperative use of the balloon-counter pulsation device is occasionally beneficial in this setting.[65]

Ventricular ectopic beats are managed with a lidocaine infusion that is begun before induction of anesthesia. Prophylactic preoperative administration of digitalis for asymptomatic cardiomegaly is no longer recommended. Myocardial systolic function can be adequately assessed using the noninvasive studies described previously. In the event that there is still uncertainty regarding cardiac function, a simple bedside right heart catheterization can be performed. The perioperative experience in patients who have asymptomatic bifascicular block has been uniformly favorable. Transvenous pacing is not recommended unless there is documented second- or third-degree heart block. Endocarditis prophylaxis is indicated for patients with valvular or congenital heart lesions in accordance with American Heart Association recommendations.[66] Most surgeries can be completed with a

Table IV. Preoperative Assessment of the Cardiac Patient

Problem	Assessment	Management
Coronary disease		
Unstable[a]		
Recent MI	MI within 6 months	Elective surgery—defer
Unstable angina	Progressive, prolonged, or recent onset angina	Urgent surgery—hemodynamic monitoring; consider balloon pump
Chronic		
Stable angina	Nondisabling angina > 2 months	Limited stress test to identify unsuspected high risk
Old MI	MI by history or EKG > 6 months	
Valvular disease	Functional Class (NYHA I–IV)	Endocarditis Class I–II-prophylaxis
		Class III–IV[a]—defer elective surgery. Hemodynamic monitoring; endocarditis prophylaxis
Arrhythmias	LV dysfunction (?)	Lidocaine preinduction
VPBs	Unstable coronary disease (?)	EKG monitoring
	Complex VPBs (?)	
Conduction disorders		
Fascicular blocks	EKG changes	Pacemaker for documented bradycardia
Sick sinus syndrome		

[a]High surgical risks.

minimum of cardiac complications if this format is followed. Close liaison among the primary physician, surgeon, and anesthesiologist will assure the best possible outcome (Table IV).

1.13. Blood Pressure and Aging

Abnormal elevation and depression of blood pressure is common in elderly patients. This section examines the interaction between the aging process and blood pressure measurement and interpretation.

1.13.1. Blood Pressure: Determinants and Effects of Age

The relationship between blood pressure, cardiac output, and total peripheral resistance is well-known. The effects of aging on the cardiovascular system and the neurohumoral modulators of this system can potentially alter blood pressure in later life.[67-70] The changes in the vasculature that affect blood pressure were alluded to earlier. The combination of less distensable vessels and baroreceptor sensitivity decline leads to a propensity for isolated systolic blood pressure elevation and greater blood pressure liability in the elderly.

1.13.1.1. Cardiac Influences

Along with total peripheral resistance, cardiac output is a major determinant of blood pressure. The decline in cardiac output with age is primarily due to stroke volume decline rather than heart rate decline. Of the three determinants of stroke volume (preload, contractility, and afterload), afterload is the most important in explaining this decline. Its rise with age results in a decline in stroke volume and cardiac output. More recent reports with careful screening of subjects suggest that, at rest, aged subjects who are healthy have no change in cardiac output.[18]

1.13.1.2. Neurohumoral Influences

Age influences the neurohumoral system that modulates the cardiovascular system and blood pressure. The renal fluid volume system is affected by the decline in blood volume with increasing age. Renal blood flow, glomerular filtration rate, and renal sodium concentrating capacity decline steadily from adulthood to late life. Plasma renin and aldosterone levels, in most reports, decline with increasing age contrary to what would have been predicted from the renal blood flow and sodium conservation data.

Young and colleagues[71] have demonstrated an increased catecholamine response in elderly subjects versus young subjects from a standard stress. Changes in synthesis, storage, metabolism, or tissue sensitivity could explain this observation and need to be investigated. It is known that sympathetic stimulation produces less of a response of cardiac beta receptors in the aged.[72] This suggests a decreased tissue sensitivity to catecholamines. Table V summarizes the changes in the cardiovascular system that affect blood pressure with age. Tobian[73,74] has reviewed the evidence in man and animals that suggests salt intake in a genetically suscep-

Table V. Age-Related Factors Affecting Blood Pressure

Increase blood pressure	Decrease blood pressure
Increased total peripheral resistance	Decreased cardiac output (?)
High plasma catecholamines	Decreased tissue sensitivity to catecholamines
	Decreased vascular volume
	Decreased plasma renin–aldosterone

tible group is a contributing factor to the development of hypertension. This may be important in the elderly since the threshold for taste detection of salt rises with age in healthy elderly subjects.[75] It is unknown whether these gustatory changes result in the elderly ingesting more salt when compared with a young or middle-aged population. Socioeconomic factors that promote consumption of high sodium "fast foods" or processed foods may play an equally important role.

1.13.2. Population Studies

Miall and Lovell[76] reported a rise in both systolic and diastolic blood pressure with increasing age. Using a cross-sectional and longitudinal study design, these findings were noted in both men and women. The results of the Framingham study are similar.[77] Systolic blood pressure increase was particularly noted in women. The diastolic blood pressure rose to the middle of the sixth decade and then plateaued or declined with advancing age. Similar findings were also reported by the U.S. National Center for Health Statistics which reported mean blood pressures of 148/86 mm Hg for the population aged 60 to 74 years.[78] Although the group as a whole was not hypertensive (W.H.O. criteria 160/95 mm Hg), subsets of patients within the population were distinctly hypertensive.

It is important to consider whether or not the blood pressures reported in these studies are related to age alone. Aging is defined as a universal, progressive, and irreversible process in any organism. Blood pressure measurements from primitive populations do not exhibit the magnitude of change that has been reported in the "more civilized" countries.[79,80] This suggests that genetic as well as environmental and nutritional variables may be important in the aging process.

1.13.3. Hypertension: Definition

It is difficult to define normal blood pressure for any population. The epidemiologic approach to this problem has been to define the risk of mortality or cardiovascular morbidity associated with any blood pressure measurement at any age. Thus, the clinician is aided in developing a rational approach to diagnosis and treatment.

The Framingham study showed that advancing age is a marker (risk factor) for mortality and cardiovascular morbidity but that hypertension increased that risk. This effect was more pronounced in the older patient. Although related to both systolic and diastolic hypertension, the correlation was stronger with elevation of systolic blood pressure. The National Cooperative Pooling Project which combined data from several large epidemiologic studies reported similar findings.[81] The risk of combined classic hypertension (diastolic > 95 mm Hg) for coronary artery disease, stroke, and mortality from all causes rose with increasing diastolic pressure. The oldest cohort reported was 60 to 64 years and was the most affected.

The risk conferred by systolic hypertension (systolic blood pressure > 160

mm Hg) is particularly germane to the geriatric population. It has been estimated that only 4.6% of white women aged 45 to 54 years have this condition, although it was seen in 33% of white women aged 75 to 79 years. Numerous studies have reported similar findings. The association of high blood pressure (either systolic or diastolic) and increased morbidity and mortality does not mean that lowering the blood pressure will necessarily lower the risk of mortality and morbidity in the elderly. Few studies have analyzed these data for the elderly patient (vide infra).

1.13.4. Approach to the Patient

Kennedy[82] has pointed out appropriately that although epidemiologic data are often used as the basis for treatment of the hypertensive patient, these data should not be used as independent criteria for managing patients. Individualization of diagnosis and therapy is required. Chronologic age is not always indicative of biologic age.

1.13.4.1. History

Communication difficulties (e.g., presbycusis) and short-term memory loss may require more time for history-taking in the elderly patient. A history of long-standing hypertension makes a secondary cause less probable. Specific questions must be directed to the patient regarding target organ damage (e.g., angina, dyspnea, transient ischemic events). The elderly tend to underreport illness as a group. History should always include detailed information about concomitant drug use. Medications such as over-the-counter cold remedies often are regarded as innocuous by the patient, but may influence blood pressure. Nonsteroidal antiinflammatory agents, corticosteroids, or estrogen promote sodium retention. Dietary histories can be time-consuming and physicians often neglect them altogether. Elderly persons with limited income or who live alone may eat large quantities of processed foods which contain generous amounts of sodium. Sexual history should be reviewed since therapy may influence sexual function.

1.13.4.2. Physical Examination

The physical examination should concentrate on signs of atherosclerosis and target organ damage. Altered mentation may suggest a multiinfarct dementia resulting from hypertension. Certain features of blood pressure measurement are important in the elderly. Spence, Sibbald, and Cape have reported a group of elderly hypertensives whose pressure normalized with intraarterial recording.[83] This finding (pseudohypertension) is attributed to an unusually stiff brachial artery which cannot be compressed adequately by the syphygmomanometer cuff. What proportion of any aged hypertensive population is pseudohypertensive is unknown. Typically these patients have no evidence of target organ damage despite elevated blood pressure. Blood pressure should be measured in recumbent and upright positions and in both upper extremities. Caird, Andrews, and Kennedy have reported that 24% of elderly patients in the community had a 20-mm or greater orthostatic drop in blood pressure without symptoms.[84] At least three independent recordings of blood pressure should be obtained before a definitive diagnosis of hypertension is made. This is particularly true of the elderly whose less distensible vessels are unable to buffer the effects of stress-related catecholamine release. Measurement of the blood pressure in the home or nursing home helps to circumvent this problem.

1.13.4.3. Laboratory Evaluation

Laboratory evaluation should be cost-effective. Data should provide information about target organ function as well as the parameters that may be influenced by treatment (see Table VI). Serum potassium levels may reflect primary or secondary mineralocorticoid abnormalities. The European Working Party on High Blood Pressure in the Elderly describes the adverse effects which diuretic therapy may have on glucose metabolism.[85] A baseline fasting blood sugar should be obtained. Similarly, thiazide diuretics are known to affect calcium and uric acid levels. Serum creatinine is used to assess renal function and aids in the choice and dose of pharmacologic agents. The electrocardiogram and to a lesser extent the chest X ray may indicate the extent of cardiovascular damage. Thyroid function tests may be justified particularly in this elderly group in whom thyroid disease presents atypically. Other tests such as catecholamine measurements, renin–aldosterone levels, dexamethasone suppression, or saralasin infusions are performed when warranted by the appropriate clinical circumstances.

Table VI.   Laboratory Evaluation
of the Hypertensive

Urinalysis

Blood chemistries
   Serum potassium
   Serum creatinine
   Serum glucose
   Serum uric acid

Electrocardiogram

Optional
   Chest X ray
   Hemoglobin or complete blood count
   Thyroid function tests
   Serum calcium

The extent to which diagnostic evaluation should be pursued in the elderly patient suspected of having renal artery stenosis is still controversial. Typically, patients with renal vascular hypertension on an atherosclerotic basis have had a poorer response to surgery than patients with fibromuscular hyperplasia. Conversely, Whitehouse et al. found no difference in results in their surgical series.[86] Transluminal angioplasty may be an effective alternative therapy. However, Grim et al. reported a disappointingly high recurrence rate of stenosis (11 of 16) in patients with atherosclerotic renal artery stenosis.[87] The diagnosis of renal artery stenosis is made using a hypertensive intravenous pyelogram, radioactive renogram, and renal angiography. The new technique of digital subtraction angiography has been shown to effectively diagnose renal artery stenosis.[88] Its role in the evaluation of hypertension of the hypertensive elderly patient is evolving. Not all patients with renal artery stenosis have hypertension related thereto. Appropriate hormonal studies including direct measurements of renin should be done before considering invasive intervention. Madias, Kwon, and Millan[89] found that renal function stabilized in patients following angioplasty. Unfortunately, most of the atherosclerotic patients so treated were middle-aged and there are insufficient reports of similar results in elderly patients. In summary, the vast majority of elderly hypertensives have essential hypertension and require a minimum of laboratory investigation.

1.13.5. Essential Hypertension in the Aged

Messerli and colleagues[90] have shown that hypertensives over age 50 years have a normal cardiac index. Total peripheral resistance is elevated. This differs from young hypertensives (less than age 30) who have a higher cardiac index, increased renal blood flow, and lower total peripheral resistance than age-matched controls. The same authors report that epinephrine levels rose significantly with age in borderline hypertensive patients but not in normotensive controls. Lake et al.[91] found high plasma norepinephrine levels in older hypertensive patients, but could establish no relationship between levels and age in either normotensive or hypertensive populations. Epinephrine levels were lower in elderly patients whether hypertensive or normotensive.

In a small study of both young and elderly hypertensives, Mandai et al. showed lower plasma renin levels in the elderly hypertensives and controls than in the younger population.[92] This study also examined urinary catecholamine response to glucagon stress and found that urinary noradrenalin and adrenalin response was significantly greater in the younger hypertensive patients than the normotensive group or the hypertensive elderly. This study suggests that sympathetic overdrive may play a smaller role in causing hypertension in the elderly.

Takeda et al. have reported that normotensive elderly patients have a decline in plasma renin and aldosterone compared to younger subjects.[93] Morimoto et al. subsequently reported similar data in elderly patients with essential hypertension.[94] They found a subpopulation who had subnormal plasma renin increase after sodium restriction and this same group had an abnormally enhanced adrenal response to angiotensin II infusion. Ogihara et al. confirmed that elderly hypertensives have suppressed plasma renin and aldosterone compared to age-matched controls and young hypertensives.[95] When an angiotensin II antagonist (saralasin) was administered, the elderly hypertensives and normotensives had greater blood pressure elevation and renin–aldosterone suppression than middle-aged hypertensives. Since angiotensin II antagonists cause an abnormal pressure response in low renin states, these data suggest that elderly controls and hypertensives are similar and that the renin–angiotensin system is not responsible for hypertension in this group.

Urinary kallikrein excretion has been reported to decrease in patients with essential hypertension. Naka et al. described the effect of aging on this endogenous vasodilator in normotensive and essential hypertensive patients.[96] Excretion declined as a function of age in normotensive subjects and correlated with a decline in urinary aldosterone excretion. In contrast, hypertensive subjects showed no decrease in urinary kallikrein excretion despite the decrease in urinary aldosterone levels. In the aged hypertensive subjects, urinary kallikrein excretion was greater than normotensive controls. The role of declining urinary kallikrein excretion in the pathogenesis of hypertension in the elderly remains to be determined.

1.13.6. Therapeutic Decision Making

Having confirmed the diagnosis of hypertension, the clinician must make a decision regarding therapy. Is there evidence that treatment improves the quality or quantity of life in the elderly hypertensive patient? Koch-Weser points out that despite the availability of an adequate population for study, only 7 of 1000 subjects reported in earlier drug studies of hypertension therapy were over 69 years of age.[97] There is still a paucity of data relative to patients over age 75 years. Systolic hypertension will be considered first.

1.13.6.1. Systolic Hypertension

A prospective randomized study to evaluate large numbers of elderly patients with isolated systolic hypertension has yet to be performed. The epidemiologic data to which we previously referred has influenced clinicians to empirically treat this population. Gifford suggests cautious treatment based on these considerations and seeks to control standing systolic pressure between 140 and 160 mm Hg.[98] Chobanian arbitrarily chose 180 mm Hg as a pressure which should be treated in "asymptomatic" patients.[99] American and Japanese authors agree that isolated systolic hypertension in the face of target organ damage is a stronger indication for therapy. The Joint National Committee on Detection, Evaluation, and Treatment of High Blood Pressure[99a] addresses this issue as follows: "Consequently, for elderly patients with isolated systolic hypertension, the decision to treat must be individualized. If the decision is made to treat isolated systolic hypertension, blood pressure should be lowered cautiously to a goal of 140 to 160 mm Hg systolic" (p. 1284).

1.13.6.2. Combined Systolic Diastolic Hypertension

There is more universal agreement as to the treatment of diastolic hypertension. The 2376 subjects over the age of 60 years in the Hypertension Detection and Follow-up Program (HDFP) were randomized to stepped-care (Table VII) or referred care for blood pressure therapy.[100,101] The stepped-care group had lower blood pressures after a 5-year follow-up. Mortality data showed improved survival in the aged even in those with mild hypertension (90 to 105 mm Hg diastolic). However, when one divides these data into subsets including sex and race, differences are apparent. Statistical benefit has not been demonstrated for elderly white women prompting some investigators to point out that therapy of diastolic hypertension is not entirely straightforward at this time.[102] At the end of the HDFP study, the oldest subject was 74 years of age. What of the patients who are older? Women outnumber men 1.5 to 1.0 in the elderly population. Doesn't the HDFP study support treatment for this large population of elderly women? Hopefully, as data on morbidity[103] become available, answers to these questions will be forthcoming. Kuramoto et al. reported results of a 4-year prospective trial

Table VII. Stepped-Care Regimens[a]

Step 1:		Diuretic[b]	
		+	
Step 2:		Adrenergic inhibiting agents[c]	
	Atenolol	Nadolol	Rauwolfia alkaloids
	Methyldopa	Prazosin[d]	Timolol
	Metoprolol	Propranolol	
		+	
Step 3:		Vasodilator[e]	
		Hydralazine	
		+	
Step 4:		Additional adrenergic inhibiting agent	
		Guanethidine[f]	

[a]Modified from the 1980 report of The Joint National Committee on Detection, Evaluation, and Treatment of High Blood Pressure.[99a]
[b]Thiazide-type diuretics are drugs of choice. Loop diuretics are reserved for selected patients. Potassium-sparing agents may be used in combination with thiazide diuretics.
[c]Adrenergic inhibiting agents are listed in alphabetical order: This does not indicate preferential order of usage.
[d]The postsynaptic alpha-receptor-blocking effects of prazosin appear to be more prominent than its vasodilator effects, thus encouraging its inclusion as a Step 2 drug. Prazosin may be used as a Step 3 drug if it has not been added in Step 2.
[e]Minoxidil is reserved only for selected patients and should not be considered as a Step 3 drug.
[f]Guanethidine is a potent agent, but may be used in small doses as a Step 2 agent.

of therapy in 91 mildly hypertensive patients (BP mean).[104] A significant reduction in cerebrovascular and cardiac complications was found in treated patients although mortality did not differ in this small study. The Joint National Committee on Detection, Evaluation, and Treatment of High Blood Pressure[99a] encourages treatment of any elderly patient with diastolic hypertension. This group also points out that cerebrovascular disease, cardiovascular disease, and impaired renal function do not constitute contraindication to treatment.

1.13.7. Treatment

There is probably as much written about how to treat the elderly patient as there is whether to treat the patient. The goal should be a symptomless patient with a systolic pressure of 140 to 160 mm Hg and diastolic pressure of less than 95 mm Hg.

1.13.7.1. Nonmedical Treatment

Treatment of hypertension with salt restriction has been recognized for many years. Parijs et al. emphasizes that diuretic efficacy is enhanced with salt restriction in the treatment of high blood pressure.[105] Patients should not be permitted to use salt indiscriminantly just because they are taking a diuretic. Along with sodium restriction, weight loss has also been advocated. There is some evidence to suggest that weight loss alone is effective and patients whose weight exceeds ideal body weight by more than 30% may benefit from weight reduction.[106] A certain amount of physician apathy frequently exists in this area. To deny patients these therapies on the basis of prejudices that the elderly are incapable of change and cannot learn new health care practices is unfair to the patient and suggests an ageistic approach.

1.13.7.2. Medical Therapy

The step-care approach to treatment is recommended. Special aspects of therapy for the elderly patient are described in Table VIII. The primary tenets of therapy should include patient education to assure compliance with treatment, simplified drug regimens, and a recognition of economic constraints and limited reimbursement for medication cost. The dictum "Start low and go slow" applies and drug therapy should be initiated with the lowest possible dose.

Diuretic therapy is the first step in the treatment of hypertension. Special considerations in the elderly include: (1) A lower extracellular fluid volume and physiologic decline in renal concentration which make the elderly more susceptible to overdiuresis. Large series of patients with heat sickness often include elderly patients who have been on some form of diuretic therapy. Drugs may need to be

Table VIII. Drug Therapy for Hypertension[a]

Drug	Usual dose	Schedule	Comments
Thiazide diuretic	Equivalent of 25–100 mg HCTZ	qd or bid	Hypokalemia common. Ineffective when glomerular filtration rate is less than 30 ml/min
Furosemide	20–100 mg	qd or bid	Effective in advanced renal disease. 40 mg = 50 mg HCTZ
Spironolactone	50–400 mg	Divided doses (bid or qid)	Weak diuretics, contraindicated in renal insufficiency, do not use with potassium supplements; hyperkalemia; effective in 1° mineralocorticoid excess
Triamterene	100–200 mg	Divided doses (bid)	
Reserpine	0.1–0.25 mg	qd	Depression, sedation, peptic ulceration, nasal congestion
Methyldopa	250–500 mg	qid or bid	Sedation, positive Coombs test, liver dysfunction, orthostatic hypotension
Propranolol	20–120 mg	qid or bid	Congestive heart failure, bronchospasm, atrioventricular block, peripheral vascular insufficiency, hypoglycemia, potential withdrawal syndrome
Nadolol	40–320 mg	qd	Adverse effects similar to those of propranolol. Renal elimination
Metoprolol	50–100 mg	bid	More cardioselective than propranolol.
Hydralazine	25–100 mg	bid	Reflex tachycardia, SLE-like syndrome, exacerbation of coronary artery disease. Use with β-adrenergic blocker
Clonidine	0.1–0.8 mg	bid or tid	Transient sedation, dry mouth, potential withdrawal syndrome.
Prazosin	1–6 mg	tid	First dose syncope 0.15%
Guanethidine	10–50 mg	qd	Frequent side effects, orthostatic hypotension
Captopril	25–150 mg	tid	Should be taken 1 hr A.C. Decrease dosage in renal failure

[a]Modified from Prosnitz, E. H., 1982, Therapy of hypertension, in: *Drug Therapy for the Elderly* (K. Conrad and R. Bressler, eds.), C. V. Mosby Company, St. Louis.

temporarily discontinued under such environmental conditions. (2) Lower total body potassium and, in some cases, poor intake of dietary potassium increase the risk of hypokalemia in the elderly. Routine potassium supplementation is not advocated.[107] A salt substitute in patients with normal renal function may promote dietary compliance and avoid hypokalemia. The European Working Party Study on Hypertension in the Elderly employs a thiazide–triamterene combination as initial therapy. Potassium-sparing agents should not be used when the patient presents with concomitant renal disease. (3) Urinary incontinence is frequent in the elderly.[108] Diuretic therapy producing nocturnal diuresis may precipitate undesirable incontinence.

Second-step therapy includes several drugs which are broadly classified as antiadrenergic agents. Centrally acting agents (clonidine and alphamethyldopa), beta-adrenergic blockers (propranolol et al.), a peripheral alpha antagonist (prazosin), and the rauwolfia alkaloids. Methyldopa and clonidine have been used successfully in the elderly hypertensive patients. Messerli et al. studied the mechanism of action of methyldopa in both young and elderly hypertensives.[109] The aged patients experienced a significant decline in cardiac output and heart rate with no change in peripheral resistance. They also had a significant fall in plasma norepinephrine levels with maintenance of plasma epinephrine and dopamine levels. Methyldopa should be used cautiously in patients with heart failure and there is a tendency to produce postural hypotension. Hepatitis secondary to Aldomet may be more frequent in older patients.[110] Clonidine is lipid-soluble and as such its volume of distribution is increased in the elderly. This feature prolongs the clearance of the drug. Sedation, dizziness, and dry mouth may be caused by either methyldopa or clonidine. Decreased first-pass hepatic metabolism of propranolol results in higher plasma levels for a given dose in older patients.[111] Reduction in beta-receptor sensitivity may reduce the effect of this drug in the elderly. The therapeutic response is not significantly different in the elderly patient, however, and this may relate to the combination of these two factors. The effects of other beta-blockers are described in Table I. Prazosin can be used alone as a Step 2 agent or in combination with a beta-blocker at Step 3. The first-dose phenomenon is characterized by hypotension, palpitation, and occasional syncope. This initial dose might best be taken at bedtime to avoid postural problems. Rauwolfia alkaloids have fallen out of favor in recent years. The long half-life and troublesome side effects of this drug have reduced its popularity. Although it was used in the V.A. Cooperative Blood Pressure Study,[111a] there is no mention of excessive problems in elderly patients.

Hydralazine and minoxidil are vasodilators used at Step 3. Hydralazine is an arteriolar smooth muscle dilator. The likelihood of a lupuslike syndrome can be reduced by keeping the dosage below 200 mg/day.

Guanethidine depletes nerve endings of norephinephrine. It is a Step 4 drug which is associated with significant orthostatic side effects in 40% of patients. Sexual dysfunction, cardiac arrhythmias, and other side effects are seen.

Captopril inhibits angiotensin-converting enzyme. This drug has been well studied.[112] There are no obvious special considerations for its use in the elderly patient. Its position in the step-care approach is to be determined.

Attention to patient education can optimize compliance. If noncompliance is suspected, consider subclinical dementia as a cause. Antihypertensive agents can cause confusion in the elderly patients through electrolyte change or primary central nervous system side effects. In general, elderly patients accept chronic illness, and if approached appropriately they will comply with recommended treatment.

1.13.8. Hypotension

To this point, the discussion has concentrated on issues concerning elevation of blood pressure. Hypotension is an equally important problem in the aged. Thomas et al. have recently reviewed the topic.[113]

1.13.8.1. Definitions

As described previously Caird[84] reported a significant orthostatic drop in blood pressure in 24% of asymptomatic elderly patients. Orthostatic hypotension has been defined by the Mayo Clinic Group[113] as "the consistent and persistent decrease of 30 mm Hg or more systolic and a decrease of 15 mm Hg or more diastolic pressure, provided that the assumption of the upright position or exercise induces clinical symptoms" (p. 118). Upright position should be maintained for a minimum of 1 min during orthostatic BP recordings. A number of clinical conditions cause postural hypotension (Table IX). When secondary causes have been excluded, a diagnosis of idiopathic orthostatic hypotension (IOH) is made. Somatic neurologic manifestations (extrapyramidal signs indistinguishable from Parkinson's disease, lax anal sphincter, pupillary abnormalities, and Horner's syndrome) which accompany IOH define the Shy–Drager syndrome or multiple system atrophy (MSA). White has reported that subjects with IOH consistently have a delayed heart rate response to standing versus controls.[114] The same is probably true for subjects with MSA. Another subpopulation of IOH patients develop a brisk tachycardia with hypotension, called sympathotonic orthostatic hypotension.

Polinsky et al. attempted to characterize postural hypotension from a neuropharmacologic standpoint.[115] Controls and patients with MSA and IOH were studied for response to infusions of norepinephrine, tyramine, and angiotensin II. The MSA and IOH groups both demonstrated abnormally high blood pressure rises for each increment of pressor added when compared to controls. The authors of this study term this an abnormality in the gain of the pressor response and attribute it to deficient baroreceptor modulation. The MSA and IOH groups differed in that the subjects with IOH demonstrated a lower plasma level of pressor (threshold) to initiate a pressor response than either the controls or the subjects with MSA. The data suggest that patients with IOH have hypersensitivity to catecholamine infusion, similar to that seen in the denervated preparation. Other data have supported the concept that this disease is due to loss of peripheral norepinephrine and nerve terminals with low baseline norepinephrine levels.[116] Patients with MSA differed in their responses to pressors. It is postulated that they have deficient baroreceptor modulation without significant hypersensitivity of peripheral receptors.

Table IX.   Secondary Orthostatic Hypotension

Endocrine abnormalities
   Diabetes mellitus
   Adrenal insufficiency
   Pheochromocytoma
   Primary aldosteronism with hyperkalemia

Metabolic disorders
   Systemic amyloidosis
   Porphyria

Central and peripheral nervous system disorders
   Parasellar and posterior cranial fossa tumors
   Multiple cerebral infarcts
   Wernicke's encephalopathy
   Parkinson's disease
   Brainstem lesions
   Tabes dorsalis
   Traumatic and inflammatory myelopathies
   Guillian–Barré syndrome
   Chronic inflammatory polyradiculopathy
   Polyneuropathy secondary to any cause (carcinoma, uremia, alcohol, etc.)

Volume depletion
   Drug induced (diuretics, cathartics, emetics)
   Blood loss
   Diarrhea
   Vomiting

Postsurgical
   Interruption of peripheral sympathetic innervation

Drugs
   Tricyclic antidepressants
   Phenothiazines
   Antihypertensives

Hyperbradykininism

Other
   Prolonged recumbency
   Physical exhaustion
   Surgical gastrectomy

1.13.8.2. Management

The management of symptomatic orthostatic hypotension is a multifaceted approach.[117,118] Extracellular fluid is expanded by increasing sodium intake. 9-α-Fluorocortisone, a mineralocorticoid, is used in doses 0.2 to 0.5 mg/day. Compressive antigravity garments have been employed to minimize peripheral venous pools. Elevation of the head of the bed to the steepest angle tolerated has been advocated by Bannister.[119] Thomas and Bannister have shown that cerebral autoregulation in these patients is capable of adjusting to the lower blood pressure levels.[120] Sympathomimetic amines have also been used. Midodrine, an alpha-adrenergic agonist, has been used on an investigational basis.[121] Limited experience with this drug suggests that it may be helpful. Its major side effect was supine hypertension which was managed with beta-adrenergic blockade. Ephedrine and tyramine have been used alone or with monoamine oxidase inhibitors and, in select patients, with other drugs including methylphenidate and phenylephrine. Kochar and Itskovitz reported the efficacy of indomethicin in a small group of patients with MSA.[122] Current studies are being conducted to explain its benefits since no changes were found in plasma volumes, circulating renin, or plasma catecholamines. Side effects were volume overload, supine hypertension, and central nervous system side effects from indomethicin. Beta-blockers have also been used in the management of these troublesome syndromes. Parenteral dihydroergotamine, an alpha-agonist, has been known for some time to be effective in treating IOH. Jennings, Esler, and Holmes recently reported large doses (greater than 20 mg/day) to be effective orally in small numbers of patients.[123] These patients are difficult to manage and an empathetic approach is required.

1.13.9. Conclusion

Late life is marked by changes in blood pressure which are both physiologic and pathologic. Controversy exists concerning many aspects of diagnosis and treatment.[124,125] If the diseases caused by atherosclerosis (e.g., stroke, heart attack, kidney disease) can be modified through the efforts of the health care team, the elderly population will be grateful beneficiaries.

References

1. Levy, R. I. and Feinleib, M., 1980, Risk factors for coronary artery disease and their management in heart disease, in: *Textbook of Cardiovascular Medicine* (E. Braunwald, ed.), W. B. Saunders Company, Philadelphia, London, and Toronto, pp. 1246–1278.
2. Kannel, W. B. and Thom, T. J., 1979, Implications of the recent decline in cardiovascular mortality, *Cardiovasc. Med.* 9:983–997.
3. Pomerance, A., 1976, Pathology of the myocardium and valves, in: *Cardiology in Old Age* (F. I. Caird, J. L. C. Dall, and R. D. Kennedy, eds.), Plenum Press, New York and London, pp. 11–55.
4. Lev, M., 1964, Anatomic basis for atrioventricular block, *Am. J. Med.* 37:742–747.
5. Dhingra, R. C., Amat-y-Leon, F., Pietras, R. J., Wyndham, C., Deedwania, P.

C., Wu, D., Denes, P., and Rosen, K. M., 1977, Sites of conduction disease in aortic stenosis, *Ann. Intern. Med.* 87:275–280.

6. Bader, H., 1967, Dependence of wall stress in the human thoracic aorta on age and pressure, *Circ. Res.* 20:354–361.

7. Gribbin, B., Pickering, T. G., Steight, P., and Peto, R., 1971, Effect of age and high blood pressure on baroreflex sensitivity in man, *Circ. Res.* 29:424–431.

8. Strandell, T., 1976, Cardiac output in old age, in: *Cardiology in Old Age* (F. I. Caird, J. L. C. Dall, and R. D. Kennedy, eds.), Plenum Press, New York and London, pp. 81–100.

9. Bethel, C. S. and Crow, E. W., 1963, Heart sounds in the aged, *Am. J. Cardiol.* 11:763–767.

10. Ostenberger, L. E., Goldstein, S., Khaja, F., and Lakier, J. B., 1981, Functional mitral stenosis in patients with massive mitral annular calcification, *Circulation* 64:472–476.

11. Kistler, J. P., Lees, R. S., Friedman, J., Pressin, M., Mohr, J. P., Roberson, G. S., and Ojemann, R. G., 1978, The bruit of carotid stenosis versus radiated basal heart murmurs differentiation by phonoangiography, *Circulation* 57:975–981.

12. Fisch, C., 1981, Electrocardiogram in the aged: An independent marker of heart disease? *Am. J. Med.* 70:4–6.

13. Chiang, B. N., Perlman, L. V., Ostrander, L. D., and Epstein, F. H., 1969, Relationship of premature systoles to coronary heart disease and sudden death in the Tecumseh Epidemiologic Study, *Ann. Intern. Med.* 70:1159–1166.

14. Camm, A. J. Evans, K. E., Ward, D. E., and Martin, A., 1980, The rhythm of the heart in active elderly subjects, *Am. Heart J.* 99:598–603.

15. Freisinger, G. C. and Smith, R. F., 1972, Correlation of electrocardiographic studies and arteriographic findings with angina pectoris, *Circulation* 46:1173–1184.

16. Ellestad, M. H., 1975, Predictive implications, in: *Stress Testing Principles and Practice,* F. A. Davis Company, Philadelphia, pp. 157–176.

17. Okada, R. D., Boucher, C. A., Strauss, H. W., and Pohost, G. M., 1980, Exercise radionuclide imaging approaches to coronary artery disease. *Am. J. Cardiol.* 46:1188–1204.

18. Port, S., Cobb, F. R., Coleman, R. E., and Jones, R. H., 1980, The effect of age in left ventricular function at rest and during exercise, *N. Engl. J. Med.* 303:1131–1137.

19. Corbett, J. R., Dehmer, G. J., Lewis, S. E., Woodward, W., Henderson, E., Parkey, R. W., Blomqvist, C. G., and Willerson, J. T., 1981, The prognostic value of submaximal exercise testing with radionuclide ventriculography before hospital discharge in patients with recent myocardial infarction, *Circulation* 64:535–544.

20. Parkey, R. W., Bonte, F. J., Lewis, S. E., Buja, C. M., and Willerson, J. T., 1980, Acute myocardial infarct imaging using Technetium-99m pyrophosphate, in: *Nuclear Cardiology for Clinicians* (J. S. Soin and H. L. Brooks, eds.), Futura Publishing Company, Mt. Kisco, N.Y., pp. 133–150.

21. Davis, K., Kennedy, J. W., Kemp, H. G., Jr., Judkins, M. P., Gosselin, A. J., and Killip, T., 1979, Complications of coronary angiography from the collaborative study of coronary artery surgery (CASS), *Circulation* 59:1105–1112.

22. Mason, J. W. and Winkle, R. A., 1980, Accuracy of the ventricular tachycardia

induction study for predicting long-term efficacy and inefficacy of antiarrhythmic drugs, *N. Engl. J. Med.* 303:1073–1077.

23. Pathy, M. S., 1967, Clinical presentation of myocardial infarction in the elderly, *Br. Heart J.* 29:190–199.

24. Epstein, S. E., Kent, K. M., Goldstein, R. E., Borer, J. S., and Rosing, D. R., 1979, Strategy for evaluation and surgical treatment of the asymptomatic or mildly symptomatic patient with coronary artery disease, *Am. J. Cardiol.* 43:1015–1025.

25. Jones, R. H., McEwan, P., Newman, G. E., Port, S., Rerych, S. K., Scholz, P. M., Upton, M. T., Peter, C. A., Austin, E. H., Leong, K., Gibbons, R. J., Cobb, F. R., Coleman, R. E., and Sabiston, D. C., Jr., 1981, Accuracy of diagnosis of coronary artery disease by radionuclide measurement of left ventricular function during rest and exercise, *Circulation* 64:586–601.

26. Beta Blocker Heart Attack Study Group, 1981, The beta-blocker heart attack trial, *JAMA* 246:2073–2074.

27. Norwegian Multicenter Study Group, 1981, Timolol-induced reduction in mortality and reinfarction in patients surviving acute myocardial infarction, *N. Engl. J. Med.* 304:801–807.

28. Frishman, W. H., 1981, Beta adrenoceptor antagonists: New drugs and new indications, *N. Engl. J. Med.* 305:500–506.

29. Antman, E. M., Stone, P. H., Muller, J. E., and Braunwald, E., 1980, Calcium channel blocking agents in the treatment of cardiovascular disorders. Part I: Basic and clinical electrophysiologic effects, *Ann. Intern. Med.* 93:875–885.

30. Stone, P. H., Antman, E. M., Muller, J. E., and Braunwald, E., 1980, Calcium channel blocking agents in the treatment of cardiovascular disorders. Part II: Hemodynamic effects and clinical applications, *Ann. Intern. Med.* 93:886–904.

31. Kawai, C., Konishi, T., Matsuyama, E., and Okazaki, H., 1981, Comparative effects of three calcium antagonists—diltiazem, verapamil, nifedipine—on sinoatrial and atrioventricular nodes, *Circulation* 63:1035–1042.

32. Proceedings of the Workshop on Platelet Active Drugs in the Secondary Prevention of Cardiovascular Events, 1980, *Circulation* 62(Suppl):V1–V135.

33. Jolly, W. W., Isch, J. H., and Schumacker, H. R., 1981, Cardiac surgery in the elderly, in: *Cardiovascular Clinics,* Volume 12, Number 2 (R. J. Noble and D. A. Rothbaum, eds.), F. A. Davis Company, Philadelphia, pp. 195–210.

34. Rahimtoola, S. H., Grunkemeier, G., Tepley, J., Lambert, L., Thomas, D. R., Yuen-Fure, S., and Starr, A., 1981, Changes in coronary bypass surgery leading to improved survival, *JAMA* 246:1912–1916.

35. Kennedy, J. W., Kaiser, G. C., Fischer, L. D., Fritz, J. K., Myers, W., Mudd, J. G., and Ryan, T. J., 1981, Clinical and angiographic predictors of operative mortality from collaborative study in coronary artery (CASS), *Circulation* 63:793–802.

36. Cines, D. B., Kaywin, P., Bina, M., Tomaski, A., and Schrieber, A. D., 1980, Heparin associated thrombocytopenia, *N. Engl. J. Med.* 303:788–795.

37. Miller, D. H. and Borer, J. S., 1982, Exercise testing early after myocardial infarction, *Am. J. Med.* 72:427–438.

38. Pomerance, A., 1965, Pathology of the heart with and without cardiac failure in the aged, *Br. Heart J.* 27:697–709.

39. Schlatmann, T. J. M. and Becker, A. E., 1977, Histologic changes in the normal

aging aorta: Implications for dissecting aortic aneurysm, *Am. J. Cardiol.* 39:13–20.

40. Wheat, M. W., 1979, Treatment of dissecting aneurysms of the aorta: Current status, *Prog. Cardiovasc. Dis.* 16:87–101.

41. Finegan, R. E., Gianelly, R. E., and Harrison, D. C., 1969, Aortic stenosis in the elderly. Relevance of age to diagnosis and treatment, *N. Engl. J. Med.* 281:1261–1264.

42. Glancy, L., Freed, T. A. O'Brien, K. P., and Epstein, S., 1969, Calcium in the aortic valve–roentgenographic and hemodynamic correlations in 148 patients, *Ann. Intern. Med.* 71:246–250.

43. Wann, L. S. and Dillon, J. C., 1978, Echocardiography of the aortic valve, in: *Handbook of Clinical Ultrasound* (M. DeVlieger, ed.), John Wiley and Sons, New York, pp. 453–463.

44. Wagner, S. and Selzer, A., 1980, Natural history of unoperated aortic stenosis: Hemodynamic progression, *Am. J. Cardiol.* 45:440 (Abstract).

45. Tresch, D. D., Siegel, R., Keelan, M. H., Jr., Gross, C. M., and Brooks, H. L., 1979, Mitral valve prolapse in the elderly, *J. Am. Geriatr. Soc.* 27:421–424.

46. Cooper, E. S., Cooper, J. W., and Schnabel, T. G., 1966, Pitfalls in the diagnosis of bacterial endocarditis, *Arch. Intern. Med.* 118:55–61.

47. Dhingra, R. C., Wyndham, C., Amat-y-Leon, F., Denes, P., Wu, D., Sridhar, S., Bustin, A. G., and Rosen, K. M., 1979, Incidence and site of atrioventricular block in patients with chronic bifascicular block, *Circulation* 59:238–246.

48. Rodstein, M., Wolloch, L., and Iuster, Z., 1979, The natural history of intraventricular conduction disturbances in the aged: An analysis of the magnitude of risk of developing second and third degree heart block with clinical pathological correlations, *Am. J. Med. Sci.* 277:179–188.

49. McAnulty, J. H. and Rahimtoola, S. H., 1981, Chronic bundle branch block—clinical significance and management, *JAMA* 246:2202–2204.

50. Ruberman, W., Weinblatt, E., Goldberg, J. D., Frank, C. W., and Shapiro, S., 1977, Ventricular premature beats and mortality after myocardial infarction, *N. Engl. J. Med.* 297:750–757.

51. DiMarco, J. P., Garan, H., Harthorne, J. W., and Ruskin, J. N., 1981, Intracardiac electrophysiologic techniques in recurrent syncope of unknown cause, *Ann. Intern. Med.* 95:542–548.

52. Lovett, J. L., Sandok, B. A., Giuliani, E. R., and Nasser, F. N., 1981, Two-dimensional echocardiography in patients with focal cerebral ischemia, *Ann. Intern. Med.* 95:1–4.

53. Dodek, A., 1979, The serum digoxin test: A clinical perspective, *Cardiol. Digest* 14:19–24.

54. Keren, A., Tzivoni, D., Gavish, D., Levi, J., Gottlieb, S., Benhorin, J., and Stern, S., 1981, Etiology, warning signs, and therapy of Torsade de Pointes, *Circulation* 64:1167–1174.

55. Leahey, E. B., Jr., Reiffel, J. A., Drusin, R. E., Heissenbuttel, R. H., Lovejoy, W. P., and Bigger, J. T., 1978, Interaction between quinidine and digoxin, *JAMA* 240:533–534.

56. Feely, J., Wilkinson, G. R., and Wood, A. J. J., 1981, Reduction of liver blood flow and propranolol metabolism by cimetidine. *N. Engl. J. Med.* 304:692–695.

57. Feely, J., Wilkinson, G. R., McAllister, C. B., and Wood, A. J. J., 1982, Increased toxicity and reduced clearance of lidocaine by cimetidine, *Ann. Intern. Med.* 96:592-594.
58. Cohn, J. N. and Franciosa, J. A., 1977, Vasodilator therapy in cardiac failure, *N. Engl. J. Med.* 297:27-31, 254-258.
59. Weber, K. T., 1982, New hope for the failing heart, *Am. J. Med.* 72:665-670.
60. Arkins, R., Smessaert, A. A., and Hicks, R. G., 1964, Mortality and morbidity in surgical patients with coronary artery disease, *JAMA* 190:485-488.
61. Goldman, L., Caldera, D. L., Southwick, F. S., Nussbaum, S. R., Murray, B., O'Malley, T. A., Goroll, A. H., Caplan, C. H., Nolan, J., Burke, D. S., Krogstad, D., Carabello, A. C., and Slater, E. E., 1978, Cardiac risk factors and complications in noncardiac surgery, *Medicine* 57:357-370.
62. Harken, D. E., 1977, Malnutrition: A poorly understood surgical risk factor in aged cardiac patients, *Geriatrics* 32:83-85.
63. Skinner, J. F. and Pearce, M. L., 1964, Surgical risk in the cardiac patient, *J. Chronic. Dis.* 17:57-72.
64. Tarhan, S., Moffitt, E. A., Taylor, W. F., and Giuliani, E. R., 1972, Myocardial infarction after general anesthesia, *JAMA* 220:1451-1454.
65. Bonchek, L. I., Olinger, G. N., Keelan, M. H., Jr., Tresch, D. D., and Siegel, R., 1977, Management of sudden coronary death, *Ann. Thoracic Surg.* 24:337-345.
66. American Heart Association Committee Report (E. L. Kaplan, Chairman), 1977, Prevention of bacterial endocarditis, *Circulation* 56(1):139A-143A.
67. Kirkendall, W. M. and Hammond, J. J., 1980, Hypertension in the elderly, *Arch. Intern. Med.* 140:1155-1161.
68. Niarchos, A. P. and Laragh, J. H., 1980, Hypertension in the elderly, *Mod. Concepts Cardiovasc. Dis.* 49:43-48.
69. Niarchos, A. P. and Laragh, J. H., 1980, Hypertension in the elderly. II. Diagnosis and treatment, *Mod. Concepts Cardiovasc. Dis.* 49:49-54.
70. Brest, A. N. and Majdan, J., 1981, Hypertension in the elderly, *Cardiovasc. Clin.* 12:161-168.
71. Young, J. B., Rowe, J. W., Pallotta, J. A., Sparrow, D., and Landsberg, L., 1980, Enhanced plasma norepinephrine response to upright posture and oral glucose administration in elderly human subjects, *Metabolism* 29:532-539.
72. Vestal, R., Wood, A. J. J., and Shand, D. G., 1979, Reduced beta-adrenoreceptor sensitivity in the elderly, *Clin. Pharm. Ther.* 26:181-186.
73. Tobian, L., 1979, Dietary salt (sodium) and hypertension, *Am. J. Clin. Nutr.* 32(Suppl 12):2659-2663.
74. Tobian, L., 1979, The relationship of salt to hypertension, *Am. J. Clin. Nutr.* 32(Suppl 12):2739-2748.
75. Weiffenbach, J. M., Baum, B. J., and Burghauser, R., 1982, Taste thresholds: Quality specific variation with human aging, *J. Gerontol.* 37:372-377.
76. Miall, W. E. and Lovell, H. G., 1967, Relation between change of blood pressure and age, *Br. Med. J.* 2:660-664.
77. Kannel, W. B., 1976, Blood pressure and the development of cardiovascular disease in the aged, in: *Cardiology in Old Age* (F. I. Caird, J. L. C. Dall, and R. D. Kennedy, eds.), Plenum Press, New York and London, pp. 143-175.
78. National Health Survey, 1975, Blood pressure of persons 18-74 years in *United*

States from 1971–1972, National Center for Health Statistics, Rockville, Maryland.

79. Sinnet, P. F. and Whyte, H. M., 1973, Epidemiological studies in a total highland population—Tukisenta, New Guinea: Cardiovascular disease and relevant clinical, electrocardiographic, radiological, and biochemical findings. *J. Chron. Dis.* 26:265–290.

80. Truswell, A. S., Kennelly, B. M., Hansen, J. D. L., and Lu, R. B., 1972, Blood pressures of Kury bushmen in northern Botswanna, *Am. Heart J.* 84:5–12.

81. Dyer, A. R., Stamler, J., Shekelle, R. B., Schoenberger, J., and Farinaro, E., 1977, Hypertension in the elderly, *Med. Clin. North Am.* 61:513–529.

82. Kennedy, R. D., 1976, High blood pressure and its management, in: *Cardiology in Old Age,* (F. I. Caird, J. L. C. Dall, and R. D. Kennedy, eds.), Plenum Press, New York and London, pp. 177–190.

83. Spence, J. D. Sibbald, W. J., and Cape, R. D., 1978, Pseudohypertension in the elderly, *Clin. Sci. Mol. Med.* 59:399s–402s.

84. Caird, R. I., Andres, G. R., and Kennedy, R. D., 1973, Affect of posture on blood pressure in the elderly, *Br. Heart J.* 35:527–530.

85. Dollery, C., Fagard, R., Forette, F., Hellemans, J., Lund-Johnsen, P., Mutsers, A., and Tuomilehto, J., 1978, Glucose intolerance during diuretic therapy: Results from the European Working Party on High Blood Pressure in the Elderly trial, *Lancet* 1:681–683.

86. Whitehouse, W. M., Kazmers, A., Zelenviu, G., Erlandson, E., Cronenwett, J., Lindenaver, S., and Stanley, J. C., 1981, Chronic total renal artery occlusion—Effects of treatment on secondary hypertension and renal function, *Surgery* 89:753–763.

87. Grim, E. E., Luft, F. C., Yune, H. Y., Klatte, E., and Weinberger, M., 1981, Percutaneous transluminal dilatation in the treatment of renal vascular hypertension, *Ann. Intern. Med.* 95:439–442.

88. Brown, J., 1982, Digital subtraction arteriography of the abdomen with emphasis on renal vasculature, in: *Digital Subtraction Arteriography and Application of Computerized Fluoroscopy* (C. Mistretta, A. Crummy, C. Strother, and J. Sackett, eds.), Year Book Medical Publishers, Inc., Chicago, pp. 69–73.

89. Madias, N. E., Kwon, O. J., and Millan, V. G., 1982, Percutaneous transluminal angioplasty: A potentially effective treatment for preservation of renal function, *Arch. Intern. Med.* 142:693–697.

90. Messerli, F. H., Frohlich, E. D., Suarez, D. H., Reisin, E., Dreslinski, G., Dunn, F., and Cole, F., 1981, Borderline hypertension: Relationship between age, hemodynamics, and circulating calectrolamines, *Circulation* 64:760–764.

91. Lake, C. R., Ziegler, M. G., Coleman, M. D., and Kopin, I. J., 1977, Age-adjusted plasma norepinephrine levels are similar in normotensive and hypertensive subjects, *N. Engl. J. Med.* 296:208–209.

92. Mandai, T., Ogihara, T., Hata, T., Okada, T., Ogasahara, S., Nikami, H., Nakamaru, M., and Kumahara, Y., 1980, Urinary catecholamine response to glucagon in young and elderly patients with essential hypertension, *J. Am. Geriatr. Soc.* 28:462–465.

93. Takeda, R., Morimoto, S., Uchida, K., Miyamori, I., and Hashiba, T., 1980,

Effect of age on plasma aldosterone response to exogenous angiotensin II in normotensive subjects, *Acta Endocrinol.* 94:552–558.

94. Morimoto, S., Uchida, K., Miyamoto, M., Kigoshi, T., Morise, T., Takimoto, H., and Takeda, R., 1981, Plasma aldosterone response to angiotensin II in sodium-restricted elderly subjects with essential hypertension, *J. Am. Geriatr. Soc.* 29:302–307.

95. Ogihara, T., Hata, T., Maruyama, A., Mikami, M., Nakamaru, M., Mandai, T., and Kumahara, Y., 1979, Studies on the renin-angiotensin-aldosterone system in elderly hypertensive patients with angiotensin II antagonist, *Clin. Sci.* 57:461–463.

96. Naka, T., Ogihara, T., Hata, T., Maruyama, A., Mikami, H., Nakamaru, M., Gotoh, S., Masuo, K., Ohde, H., Iwanaga, K., and Kumahara, T., 1981, The effect of aging on urinary kallikrein excretion in normotensive subjects and in patients with essential hypertension, *J. Clin. Endocrinol. Metab.* 52:1023–1026.

97. Koch-Weser, J., 1979, Treatment of hypertension in the elderly, in: *Drugs and the Elderly,* (J. Crooks and I. H. Stevenson, eds.), University Park Press, Baltimore, pp. 247–262.

98. Gifford, R., 1982, Isolated systolic hypertension in the elderly: Some controversial issues, *JAMA* 247:781–785.

99. Chobanian, A. V., 1981, Therapeutic decision making in systolic hypertension, *Geriatrics* 36(3):36–41.

99a. The Joint National Committee in Detection, Evaluation, and Treatment of High Blood Pressure, 1980, The 1980 report of The Joint Committee in Detection, Evaluation, and Treatment of High Blood Pressure, *Arch. Intern. Med.,* 140:1280–1285.

100. Five year findings of the Hypertension Detection and Follow-up Program. I. Reduction in mortality of persons with high blood pressure including mild hypertension, 1979, *JAMA* 242:2562–2571.

101. Five year findings of the Hypertension Detection and Follow-up Program. II. Mortality by race, sex, and age, 1979. *JAMA* 242:2572–2577.

102. Libow, L. and Butler, R. N., 1981, Treating mild diastolic hypertension in the elderly: Uncertain benefits and possible dangers, *Geriatrics* 36(11):55–62.

103. Amery, A. and DeSchaepdryver, A., 1973, European Working Party on High Blood Pressure in the Elderly (EWPHE). Organization of double-blind multicentre trial on antihypertensive therapy in elderly patients, *Clin. Sci. Mol. Med.* 45:71s–73s.

104. Kuramoto, K., Matsushita, S., Kuwajima, I., and Mvrakami, M., 1981, Prospective study on the treatment of mild hypertension in the aged, *Jap. Heart J.* 22:75–85.

105. Parijs, J., Joossens, J. V., VanderLinden, L., Verstreken, G., and Amery, A., 1973, Moderate sodium restriction and diuretics in the treatment of hypertension, *Am. Heart J.* 85:22–34.

106. Reisin, E., Abel, R., Modan, M., Silverberg, D., Eliahou, H., and Modan, B., 1978, Effect of weight loss without salt restriction on the reduction of blood pressure in overweight hypertensive patients, *N. Engl. J. Med.* 298:1–6.

107. Navarro, R., O'Brien, D. L., Nuffort, P., and Spencer, D. L., 1982, Diuretic induced hypokalemia in the elderly, *J. Fam. Prac.* 14:685–689.

108. Ouslander, J. G., 1981, Urinary incontinence in the elderly, *West. J. Med.* 135:482–491.

109. Messerli, F. H., Dreslinski, G. R., Husserl, R. E., Svarez, D., MacPhee, A., and Frohlich, E., 1981, Antiadrenergic therapy: Special aspects in hypertension in the elderly, *Hypertension* 3(Suppl. II):226–229.

110. Sotaniemi, E. A., Hukkanen, O. T., Akokas, J. T., Pelkonen, R. O., and Ahlqvist, J., 1977, Hepatic injury and drug metabolism in patients with alpha-methylodopa induced liver damage, *Eur. J. Clin. Pharm.* 12:429–435.

111. Castelden, C. M. and George, C. F., 1979, The effect of age on the hepatic clearance of propranolol, *Br. J. Clin. Pharm.* 7:49–54.

111a. Veteran's Administration Cooperative Study Group on Antihypertensive Agents, 1967, Effects of treatment on morbidity in hypertension: Results in patients with diastolic blood pressures averaging 115 through 129 mm Hg, *JAMA* 202:1028–1034.

112. Vidt, D. G., Bravo, E. L., and Fouad, F. M., 1982. Drug therapy—Captopril. *N. Engl. J. Med.* 306:214–219.

113. Thomas, J. E., Schirger, A., Fealey, R. D., and Sheps, S. G., 1981, Orthostatic hypotension, *Mayo Clin. Proc.* 56:117–125.

114. White, N. J., 1980, Heart rate changes on standing in elderly patients with orthostatic hypotension, *Clin. Sci.* 58:411–413.

115. Polinsky, R. J., Kopin, I. J., Ebert, M. H., and Weise, V., 1981, Phamacologic distinction of different orthostatic hypotension syndromes, *Neurology (New York)* 31:1–7.

116. Lake, C. R., 1979, Relationship of sympathetic nervous system tone and blood pressure, *Nephron* 23:84–90.

117. Management of orthostatic hypotension (Editorial), 1981, *Lancet* 2:963–964.

118. Ziegler, M. G., 1981, Choosing therapy for postural hypotension, *Drug Ther.* 10:97–114.

119. Bannister, R., 1979, Chronic autonomic failure with postural hypotension, *Lancet* ii:404–406.

120. Thomas, D. J. and Bannister, R., 1980, Preservation of autoregulation of cerebral blood flow in autonomic failure, *J. Neurol. Sci.* 44:205–212.

121. Schirger, A., Sheps, S. G., Thomas, J. E., and Fealey, R. D., 1981, Midodrine: A new agent in the management of idiopathic orthostatic hypotension and Shy–Drager syndrome, *Mayo Clin. Proc.* 56:429–433.

122. Kochar, M. and Itskovitz, H., 1978, Treatment of idiopathic orthostatic hypotension (Shy–Drager syndrome) with indomethicin, *Lancet* i:1011–1014.

123. Jennings, G., Esler, M., and Holmes, R., 1979, Treatment of orthostatic hypotension with dihydroergotamine, *Br. Med. J.* 2:307.

124. Relman, A., 1980, Mild hypertension: No more benign neglect, *N. Engl. J. Med.* 302:293–294.

125. Kaplan, N. M., 1981, Whom to treat: The dilemma of mild hypertension, *Am. Heart J.* 101:867–870.

Pulmonary Aspects of Aging

Donald A. Mahler

2.1. Introduction

This chapter focuses on four topics concerning respiratory function and disease in the elderly population. First, understanding the effects of aging on lung function and gas exchange provides the basis for distinguishing between age-related alterations and dysfunction. Health, at whatever age, is most often determined by the ability of an individual to perform activities of daily living, to work, and/or to participate in recreational interests. In order to achieve these objectives, the elderly person must develop and maintain a minimal level of exercise tolerance. Accordingly, the physiologic interactions affecting exercise performance in the elderly will be discussed.

The fourth and fifth sections involve chronic obstructive pulmonary disease (COPD) and pneumonia, which are the two leading respiratory causes of morbidity and mortality in the United States. Due to the combined effects of cigarette smoking and the decline in lung function with age, nearly 500,000 people are disabled with advanced COPD. In most instances, the disease is diagnosed between the ages of 55 and 65 years, while complications frequently develop as dysfunction progresses with time. Pneumonia is a common malady in the elderly. Colonization of the oropharynx is increased in the aged, and predisposing factors contribute to aspiration problems. Also, host responses may vary considerably in the geriatric patient so that clinical manifestations of pneumonia may not be completely expressed.

DONALD A. MAHLER • Pulmonary Function Laboratory, and Pulmonary Section, Department of Medicine, Dartmouth Medical School, Hanover, New Hampshire 03756.

2.2. The Aging Lung

2.2.1. Introduction

In general, lung function deteriorates progressively with increasing age after maturation (age 25 years in men and 20 years in women). Changes in respiratory function may not be truly linear as the rate of decline in expiratory flow rates is small in the earlier years and accelerates with advancing age.

Although the mechanisms leading to diminished respiratory function are not completely understood, three predominant factors are important: (1) decreased elasticity of the lungs; (2) decreased strength of the respiratory muscles; and (3) increased stiffness of the thoracic cage. Most age-related physiologic changes of the respiratory system can be explained, at least in part, by these three alterations in the mechanics of breathing.

As a result of these changes in older persons, it may be difficult to determine whether results of physiologic testing merely reflect advanced age or indicate disease. Furthermore, caution is necessary in evaluating pulmonary function data in the elderly since many values considered normal for older people have been derived from relatively small numbers of subjects and the standard deviation from normal values is proportionately greater for older than younger individuals.[1] Thus, knowledge of the physiologic changes of the respiratory system associated with aging should help to distinguish between advanced age and disease.

2.2.2. Physiologic Changes

2.2.2.1. Lung Volumes

For over a century it has been known that forced vital capacity (FVC) of the lung decreases with age.[2] The decline in FVC ranges between 19 and 35 ml/year in men and between 15 and 29 ml/year in women.[3] Since loss of elastic recoil in the lung contributes to airway closure during expiration at higher lung volumes, residual volume (RV) increases with age. In contrast, total lung capacity (TLC) remains virtually constant throughout life.[3]

2.2.2.2. Flow Rates

All measurements of expiratory flow decrease with advancing age. The decline in forced expiratory volume in 1 sec (FEV_1) is approximately 30 ml/year for men and 23 ml/year for women[4-6]; however, the rate of decline is smaller in the earlier years and accelerates with advancing years.[7]

In addition, peak expiratory flow rate (PEFR) and maximal expiratory flow at 50% of FVC (MEF50) decrease with age. The FEV_1:FVC ratio also declines during aging, approaching 65% in the elderly. With this in mind, further evaluation of the patient is often necessary so that results of pulmonary function tests are not mistakenly attributed to obstructive airway disease. Age-related decreases in flow rates lead to an increasingly concave shape of the maximal expiratory flow-volume (MEFV) curve.[8]

2.2.2.3. Respiratory Mechanics

After maturity, elastic recoil of the lungs gradually diminishes resulting in increased static lung compliance.[9] This diminution in lung elasticity may explain the age-related changes in lung volumes (FVC and RV) and expiratory flow rates. Due to fixation of the intercostal joints, the thorax becomes more rigid, and compliance or distensibility of the chest wall is reduced.

2.2.2.4. Gas Exchange

The purpose of breathing is to provide for the uptake of oxygen from the air and elimination of carbon dioxide. To achieve these objectives, ventilation must be matched with perfusion in the lungs. Clinically, gas exchange can be evaluated by measuring gas tensions and pH of arterial blood. Although age does not influence arterial pH (normal range, 7.42 ± 0.02) or arterial carbon dioxide tension [($PaCO_2$), normal range, 40 ± 2 Torr], aging of the lung results in a progressive reduction in arterial oxygen tension (Fig. 1). The following regression equations may be used to predict arterial oxygen tension (PaO_2) at sea level in the adult:

$$\text{Seated}^{10}\text{: } PaO_2(\text{Torr}) = 104.2 - 0.27 \times \text{age (years)}$$
$$\text{Supine}^{11}\text{: } PaO_2(\text{Torr}) = 103.5 - 0.42 \times \text{age (years)}$$

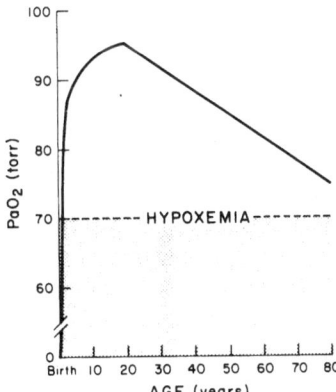

Figure 1. The change in arterial oxygen tension (PaO_2) with increasing age. Hypoxemia is arbitrarily defined as PaO_2 less than 70 Torr.

In evaluating a measured PaO_2 level, two questions should be addressed: (1) Is the PaO_2 normal? and (2) Is the PaO_2 adequate? To assess the first question, both $PaCO_2$ and the alveolar–arterial oxygen difference [(A–a) DO_2] must be considered. Even though the PaO_2 may be in the normal range ($\geq$ 90% of predicted), this may be at the expense of increased ventilation as indicated by a low $PaCO_2$. To further assess impaired gas exchange, the (A–a)DO_2 should be calculated. Generally, the *alveolar* oxygen tension (PAO_2) can be estimated at sea level by the equation[10]:

$$PAO_2 = 150 - 1.25(PaCO_2)$$

Then, the difference between alveolar and arterial oxygen tension can be determined by subtracting PaO_2 from PAO_2. According to Mellemgaard,[10] the regression formula for the ideal (A–a) DO_2 for a given age is:

$$(A-a)DO_2(Torr) = 2.5 + 0.21 \times age\ (years)$$

Thus, for a 50-year-old person, the (A–a)DO_2 would be 13 Torr, while for a 70-year-old individual, the gradient would increase to 17 Torr. As a guideline, if the (A–a)DO_2 is greater than 20 Torr despite a "normal PaO_2," there is impairment of gas exchange.

The physiologic consequences of hypoxemia determine whether oxygenation is adequate or not. Arterial oxygen content (CaO_2) can be calculated by the following equation[12] [(gHb) grams hemoglobin; (SaO_2) arterial oxygen saturation]:

$$CaO_2(ml/100\ ml) = gHb \times 1.34\ ml/gHb \times SaO_2 + (0.0031 \times PaO_2)$$

To estimate the amount of oxygen available for use by the tissues, systemic oxygen transport (SOT) can be determined by the formula[12]:

$$SOT(ml/min) = CaO_2 \times cardiac\ output$$

Since the majority of O_2 carried in the blood is bound to hemoglobin, while only a small amount is dissolved in plasma, SOT is primarily influenced by hemoglobin level, oxygen saturation, and cardiac performance. Based on the oxyhemoglobin dissociation curve (Fig. 2), an O_2 tension of 60 Torr indicates that approximately 90% of hemoglobin will be saturated with oxygen. As the PaO_2 increases above 60 Torr, the increment in SaO_2 is relatively small; in contrast, with a PaO_2 below 60 Torr, there is a more linear reduction in arterial oxygen saturation. Considering the determinants of SOT, a $PaO_2 \geq 60$ Torr is generally considered acceptable. With increasing age, SOT is reduced due to decreases in oxygen saturation and cardiac output.

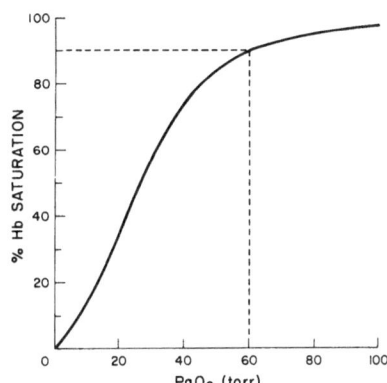

Figure 2. Oxyhemoglobin dissociation curve. Note that a PaO_2 of 60 Torr corresponds to a hemoglobin saturation of 90%.

2.2.2.5. Diffusing Capacity

Diffusing capacity of the lung reflects the passive exchange of gases between alveoli and capillary blood. For oxygen, molecules must diffuse through the alveolar space, cross the air–blood barrier, and traverse the plasma and red blood cell to combine with hemoglobin. Diffusion of carbon dioxide occurs in a reverse direction.

With increasing age there is a progressive reduction of diffusing capacity of the lung ranging from 0.20 to 0.32 ml/min per mm Hg per year of adult life for men and 0.06 to 0.18 ml/min per mm Hg per year for women.[3] These changes are largely due to a loss of lung tissue with a resulting reduction in alveolar-capillary surface area.

2.2.2.6. Respiratory Muscle Function

Both respiratory muscle strength and endurance diminish as a result of the aging process. Black and Hyatt[13] have shown that maximal inspiratory (PIMAX) and expiratory (PEMAX) pressures remain stable until 55 years of age, at which time both PIMAX and PEMAX begin to decrease with age. Maximal voluntary ventilation (MVV), which is the maximal volume of air exhaled during voluntary hyperventilation for 12 to 15 sec, reflects respiratory muscle endurance. Due to multiple factors, including decreases in expiratory flow rates and respiratory muscle strength, MVV is reduced during aging.

2.2.2.7. Control of Breathing

In the elderly population there is approximately 50% diminution in the ventilatory responses to both hypoxic and hypercapnic stimuli.[14] It appears that a reduction in neuromuscular inspiratory output may be the major factor in the attenuation of ventilatory drive.[15] These findings suggest that the respiratory drive of the older individual may not be appropriate to maintain adequate gas exchange when stressed by hypoxia associated with either acute or chronic disease.

2.2.3. Effects of Cigarette Smoking

Acute inhalation of tobacco smoke leads to an immediate rise in airway resistance and carboxyhemoglobin levels while decreasing ciliary and alveolar macrophage function. Individuals who smoke have increased nonspecific bronchial reactivity which may contribute to the development of airway obstruction in smokers.[16] Even long-term passive smoking (involuntary inhalation of tobacco smoke) can lead to dysfunction of the small airways in nonsmokers.[17]

Cigarette smoking accelerates the decline in pulmonary function with age. In a longitudinal study, Bossé and colleagues[18] found that the age-related decrease in FEV_1 and FVC over a 5-year period were greater in current smokers than those who quit smoking. Cessation of smoking can result in definite and immediate improvement in both FEV_1 and FVC which may continue for several months.[19] In fact, greater improvement can occur in persons who have more severe dysfunction prior to stopping smoking. An appreciation that smoking and aging have combined adverse effects on lung function is important in caring for and advising older patients who continue to smoke despite respiratory complaints.

2.3. Aging and Physical Performance

Action may not always bring happiness; but there is no happiness without action.
BENJAMIN DISRAELI (1804–1881)

2.3.1. Introduction

Any physical activity depends on the interaction or coupling of the respiratory, cardiovascular, and musculoskeletal systems for the uptake and transport of O_2 to the mitochondria and elimination of CO_2 (Fig. 3). With increased requirements for oxygen, as occur with exercise, greater demands are placed on gas exchange and transport. Accordingly, a defect in either the respiratory, cardiovascular, or musculoskeletal systems can adversely affect or limit exercise capacity.

Most individuals are aware by observation that diminished physical fitness and performance are a consequence of aging. Before the age-related physiologic changes in exercise performance are described, a brief summary of the physiologic responses to exercise is relevant.

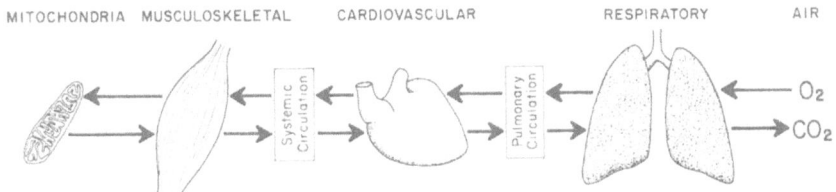

Figure 3. Interaction of the respiratory, cardiovascular, and musculoskeletal systems for transport and exchange of oxygen and carbon dioxide.

2.3.2. Normal Physiologic Responses to Exercise

The physiologic responses to progressive work in healthy individuals are illustrated in Fig. 4. Oxygen consumption ($\dot{V}O_2$) increases linearly as the workload increases until a plateau is reached; this represents maximal oxygen consumption ($\dot{V}O_2$max). There is a linear increase in both minute ventilation ($\dot{V}_E$) and carbon dioxide production ($\dot{V}CO_2$) until the onset of anaerobic metabolism (increased lactic acid production) at which time further augmentation of $\dot{V}_E$ and $\dot{V}CO_2$ occurs. Cardiac output also increases progressively with the intensity of exercise.

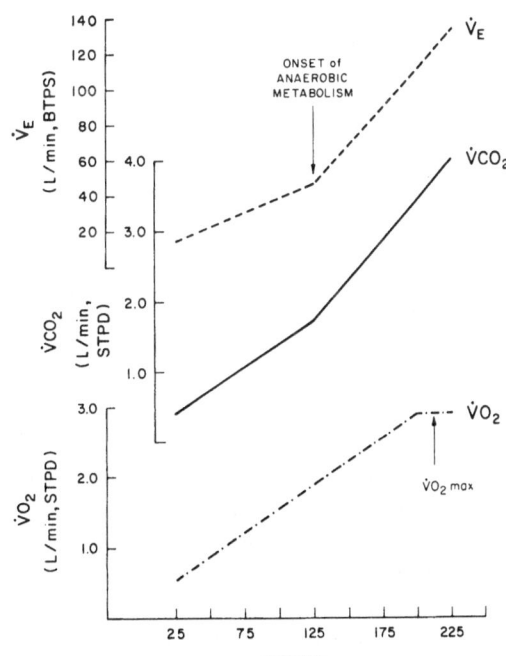

Figure 4. Physiologic responses of minute ventilation ($\dot{V}_E$), carbon dioxide production ($\dot{V}CO_2$), and oxygen consumption ($\dot{V}O_2$) to progressive work in healthy individuals.

In healthy subjects, increased ventilation at low levels of exercise is primarily due to tidal volume, which increases to 60 to 70% of the FVC. As exercise continues, further augmentation in ventilation is related to the respiratory rate.[20] In a similar manner, stroke volume of the heart reaches a maximum at approximately 40% of $\dot{V}O_2$max; subsequent increases in cardiac output are due to the heart rate response.[21]

The cardiovascular system has been considered to impose the upper limit on oxygen uptake and exercise capacity.[22,23] Since exercise heart rate does not exceed 180 to 200 beats/min, maximal cardiac performance may be ultimately affected by cardiac frequency. However, it remains to be determined whether the central circulation or peripheral perfusion is the critical factor limiting maximal oxygen consumption.[22]

Concerning the respiratory system, lung function does not apparently limit exercise capacity in normal individuals.[22] However, we have recently demonstrated that vital capacity is decreased after prolonged exercise in trained athletes.[24,25] Furthermore, fatigue of the respiratory muscles can develop after marathon running.[26] Despite these findings, it is unclear whether respiratory factors may actually limit exercise ability in healthy individuals.

2.3.3. Effects of Age on Exercise Performance

Studies that have evaluated the effects of aging on physical ability have involved both maximal and submaximal work intensities. Most physiologic parameters at *maximal* exercise decline with age. However, during *submaximal* levels of exercise, these variables are generally higher in the elderly population. These age-related changes reflect both the decrease in maximal work capacity as well as less efficiency in gas exchange and transport. In order to appreciate the effects of age on exercise performance, it is important to distinguish the level of exercise at which the physiologic alterations occur. In addition, most of the available information on aging and exercise have been obtained in men, and thus comparisons with women may not be appropriate.

2.3.3.1. Oxygen Consumption

Oxygen consumption ($\dot{V}O_2$, ml/min) during submaximal exercise is not affected by age (Fig. 5). That is, individuals of the same weight but different ages require the same $\dot{V}O_2$ for a given workload. However, the overall efficiency of the gas exchange mechanisms is diminished in the elderly.

Maximal oxygen consumption (ml/kg per min) is a standard measure of fitness or aerobic capacity. Longitudinal studies have demonstrated a progressive reduction in $\dot{V}O_2$max with aging.[27-29] Paired observations in 40 men taken 2.3 years apart showed a mean decline of -0.04 ml/kg per min/year.[28] Of interest, the decrease in $\dot{V}O_2$max parallels the decline in work capacity.

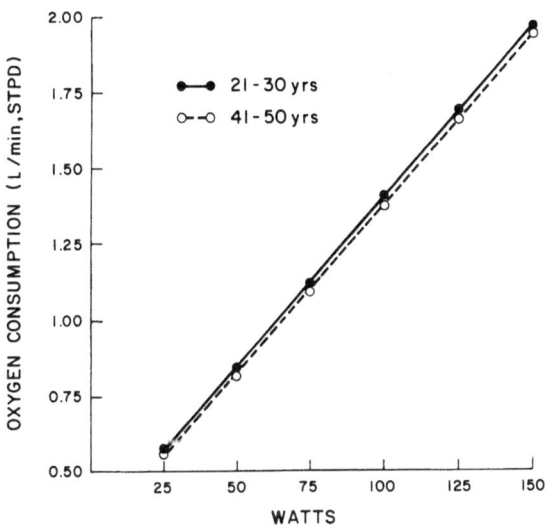

Figure 5. Relationship between oxygen consumption and progressive work (watts) in men of different age groups.

2.3.3.2. Cardiac Function

2.3.3.2a. Cardiac Output. Resting cardiac output decreases approximately 1% per year.[30] With submaximal exercise at identical workloads and $\dot{V}O_2$, cardiac output increases progressively from the second to the seventh decades of life.[31] In contrast, maximal cardiac output declines with aging.[32-34]

2.3.3.2b. Heart Rate and Stroke Volume. Heart rate and stroke volume combine to determine cardiac output. Both resting and maximal heart rate and stroke volume are lower in the older as compared to a younger population. Predicted maximal heart rate (pred HRmax) is useful for estimating the relative level of exercise during testing or as part of a training program. It can be determined using the formula[35]:

$$\text{pred HRmax} = 210 - 0.65 \times \text{age (years)}$$

Results in our laboratory (Fig. 6) confirm previous findings[31] that at the same level of oxygen consumption, submaximal heart rate is lower with increased age.

2.3.3.2c. Left Ventricular Ejection Fraction. The effect of age on left ventricular performance has been evaluated noninvasively using radionuclide angiocardiography. Although age did not influence left ventricular ejection fraction (LVEF) at rest, there was a decline in the exercise response of the LVEF with increasing age.[36] These findings are consistent with an age-related decrease in left ventricular exercise reserve.

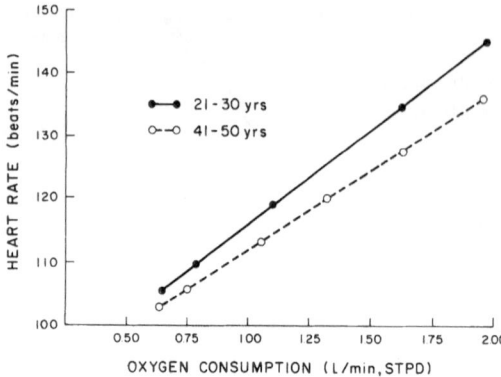

Figure 6. Relationship between heart rate and oxygen consumption in men of different age groups.

2.3.3.3. Ventilation

During submaximal exercise, $\dot{V}_E$ is greater at a given level of oxygen consumption with advancing age (Fig. 7).[31,37] This reflects a decrease in ventilatory efficiency during aerobic performance in the elderly. On the other hand, with exhaustive work, maximal exercise ventilation ($\dot{V}_E$max) is lower as age advances, which is related to the known decline in pulmonary function.

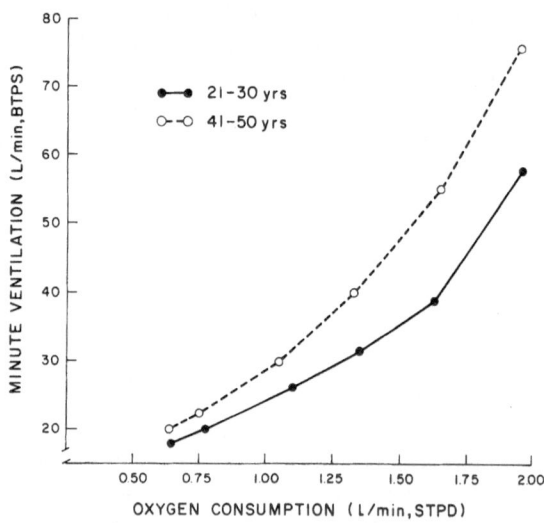

Figure 7. Relationship between minute ventilation and oxygen consumption in men of different age groups.

2.3.3.4. Oxygen Extraction

The arteriovenous oxygen difference $(a-\bar{v})O_2$ reflects the extraction of O_2 from the circulation and utilization by the tissues. As has been observed in other parameters of cardiovascular function, exercise $(a-\bar{v})O_2$ is decreased with age.[31]

2.3.4. Physical Conditioning and Aging

Despite the decline of a multitude of physiologic parameters with age, several investigations have shown that physical fitness can provide a sense of well-being and retard physiologic aging.[38-41] Fitness implies an optimal usage of oxygen, and can be assessed by measurement of maximal oxygen consumption. In healthy, sedentary middle-aged men, physical training can increase aerobic work capacity ($\dot{V}O_2$max) by approximately 10 to 20% and reduce circulatory and respiratory strain during submaximal work.[38-40] In a group of eight men and women with an average age of 70 years (range: 55-78), Barry and colleagues[41] found that $\dot{V}O_2$max increased by 40% after 3 months of light training on a bicycle ergometer. This large percentage increase in aerobic capacity may be explained by the very low levels of fitness prior to conditioning.

Improvements with physical conditioning relate to greater efficiency of the respiratory, cardiovascular, and musculoskeletal systems. Both minute ventilation and heart rate are lower at the same workload after training (Fig. 8).[37] Furthermore, physical conditioning leads to a higher stroke volume at rest and during submaximal exercise, while prolonged inactivity reduces the stroke volume.[22] Also, regular exercise increases the volume of mitochondria and enzyme levels in trained muscles, which can further augment aerobic energy capacity.[42]

The benefits of physical activity continue despite the aging process as long as

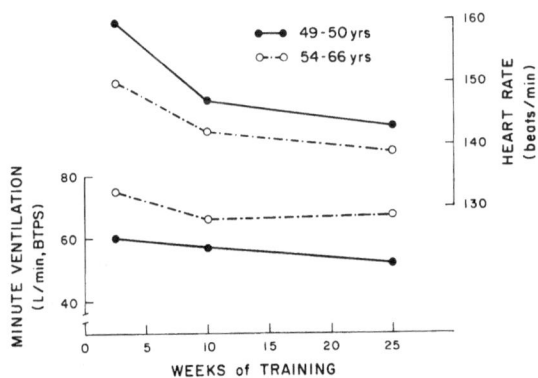

Figure 8. Minute ventilation and heart rate are decreased in healthy male subjects with progressive exercise training (adapted from Norris, Shock, and Yiengst[37]).

participation is maintained. Depending on the intensity of exercise, participants in regular and vigorous activities, such as tennis, swimming, skiing, and jogging, experience a smaller decrement in $\dot{V}O_2$max over the years.[28,29]

2.4. Chronic Obstructive Pulmonary Disease

2.4.1. Introduction

Chronic obstructive pulmonary disease (COPD) refers to three disorders (asthma, chronic bronchitis, and emphysema) that are characterized by obstruction to air flow. Chronic bronchitis and emphysema are strongly related to cigarette smoking, and symptoms usually become manifest by middle age. The natural decline in respiratory function with advancing age along with continued cigarette smoking can contribute to increased symptoms, especially dyspnea, in the elderly. Although asthma is more common in childhood than in the aged, airway hyperreactivity and bronchospasm, which are characteristic of asthma, may exist to varying degrees in chronic bronchitis as well as emphysema.

Recent developments have provided greater insights into the mechanisms limiting exercise tolerance in COPD patients. As a result, respiratory muscle training and pulmonary vasodilator therapy offer new therapeutic approaches. Also, evaluation of COPD patients during sleep has demonstrated the role of nocturnal hypoxemia in the pathogenesis of pulmonary hypertension and cardiac arrhythmias. To prevent these complications, supplemental oxygen, either continuous or nocturnal, must be considered.

2.4.2. Definition and Differentiation of Diseases

2.4.2.1. Asthma

Asthma is a disease characterized by intermittent episodes of bronchospasm alternating with symptom-free periods.[43] It can be divided into two basic types: (1) *extrinsic asthma* which occurs in atopic individuals and usually has its onset in infancy or early childhood; and (2) *intrinsic asthma* which is not related to atopy, usually occurs in adulthood, and is often associated with a history of recurrent respiratory infections.

Airway tone or reactivity is increased in asthma, and release of mediators, e.g., histamine, slow-reacting substance of anaphylaxis (SRS-A), and eosinophilic chemotactic factor of anaphylaxis (ECF-A), leads to bronchial smooth muscle contraction. Both allergens and respiratory infections can trigger mediator release; however, at times no precipitating factor can be identified. In addition to bronchoconstriction, bronchial mucosal edema, mucous secretion, and eosinophilic infiltrates contribute to airway obstruction.

Clinical features include wheezing and breathlessness that are due to airway narrowing. In atopic individuals, for example those who have experienced hay fever or eczema, serum IgE and blood eosinophils are increased. Many asthmatic patients develop bronchospasm with exertion, especially when the air is dry and cold.[44] Aspirin use and occupational exposure, especially isocyanates, formaldehyde, detergent enzymes derived from *Bacillus subtilis,* fungal antigens, animal products, and grain contaminants, can cause acute symptoms. Although typically the asthmatic response to exposure of an allergen is immediate, in many cases the reaction may be delayed by 4 to 6 hr.

2.4.2.2. Chronic Bronchitis

Chronic bronchitis, which occurs predominantly in cigarette smokers, is a disorder in which excessive mucous secretion occurs in the bronchial tree. The primary manifestation is chronic or recurrent cough productive of mucoid or mucopurulent sputum. The American Thoracic Society has arbitrarily defined chronic bronchitis as daily sputum production for at least 3 months in the year for 2 successive years.[43] Since other diseases, e.g., tuberculosis, lung abscess, and bronchiectasis, can produce identical symptoms, the diagnosis of chronic bronchitis can be made only after these other disorders are excluded.

Histopathologic changes include hypertrophy and hyperplasia of the mucus-secreting bronchial glands throughout the tracheobronchial tree. Physiologic manifestations consist primarily of increased airway resistance with evidence of obstruction to air flow on pulmonary function testing.

With progression of disease, hypoxemia and CO_2 retention may develop. Patients with chronic bronchitis have been called "blue bloaters" because both cyanosis and right heart failure are frequent complications.

2.4.2.3. Emphysema

In contrast to the clinical diagnoses of asthma and chronic bronchitis, the definition of emphysema is based on anatomic alterations characterized by enlargement of air spaces distal to the terminal, nonrespiratory bronchiole with associated destruction of the alveolar walls.[43] According to the distribution of pathologic involvement, emphysema can be classified as centrilobular or panlobular. In centrilobular emphysema, destructive changes are localized to the region of the respiratory bronchiole, develop most frequently in the upper zones of the lung, and usually occur in patients with a long history of cigarette smoking. In panlobular emphysema, the entire acinus is involved, including the respiratory bronchiole, alveolar ducts and sacs, and the alveolar wall. Lesions are often more severe in the lower zones of the lungs, and an association with α_1-antitrypsin deficiency may exist.

Table I.   Distinguishing Characteristics between Chronic
Bronchitis and Emphysema

Characteristic	Chronic bronchitis	Emphysema
Symptom	Cough; sputum	Dyspnea
Habitus	Normal or stocky	Thin
Total lung capacity	Normal	Increased
Diffusion capacity	Normal	Decreased
Arterial CO_2 tension	Increased	Normal or decreased
Right heart failure	Common	Uncommon

Distinguishing characteristics between chronic bronchitis and emphysema are listed in Table I.

Although patients with emphysema may be asymptomatic, exertional dyspnea is generally the first and most pronounced symptom. Vital capacity of the lungs may be diminished, while residual volume and total lung capacity are increased, indicating air trapping and hyperinflation, respectively. As a result of anatomic destruction, both elastic recoil and diffusion capacity (D_LCO) of the lungs are reduced. Patients with emphysema have been labeled "pink puffers" since oxygenation is generally preserved at an increased level of ventilation.

Even though the diagnosis of emphysema is based strictly on pathologic changes, it should be highly suspected in a patient with chronic airway obstruction, absence of sputum production, hyperinflation of the lungs, and a marked decrease in D_LCO.

2.4.3. Diagnosis of Airway Obstruction

2.4.3.1. Pulmonary Function Testing

Diminished expiratory flow rates are the *sine qua non* of airway obstruction. A FEV_1:FVC ratio of less than 70% indicates obstruction to air flow.[45] The severity of impairment is dependent on the measured FEV_1 as the percentage of the predicted value (Table II).[46] Usually, the lower the FEV_1, the greater the patient's respiratory symptoms. Decreases in peak expiratory (PF) and midexpiratory (MEF50) flow rates also occur in obstructive pulmonary disease.

Asymptomatic individuals who smoke cigarettes may have diminished air flow in the small or peripheral airways of the lungs (airways < 2 mm internal diameter). Although it has been suggested that these changes may antedate or help identify those who might develop obstructive airway disease, this remains speculative at the present time.

In patients with advanced COPD, progression of airway disease occurs at a predictable rate. Although individual variation exists, FEV_1 decreases 60 to 80 ml/year, or 2 to 3 times the normal decline associated with aging.[47]

Table II. Grading of Pulmonary Function
Impairment[a]

Impairment	FEV_1 (percent of predicted)
Normal	> 80
Mild	65–79
Moderate	50–64
Severe	< 50

[a]From Snider, Kory, and Lyons.[46]

2.4.3.2. Assessment of Airway Reversibility

Inhalation of a bronchodilator spray has been used to assess reversibility of airway obstruction. In contrast to "fixed" airway disease, the demonstration of reversibility strongly suggests that bronchodilator or corticosteroid therapy will improve lung function. On the other hand, the lack of a response to an inhaled bronchodilator does not indicate irreversibility, since response to treatment may take weeks to months.

Although isoproterenol is considered the classic bronchodilator for evaluating airway reversibility, newer and more selective β-adrenergic agents, such as isoetharine and metaproterenol, cause less cardiac stimulation and are safe to use in elderly patients. Generally, there is minimal risk or side effects associated with such testing. Spirometry is performed before, and 15 to 20 min after, inhalation of a nebulized bronchodilator; generally, reversibility is defined as at least 15% improvement in two of the following three tests: FVC, FEV_1, and MEF50.[48] Since any dilation of airway tone by previous medication may diminish acute responsiveness to an inhaled bronchodilator,[49] therapy should be discontinued for 24 to 48 hr prior to assessment of reversibility.

2.4.4. Physical Examination

Depending on the severity of airway obstruction, examination of the patient may reveal an increased respiratory rate, increased anterior–posterior diameter of the chest, and hypertrophy of the accessory muscles of respiration. Percussion of the posterior chest at full inspiration and full expiration may reveal limited excursion of the diaphragm consistent with hyperinflation of the lungs.

On auscultation, expiration is generally prolonged, and the intensity of breath sounds may be diminished, especially in emphysema. Inspiratory and expiratory wheezing is a common finding in acute bronchospasm, however expiratory wheezing alone may be present to variable degrees in chronic bronchitis and emphysema.

2.4.5. Laboratory Studies

2.4.5.1. Blood Tests

An increased number of eosinophils in the blood and an elevated level of seum IgE support the diagnosis of asthma in a patient with obstructive airway disease. A deficiency in serum α_1-antitrypsin is associated with development of emphysema, especially involving the lower lobes.

2.4.5.2. Sputum Analysis

In asthma, eosinophils and Charcot-Leyden crystals may be seen on smear of the sputum. In evaluating the lower respiratory infections, a Gram stain of the sputum should be obtained; the presence of polymorphonuclear cells and a predominant organism are suggestive of a bacterial etiology. The presence of epithelial cells indicates that the specimen has been contaminated with upper respiratory secretions. Ideally, the results of the sputum culture should confirm or support the findings on the Gram stain.

2.4.5.3. Arterial Blood Gases

Ventilation–perfusion inequality is present in obstructive airway disease leading to hypoxemia with or without retention of CO_2. Typically, the patient with emphysema has only moderate hypoxemia (PaO_2 = 60 to 70 Torr), and a normal or diminished $PaCO_2$. By contrast, in chronic bronchitis, hypoxemia may be severe (PaO_2 < 60 Torr), and $PaCO_2$ may be increased (> 43 Torr).

In asymptomatic asthmatic individuals arterial gas tensions may be normal. With acute episodes of bronchospasm, hypoxemia is common and carbon dioxide retention begins to occur when the FEV_1 is decreased to 15% of the predicted value.[50] Since $PaCO_2$ reflects the adequacy of alveolar ventilation, a sudden increase in $PaCO_2$ in a patient with symptomatic airway obstruction indicates marked impairment of gas exchange. At this point, further respiratory support, including mechanical ventilation, should be considered.

2.4.5.4. Chest Radiography

The chest radiograph is insensitive for the early diagnosis as well as differentiation of COPD. In fact, the chest film may be normal in patients with severe asthma and chronic bronchitis. Loss of vascular markings, especially in the periphery of the lung, flattening of the diaphragm, and an increased retrosternal air space are consistent with emphysema.

The presence of pulmonary artery hypertension (mean pulmonary artery pressure > 20 mm Hg) can be identified in patients with chronic bronchitis or emphysema by measuring the widest diameter of the right and left descending pulmonary arteries on the chest radiograph. Increased pulmonary artery pressures can be expected if the right descending pulmonary artery exceeds 16 mm and/or the left descending pulmonary artery diameter is greater than 18 mm.[51]

2.4.6. Mechanisms Limiting Exercise Performance

2.4.6.1. Diminished Ventilatory Capacity

In patients with obstructive lung disease, both altered gas mixing and gas transfer are present at rest and during exercise. With physical activity, ventilation must increase in order to meet increased oxygen requirements. However, the patient with COPD may not be able to generate adequate flow rates and/or maintain increased exercise ventilation due to diminished ventilatory capacity.[52,53] In fact, in some individuals, there may be no expiratory flow reserve even during tidal breathing at rest (Fig. 9). Thus, the mechanical properties of the respiratory system can limit exercise without the development of hypoxemia.

2.4.6.2. Hypoxemia

Based on previous studies, it is difficult to predict which patients with chronic airflow obstruction will develop exertional hypoxemia.[54] Furthermore, the cause of exercise hypoxemia is not completely understood in COPD, although it has been shown that oxygen desaturation may be related to a failure to decrease venous admixture.[54] Nevertheless, hypoxemia contributes to decreased systemic oxygen delivery and impaired cellular function.

2.4.6.3. Respiratory Muscle Fatigue

Inspiratory muscle fatigue, as demonstrated by surface electromyography, can occur during exercise in patients with COPD.[55] In addition, asynchronous or

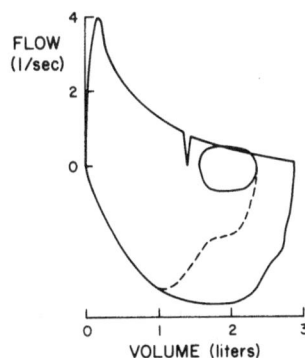

Figure 9. Resting and maximal flow-volume loops in a patient with severe obstructive airway disease. The resting flow-volume loop is represented by the small oval, while the dashed line connects the resting loop with the maximal flow-volume loop. Note that there is no flow reserve during expiration between rest and maximal effort.

paradoxical respiratory patterns have been observed during exercise,[56] further suggesting that diaphragmatic dysfunction may contribute to exercise limitation. In support of this, it has been shown that training of the inspiratory muscles in patients with COPD improved exercise performance only in those who demonstrated electromyographic changes heralding inspiratory muscle fatigue during exercise.[57]

2.4.6.4. Right Ventricular Dysfunction Secondary to Pulmonary Hypertension

It has been suggested that right ventricular dysfunction in association with pulmonary hypertension may adversely affect exercise capacity in COPD patients.[58,59] The usual course of chronic obstructive pulmonary disease is slow, progressive deterioration in lung function resulting in dyspnea on exertion. Over time, pulmonary hypertension may develop, leading to right heart failure. However, prior to the onset of overt pulmonary hypertension and cor pulmonale, patients with COPD develop increased pulmonary artery pressure and pulmonary vascular resistance *with physical exertion* (Fig. 10). The increased afterload may limit right ventricular output and adversely affect exercise performance in patients with COPD.[60,61]

2.4.7. Therapeutic Strategies

Therapy for chronic obstructive pulmonary disease should be directed at the mechanism(s) that limit gas exchange and produce symptoms. Although the

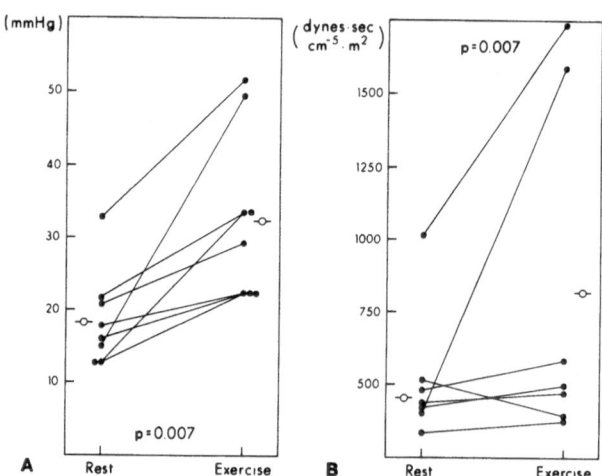

Figure 10. Mean pulmonary artery pressure (A) and pulmonary vascular resistance index (B) at rest and during steady-state exercise in patients with chronic obstructive pulmonary disease. Closed circles connected by a line indicate an individual patient. Open circles with horizontal bars represent mean values.

majority of patients breathe comfortably at rest, they commonly develop dyspnea with physical exertion. The primary goal for the physician should be to improve or relieve the patient's breathlessness. Ideally, the various mechanisms that limit exercise tolerance in COPD should be specifically evaluated, and then appropriate treatment instituted. Unfortunately, technical aspects may prevent assessment of respiratory muscle fatigue and right ventricular function except at specially equipped laboratories.

In order to determine whether specific therapy is beneficial, it is important to establish baseline measurements prior to treatment. Both objective (lung function and exercise performance) and subjective (dyspnea rating) parameters are useful to assess therapeutic efficacy.[62]

2.4.7.1. Smoking Cessation

Cessation of cigarette smoking is the single most important factor in the treatment of obstructive airway disease. When a patient stops smoking, lung function and ciliary clearance improve.[19] Furthermore, since cigarette smoking accelerates the age-related decline in respiratory function, quitting smoking is also beneficial for long-term preservation of lung function.[18]

2.4.7.2. Bronchodilator Therapy

Prescription of bronchodilators is the primary therapeutic modality for obstructive pulmonary disease. For asthma, a reversible airway disease, bronchodilators have been extremely beneficial in relieving bronchospasm.[63] Despite the widespread use of such therapy in patients with chronic bronchitis and emphysema, which are frequently characterized by nonreversible air-flow obstruction ($<15\%$ improvement in FEV_1 after inhalation of a bronchodilator), there is presently no evidence that administration of bronchodilators improves dyspnea or exercise tolerance[64] or alters the natural history of stable chronic air-flow obstruction.[65] Furthermore, side effects may also limit their usefulness.

A reasonable approach to the use of bronchodilator therapy in COPD is to first assess airway responsiveness to an inhaled agent (e.g., metaproterenol or isoetharine) in the pulmonary function laboratory. Ideally, all oral bronchodilators should be stopped for 24 to 48 hr prior to testing. If airway reversibility is demonstrated, therapy is clearly indicated. On the other hand, if no reversibility is evident, a trial of bronchodilator therapy is appropriate; however, it is important to establish pretreatment measurements of dyspnea, lung function, and exercise performance in order to assess efficacy of therapy at a later date.

2.4.7.2a. Sympathomimetic Drugs. These agents cause bronchodilatation by stimulation of adenyl cyclase which produces an increase in intracellular cyclic AMP concentration. All of the sympathomimetic agents have a phenylethylamine nucleus, and alterations of this structure produce variations in the degree of α- and β-adrenergic activity (Table III). The newer drugs in this class, especially

Table III. Selected Pharmacologic Properties of Adrenergic Activity

Sites of pharmacologic activity	α-Effect	β_1-Effect	β_2-Effect
Smooth muscle			
Bronchi and uterus	Constriction (?)		Relaxation
Alimentary tract	Decreased motility and tone	Decreased motility and tone	
	Constriction of sphincters		
Blood vessels	Constriction	Dilatation (coronary)	
Skeletal muscle			Affects skeletal muscle twitch response
Cardiac muscle	Very small increase in rate and force of contraction	Increase in force and rate of contraction	

β_2-agonists, provide the advantages of greater specificity, longer duration of action, and greater absorption by the gastrointestinal tract.

Although sympathomimetics can be administered by the oral, parenteral, and inhaled routes (Table IV), the rapid onset of action, peak effect, and acceptability by the patient of metered-dose inhalers of aerosolized medication are important for both acute and chronic therapy. Sequential administration of aerosolized bronchodilators every 10 to 20 min may be an effective method of treatment for acute bronchospasm.[66] Generally, side effects are minimal with an aerosol compared to oral medication.[67] Appropriate use of metered-dose inhalers requires that the patient be instructed how to inhale the aerosol properly and warned of the hazards of overuse. The clinical usefulness of aerosolized isoproterenol is limited because

Table IV. Pharmacologic Characteristics of Selected Sympathomimetic Bronchodilators

Drug	Receptor activity	Routes of administration	Effective dose ranges (mg)	Duration of action (hr)
Epinephrine	$\alpha = \beta_1 = \beta_2$	Subcutaneous	0.25 to 0.5	0.5 to 2
Isoproterenol	$\beta_1 = \beta_2$	Inhaled	0.08 to 0.16	0.5 to 2
Isoetharine	$\beta_1 < \beta_2$	Inhaled	0.5 to 1.0	1 to 4
Metaproterenol	$\beta_1 < \beta_2$	Inhaled	0.65 to 1.3	1 to 4
		Oral	10 to 20	3 to 4
Terbutaline	$\beta_1 < \beta_2$	Subcutaneous	0.25 to 0.5	1 to 4
		Oral	2.5 to 5	3 to 4
Albuterol	$\beta_1 \ll \beta_2$	Inhaled	0.1 to 0.24	4 to 6

of its short duration of action and cardiac stimulation. Instead, more selective β_2-agonists, such as metaproterenol, isoetharine, albuterol, and fenoterol, provide greater bronchodilatation and less tachycardia.

Currently, ephedrine, metaproterenol, terbutaline and albuterol are the oral sympathomimetic agents available in the United States. The effectiveness of oral sympathomimetic bronchodilators can be limited by skeletal muscle tremors, which may appear even at doses required for moderate degrees of bronchodilation.[68] In the elderly patient, the tremor may interfere with activities of daily living and should be carefully evaluated. By starting with a low dose and increasing the dosage gradually, patients may develop tolerance for the tremor.

Although subcutaneous administration of epinephrine has been highly effective in the treatment of acute bronchospasm, terbutaline, a more selective β_2-agent, at a dose of 0.25 mg subcutaneous provides nearly twice the bronchodilation as epinephrine and has a longer duration of action.[69] However, terbutaline does increase heart rate, and its benefit should be weighed against cardiac stimulation in the elderly.

2.4.7.2b. Theophylline Preparations. These agents are methylated xanthines that relax bronchial smooth muscle. Theophylline also stimulates the central nervous system, acts on the kidney to produce diuresis, and stimulates cardiac muscle. Intravenous aminophylline (theophylline diethylenediamine) has been used for relief of acute exacerbations of air-flow obstruction, although the development of oral sustained-release formulations has led to "prophylactic" therapy for controlling the chronic symptoms of obstructive airway disease.

The bronchodilator effect of theophylline is approximately proportional to the logarithm of serum concentrations within the range of 5 to 20 μm/ml.[70] The frequency and severity of asthmatic symptoms are minimized when serum theophylline concentrations are continuously maintained between 10 and 20 μm/ml.[71] Although there is no evidence that theophylline improves breathlessness in nonreversible obstructive airway disease,[64] aminophylline may provide a protective effect on the development of diaphragmatic fatigue.[72] Adverse effects of theophylline include nausea, vomiting, headache, decreased appetite, and irritability, and are generally associated with serum concentrations about 20 μg/ml. At higher serum levels (> 35 μg/ml), seizures, cardiac arrhythmias, and death have occurred.[73]

Guidelines for both intravenous and oral administration of theophylline preparations have been established in order to achieve therapeutic blood levels (Table V). However, individual dose requirements depend on variability in rate of elimination which is related to biotransformation into inactive metabolites in the liver. For acute therapy, a loading dose of intravenous aminophylline is given if no theophylline was taken within the previous 12 hr; this is followed by a maintenance dose in order to provide a steady and continuous therapeutic effect. With intravenous therapy, theophylline blood levels should be measured at 1, 12, and 24 hr until stabilization and then at 48-hr intervals.[74]

Table V. Guidelines for Theophylline Administration[a]

---

1. *Intravenous* (aminophylline)
   A. Loading dose
      1. No recent theophylline—5.6 mg/kg over 20 to 30 min
      2. Theophylline within 12 hr—¾ of above loading dose
   B. Maintenance dose (via infusion pump)
      1. Young patients—0.9 mg/kg per hr
      2. Older patients (> 50 yr)—0.68 mg/kg per hr
      3. Patients with congestive heart failure or liver disease—0.45 mg/kg per hr

2. *Oral* (sustained-release theophylline preparation)
   A. Otherwise healthy, nonsmoking adult—13 mg/kg per day in divided dose (q 8 hr to q 12 hr)
      1. Maximal starting dose—not to exceed 900 mg/day
      2. Minor adverse effects can be minimized by starting with a small initial dose with gradual increase to 13 mg/kg per day
   B. Older patients (> 50 yr)—25% reduction
   C. Patients with congestive heart failure or liver disease—50% reduction

---

[a]Theophylline dosages are based on ideal or lean body weight. Adapted from Weinberger, M., et al.[71] and Jusko, W. J., et al.[74]

Sustained-release oral preparations are preferred for maintenance theophylline therapy in ambulatory patients. Theo-Dur® and Sustaire® formulations provide reliable absorption and adequate dosage strengths and permit 12-hr dosing for most patients. If oral therapy is well-tolerated by the patient, a theophylline level should be obtained under steady-state conditions, which is 4 to 5 half-lives following initiation of treatment. This is approximately 2 days in otherwise healthy adults and 5 days in patients with prolonged elimination, e.g., congestive heart failure or liver disease. Once a therapeutic theophylline level has been obtained, dosage requirements are generally stable unless physiological changes occur.

In patients over 50 years old and those with congestive heart failure or liver disease, elimination of theophylline is prolonged, and the predicted dose should be reduced.[74,75] Cimetidine, an H_2 antagonist used to decrease gastric acid secretion, prolongs the half-life of theophylline[76] and blood levels should be monitored closely to prevent theophylline toxicity. Conversely, theophylline enhances clearance of phenytoin, which could lead to increased frequency of seizures if phenytoin levels are not measured and the dose adjusted during concurrent administration.[71] Also, theophylline clearance is increased in individuals who smoke, and thus, higher dosages may be required.

2.4.7.2c. Corticosteroids. Although corticosteroids produce multiple cellular effects, the mechanisms contributing to bronchodilatation in patients with airway obstruction appear related to potentiation of catecholamine stimulation of cyclic AMP synthesis, inhibition of prostaglandin synthesis or release, and antiinflammatory effects.[71] Intravenous therapy with corticosteroids has been proven beneficial in reversing bronchospasm in asthmatics and in improving air-flow obstruction associated with acute respiratory insufficiency in patients with chronic bronchitis.[77,78] Short-term use ($<$ 2 weeks) of daily oral or parenteral corticosteroids is not associated with serious toxicity; however, prolonged daily administration can lead to adrenal suppression, Cushingoid appearance, suppression of growth, cataracts, osteoporosis, and increased susceptibility to infections.

Prednisone, prednisolone, and methylprednisolone are the most commonly used systemic corticosteroids for the treatment of bronchospasm. Although the optimal dosage of intravenous corticosteroids has not been determined, 0.5 mg/kg of methylprednisolone, which has no sodium-retaining properties, or its equivalent in another glucocorticoid preparation is an appropriate dose that has been shown to be clinically effective.[78] Prednisone is the most commonly used oral preparation after intravenous medication is discontinued and for outpatient management of bronchospasm that is difficult to control with sympathomimetic and theophylline agents. The adverse effects of prolonged corticosteroid therapy can be minimized by using a single morning dose every other day. Although the efficacy of this approach remains controversial, the apparent lack of effectiveness may be the result of using inadequate doses.[71] Doses of 20 to 40 mg of prednisone have been required on alternate days to control symptoms, and few side effects occur.[79]

Beclomethasone dipropionate is an inhaled corticosteroid preparation which can provide potent local activity in the airways with minimal systemic side effects. Studies have demonstrated that beclomethasone aerosol is effective in asthmatic patients who are dependent on oral steroids and those whose symptoms are poorly controlled by nonsteroidal regimens.[80] Clinical experience indicates that beclomethasone is also useful in nonasthmatic patients with chronic pulmonary disease who have reversible airway obstruction. Most patients who require 20 mg/day or less of prednisone for control of asthma can be transferred to beclomethasone with maintenance of satisfactory respiratory function and disappearance of side effects related to systemic corticosteroids.[80] In patients who have received oral corticosteroids for prolonged periods, systemic steroid therapy must be tapered very carefully while controlling the airway disease with beclomethasone; in fact, it may be important to evaluate adrenal function during the tapering process.[81] Guidelines are provided in Table VI for decreasing oral prednisone during concomitant use of beclomethasone.[82]

Similar to oral and intravenous agents, steroid aerosols improve lung function within 2 hr of administration although the full effect is achieved in 8 hr.[83] The usual dose of beclomethasone is 2 puffs 4 times a day (400 μg/day), which is considered to be as effective as 7.5 mg of oral prednisone.[84] For severe air-flow obstruction, therapy can be initiated with 10–12 puffs/day; 1600 mg of beclomethasone is considered the minimal daily dose that might be expected to cause adrenal suppression.[80] In order to optimize delivery of the steroid aerosol, the

Table VI. Guidelines for Tapering Oral Prednisone during
Concomitant Use of Beclomethasone Dipropionate[a]

Condition	Beclomethasone dipropionate	Prednisone
First week	2 puffs qid (400 µg)	Maintain current dose
If adrenal stimulation is normal	Same	↓ by 2.5 mg/week
If evidence of adrenal suppression	Same	↓ by 1.0 mg/month

[a]Adapted from Hodson, M. E., et al.[82]

patient should inhale an adrenergic bronchodilator 5 to 10 min prior to using beclomethasone.

2.4.7.3. Oxygen Therapy

Supplemental oxygen is clearly indicated for patients with diminished oxygenation that may be manifested by dyspnea, impaired mental status, and/or restlessness and agitation. Applying the criteria used by the Nocturnal Oxygen Therapy Trial Group,[85] low flow oxygen should be prescribed when $PaO_2 \leq 55$ Torr or $PaO_2 \leq 59$ Torr plus one of the following: edema, hematocrit $\geq 55\%$; and P pulmonale on electrocardiogram. In this multicenter study in the United States, continuous O_2 therapy was associated with a lower mortality than was nocturnal O_2 therapy; however, the reason for this difference was unclear.[85]

In some patients arterial oxygen tension may be adequate at rest, but desaturation can develop with physical exertion, causing shortness of breath and limiting exercise capacity. To evaluate this situation, either O_2 tension (PaO_2) or saturation (SaO_2) should be measured during an exercise test; work loads should be selected that are comparable to the patient's daily activities. If a significant decrease in oxygenation occurs (PaO_2 falls more than 5 Torr, SaO_2 falls more than 3%, and/or $PaO_2 < 60$ Torr), a portable ambulatory system for delivering oxygen is indicated. Ideally, the exercise test should be repeated with the patient breathing oxygen in order to demonstrate improvement in exercise tolerance and to ascertain the appropriate flow rates of O_2.

In addition, COPD patients may experience severe hypoxemia while sleeping, which can cause episodic pulmonary vasoconstriction and pulmonary hypertension[86] as well as cardiac arrhythmias.[87] Oxygen therapy has been shown to reduce nocturnal pulmonary hypertension[86] and improve electrocardiographic abnormalities[87] in these patients. Also, a recent, multicenter study in Great Britain found that oxygen therapy for 15 hr a day prolonged life in patients with hypoxemic chronic obstructive pulmonary disease.[88] Although nocturnal oxygen desaturation is very common in COPD patients, the cost of treating all of these patients would be enormous. A reasonable approach in dealing with this problem is to prescribe nocturnal oxygen for patients who desaturate during the night and also have developed an associated ill effect, such as cor pulmonale, pulmonary hypertension, secondary polycytemia, nocturnal arrhythmias, and nocturnal cardiac ischemia.[89]

2.4.7.4. Respiratory Muscle Training

Although exercise training programs increase physical endurance in patients with COPD, the mechanism(s) by which improvement occurs has not been determined.[90] Inspiratory muscle fatigue can occur during exercise in patients with chronic airway obstruction and may limit exercise performance.[91] In fact, ventilatory muscle training using either isocapnic hyperpnea[92] or inspiratory resistances[57] has been shown to increase exercise capacity in these patients. At the present time, a practical approach for respiratory muscle training is for the patient to use an incentive spirometry or inspiratory resistance device at home. Several training runs should be performed daily with each run consisting of five to ten inspiratory efforts. To achieve a training effect, the duration of a maximal inspiratory force should be progressively increased.

2.4.7.5. Pulmonary Vasodilator Therapy

Since pulmonary hypertension develops during exercise in patients with COPD and can lead to right ventricular dysfunction, pulmonary vasodilating agents may be useful by unloading the right ventricle and thereby augmenting cardiac output.[93] This type of therapy is similar to the use of vasodilator therapy for left ventricular failure. Both hydralazine[94] and nifedipine[95,96] have been shown to decrease pulmonary artery pressure and improve cardiac performance in COPD. At the present time, both acute and long-term studies are needed to further evaluate the efficacy of pulmonary vasodilating agents in the treatment of obstructive airway disease.

2.4.8. Management of Complications

2.4.8.1. Upper Respiratory Infections

Both upper respiratory infections and episodes of chronic bronchitis can exacerbate air-flow obstruction in patients with COPD and lead to increased breathlessness and diminished exercise tolerance. Although these infections are frequently due to viruses, broad-spectrum antibiotics (e.g., ampicillin or tetracycline) are often prescribed empirically, especially when purulent sputum is expectorated.

Evaluation and treatment of pneumonia in the elderly will be discussed in the next section.

2.4.8.2. Pulmonary Hypertension and Cor Pulmonale

Pulmonary artery hypertension, which is the principal cause of right ventricular enlargement and failure in COPD, has five potential causes: (1) increased pulmonary vascular resistance; (2) increased cardiac output; (3) increased pulmonary blood volume; (4) increased viscosity of blood; and (5) elevated pulmonary venous pressure.[97] Hypoxia, however, is the most potent pulmonary vasoconstrictor that reduces the functional pulmonary bed. Due to increased pulmonary artery pressures, the load that the right ventricle bears, an adaptive right ventricular enlargement may develop (cor pulmonale). Over time and with progression of disease, right heart failure occurs, as manifested by distended neck veins, enlarged liver, and peripheral edema.

2.4.8.2a. Oxygen. The major goal of therapy is to decrease the work load of the right ventricle by decreasing pulmonary artery pressure. Oxygen therapy in patients with cor pulmonale reduces pulmonary artery pressure, augments right ventricular ejection fraction, and reduces hematocrit.[98,99] In fact, 15 hr/day of oxygen improved survival in patients with cor pulmonale compared to those who received no O_2 therapy.[88] In the Nocturnal Oxygen Therapy Trial involving stable COPD patients with hypoxemia, mortality in the group receiving 12 hr of nocturnal oxygen was nearly twice that of the continuous (24-hr) oxygen group.[85]

2.4.8.2b. Diuretics. Increased lung fluid compromises pulmonary gas exchange. Initial diuretic therapy decreases pulmonary artery pressure by decreasing total blood volume.[100] However, overzealous use of diuretics can lead to volume depletion, resulting in a decrease in cardiac output, as well as hypokalemic metabolic alkalosis, which diminishes the drive to breathe. Careful monitoring of fluid status and serum electrolytes is important when managing patients with right heart failure. Bed rest and modest salt restriction are beneficial during long-term care.

2.4.8.2c. Digitalis. The use of digitalis in COPD patients with cor pulmonale is controversial. In general, there is no definitive evidence supporting the use of cardiac glycosides in patients with cor pulmonale unless left ventricular failure or a supraventricular tachyarrhythmia are also present.[101] In a double-blind, digoxin–placebo trial in patients with pulmonary heart disease, right ventricular ejection fraction improved after 8 weeks of digoxin therapy only when the left ventricular ejection fraction was also initially abnormal.[102] At the present time, digitalis is indicated for COPD patients with coexisting left heart failure, a supraventricular tachyarrhythmia, or overt right heart failure that does not respond to extensive application of other therapy to relieve pulmonary artery hypertension.

2.5. Pneumonia in the Elderly

> *Pneumonia is the captain of the men*
> *in death, and tuberculosis is the*
> *handmaiden.*
> SIR WILLIAM OSLER (1849-1919)

2.5.1. Introduction

The development of pneumonia is dependent on two opposing factors: the virulence of the organism and the host's defense system. In general, a "more virulent" organism is necessary to cause pneumonia in a healthy individual, although a "less virulent" microbe can become established in the lower respiratory tract of those with impaired defenses. Even though penicillin has reduced the mortality of pneumococcal pneumonia from 40% to between 5 and 10%, pneumonia remains the most common infectious cause of death in the United States.[103] In fact, influenza and pneumonia constitute the fourth most common cause of death among the elderly.[104]

In the aged, multiple factors contribute to the development of pneumonia. In a general hospital, 82% of adult patients with pneumonia had some associated condition, such as heart disease, alcoholism, chronic lung disease, or diabetes mellitus.[105] Although there are conflicting data on whether aging is associated with changes in host defenses,[106-108] defense mechanisms are impaired in those with chronic diseases, especially airway obstruction, neurologic dysfunction, and patients receiving radiation or immunosuppressive therapy.

Recent studies have shown that the incidence of Gram-negative bacillary pneumonia is higher in elderly persons living at home or in an extended-care facility.[109-110] This may, in part, be related to the observation that elderly persons living independently in apartments have increased oropharyngeal colonization of Gram-negative bacilli compared to younger control subjects.[111] Also, the use of broad-spectrum antibiotics can cause a change in the flora of the oropharynx; any pneumonia that may develop in such a patient will likely be due to resistant organisms that can lead to a high morbidity and mortality.

In this section, emphasis will be directed toward features or specific conditions associated with pneumonia in the elderly. Comprehensive reviews of the epidemiology, diagnosis, and treatment of pneumonia in the general population are available in medical textbooks.

2.5.2. Pathogenesis of Pneumonia

In most instances, pneumonia is due to aspiration of organisms that have colonized the oropharynx. The incidence of upper airway colonization with

Gram-negative bacilli is twice as great in healthy elderly people (19%) than in young healthy controls (8%) and is further increased in those elderly subjects requiring nursing care.[111] Although the mechanism of control of the oropharyngeal flora is poorly understood, underlying disease, the selective effect of antibiotics, or simply the aging process may be important.

After colonization, the next stage is microaspiration of upper airway secretions into the bronchi.[112] Although microaspiration probably occurs in all individuals, especially during sleep, the elderly are particularly predisposed to aspiration. Predisposing conditions include altered mental status, seizures, sedative use, general anesthesia, dysphagia from esophageal or neurologic dysfunction, tracheal intubation, use of a nasogastric tube, and forced feeding of patients with diminished oropharyngeal protective reflexes. Once a microbe has entered the tracheobronchial tree, pulmonary defense mechanisms attempt to clear or sterilize the lower respiratory tract.

2.5.3. Respiratory Defenses

In healthy individuals, aspirated bacteria are cleared from the tracheobronchial tree by mucociliary clearance. The complex mechanism extends from the respiratory bronchiole to the larynx and includes a sol/gel mucus system along with the coordinated activity of the ciliated epithelium.[113] Organisms or particles that are aspirated or inhaled into the airways are removed by the mucociliary blanket toward the larynx, and then expectorated or swallowed. The elderly have decreased mucociliary clearance compared with the young, although this impairment is minimal compared with those who smoke or have chronic obstructive pulmonary disease.[113]

Organisms that extend beyond the respiratory bronchiole and enter terminal bronchioles and alveoli are cleared by alveolar macrophages. Macrophages ingest the microorganisms and then ascend or migrate to the mucociliary layer.[114] Alternatively, they may enter the lymphatic system and migrate to regional lymph nodes.[114] Specific immunoglobins, especially IgA, are secreted into the airways to aid in elimination of pathogens.

When the clearance mechanisms are overwhelmed by an inoculum of bacteria, an inflammatory cellular response ensues consisting mainly of polymorphonuclear leukocytes. Due to increased regional blood flow and capillary permeability, fluid develops in the alveoli. With organisms that multiply rapidly, exudation of fluid may provide a culture medium and contribute to local spread of the bacteria.[115]

Whether the aging process alters immunologic function is unclear. Investigators have reported that immunoglobin levels and cellular response diminish with age,[107-108] although others have stated that no immunologic impairment results from aging alone.[106]

2.5.4. Clinical Pneumonia Syndrome

Infectious pneumonia is generally characterized by an acute febrile illness, respiratory symptoms, especially purulent sputum production, and a pulmonary infiltrate on the chest radiograph. However, in the geriatric patient, the clinical picture may not always be completely expressed. Sputum may not be produced because of an ineffective cough or dehydration. Symptoms may be subtle, such as general malaise or confusion. Also, fever may be mild or even absent. Physical examination may not reveal the typical findings of pneumonitis, particularly in patients with obstructive pulmonary disease. In older patients, the chest radiograph can demonstrate a mottled-appearing infiltrate rather than dense consolidation.[116]

2.5.4.1. Typical Bacterial Pneumonias

Streptococcus pneumoniae has been considered the most common pathogen causing "typical" bacterial pneumonia in the adult. The onset of symptoms is generally sudden and classically associated with a shaking chill, pleuritic chest pain, and greenish or blood-tinged sputum. However, recent studies and reports have shown that Gram-negative bacilli, including *Escherichia coli, Klebsiella,* and *Enterobacter,* are more common infecting agents in elderly patients who acquire pneumonia at home.[109-110] This is consistent with the increased oropharyngeal colonization of Gram-negative organisms in elderly individuals who live independently.[111] In addition, *Hemophilus influenzae* and *S. Aureus* may cause typical bacterial pneumonia in older patients.

2.5.4.2. Aspiration Pneumonia

Aspiration pneumonia is a general term referring to three clinical syndromes due to the abnormal entry of endogenous secretions or exogenous substances into the lower respiratory tract.[117] Although normal individuals may aspirate oral secretions, usually this is benign and self-limited. In patients who develop pulmonary sequelae, the frequency, volume, and character of the inoculum as well as host defenses, such as glottic closure and cough reflex, are important. The type of aspiration syndrome that develops is dependent on the substance or material aspirated.

2.5.4.2a. Chemical Pneumonitis. Various toxic fluids, including acids, mineral oil, alcohol, and hydrocarbons, can initiate an inflammatory response in the lungs independent of bacterial infection. Aspiration of gastric acid is the most frequently encountered and has been called "Mendelson's syndrome."[118] Generally, the aspiration process is observed, and patients develop dyspnea and bronchospasm soon afterward. Experimental studies in animals have shown that the pH of the liquid acid must be 2.4 or less in order to cause pathologic changes.[119]

The predominant physiologic feature is hypoxemia which may progress to the adult respiratory distress syndrome. The chest radiograph typically shows parenchymal infiltrates in the dependent areas of the lungs.

2.5.4.2b. *Bacterial Pneumonitis.* Aspiration of pathogenic bacteria may lead to acute or insidious development of infectious pneumonia. Usually, the actual episode of aspiration is not observed. If the patient has mild symptoms and does not receive antibiotic therapy, the initial pneumonitis may progress to abscess formation within 8 to 14 days. Frequently, posterior segments of the upper lobes or superior segments of the lower lobes are involved due to their dependent position.

The aspirated oropharyngeal secretions contain bacteria from the tongue, gingiva, buccal mucosa, and pharynx. In community-acquired aspiration pneumonia, the predominant organisms are anaerobic Gram-positive cocci, *Bacteroides melaninogenicus,* and *Fusobacterium nucleatum;* among patients who are hospitalized, enteric Gram-negative bacilli, *Pseudomonas,* or *S. aureus* are more common pathogens.[117]

2.5.4.2c. *Aspiration of Inert Substances.* Aspiration of large volumes of fluids or particulate material can cause variable degrees of mechanical obstruction of the airways. Large objects can cause sudden respiratory distress and suffocation; smaller objects that reach segmental bronchi or peripheral airways can cause cough, wheezing, and dyspnea. Chest radiographs may show atelectasis or airway obstruction.

2.5.4.3. Atypical and the "New" Pneumonias

This type of pneumonia is characterized by gradual onset of malaise, headache, sore throat, myalgias, and dry cough. Early in the course, the cough is usually nonproductive, but scant, mucoid sputum may develop later. Pleuritic chest pain is uncommon, although coughing may lead to chest wall soreness. The patchy segmental infiltrates, which may be unilateral or bilateral, seen on the chest radiograph are frequently more extensive than would be suspected by either the patient's symptoms or physical examination.

The atypical pneumonia syndrome is commonly caused by *Mycoplasma pneumoniae, Legionella pneumophila,* and influenza viruses. Although the incidence of these types of pneumonias in the elderly is not well-known, *Mycoplasma* is *not* considered a frequent pathogen in the elderly. Legionnaires' disease, an acute bacterial infection commonly manifested as pneumonia, has been recognized in outbreaks and sporadic cases. Most documented cases have occurred during the summer and in middle-aged or older persons.[120] Patients may experience abdominal pain, pleuritic chest pain, diarrhea, and confusion.[120] The chest radiograph may demonstrate a nodular consolidation pattern. Diagnosis may be established by culture of the Gram-negative bacillus from pleural fluid or lung tissue, direct fluorescence of the organism in lung tissue, or by a significant rise in serum titer by indirect fluorescence.[120] About 15% of cases have been fatal.[114] Conditions that might suggest the possibility of Legionnaires' disease are a history of close contact with or exposure to the water from the cooling towers of air conditioners or residence in an area where soil is turned over during construction.[121]

Pneumonia associated with influenza infection may be either a primary influenza pneumonia, a secondary bacterial pneumonia, or of a mixed etiology.[122] Patients with influenza pneumonia may have an unrelenting fever, dyspnea, hypoxemia, and cyanosis which coexist with the classic influenza syndrome. In fact, the patient never appears to rally or improve from the initial symptoms, i.e., headache, malaise, and myalgia.[122] In contrast, secondary bacterial pneumonia generally occurs at 7 to 10 days after the onset of influenza, at which time the patient has begun to feel better. Shaking chills, fever, and chest pain develop suddenly, and sputum may be abundant. The usual bacterial organisms are *S. pneumoniae, S. aureus,* and *H. influenza.* The chest radiograph often shows a lobar infiltration. The mixed viral–bacterial etiology reflects an intermediate type between primary influenza and secondary bacterial pneumonia. Generally, the onset may be difficult to determine as with influenza pneumonia.

The "new" pneumonias refer to several infectious pulmonary entities that have apparently been present for many years, but the specific etiologic agents, a group of Gram-negative bacilli, have only recently been identified.[123] The clinical features appear similar to Legionnaires' disease. Generally, a unique or different epidemiologic setting may direct attention to the organism for which no diagnosis has been made by conventional microbiologic techniques. These diseases have been named WIGA, OLDA, HERBA, TATLOCK, and Pittsburgh pneumonia based on identifying characteristics of the organism or by the city where the illness developed.[123] At the present time, the incidence of these "new" pneumonias in the elderly population is unknown.

2.5.5. Diagnostic Approach

2.5.5.1. Sputum

The diagnosis of pneumonia is confirmed by sputum examination and cultures of sputum and blood. The sputum Gram-stain is the most important initial technique for preliminary assessment of the etiologic organism. An appropriate specimen from the lower respiratory tract should contain alveolar macrophages, but not be contaminated by epithelial cells of the oropharynx. Acid-fast stains should be performed in order to evaluate for tuberculosis. Culture of the sputum for bacteria should be sent in all cases. If the patient cannot produce sputum, transtracheal aspiration or fiberoptic bronchoscopy with a double lumen sterile catheter should be considered, although either procedure has associated risks. If the sputum Gram stain demonstrates a predominant organism, a bacterial pneumonia should be highly suspected. In influenza pneumonia, the Gram-stain will have numerous leukocytes, but no organisms. Direct immunofluorescence examination of respiratory tract secretions should be performed to identify *L. pneumophila.*[124]

2.5.5.2. Blood

Culture of the blood is important in order to help identify the organism. Serologic studies are appropriate when viral or influenza pneumonia, legionnaires' disease, and atypical or unusual agents are suspected.

2.5.5.3. Other Fluids and Tissue

Any pleural fluid should be aspirated, stained, and cultured. Charcoal yeast extract medium (CYE) should be used to culture *L. pneumophila* and the "Pittsburgh pneumonia agent" from specimens of lung, blood, or pleural fluid.[121,125] In an immunocompromised host, fiberoptic bronchoscopy with transbronchial brushings and biopsy may be very useful in establishing a specific diagnosis. In general, the risk and complications associated with an open lung biopsy in an elderly patient may outweigh the potential benefits.

2.5.6. Antibiotic Therapy

General therapy should be directed to correcting any hypoemia, maintaining a clear airway, and preventing further aspiration of secretions or material. Guidelines for specific antimicrobial therapy are provided in recent reviews and textbooks.[125a,125b] Obviously, the initial selection of an antibiotic depends on several factors, including the results of sputum Gram-stain, whether the pneumonia was acquired in the community or in the hospital, and how sick or toxic the patient appears. *Any elderly patient who develops pneumonia should be hospitalized for initial parenteral antibiotic treatment and supportive care.*

2.5.6.1. Typical Bacterial Pneumonias

If the Gram stain of the sputum is diagnostic, i.e., a predominant organism is present and no epithelial cells are evident, specific antibiotic treatment is indicated. However, if the Gram stain is nondiagnostic and a mixture of Gram-positive and Gram-negative organisms is seen, then broad-spectrum coverage is important. This would include an aminoglycoside *and* either a semisynthetic penicillin or a cephalosporin. Also, if the patient is extremely ill and appears toxic, broad antibiotic coverage is necessary until a cause is identified. Since Gram-negative bacilli are frequent causes of pneumonia in the geriatric population, initial treatment for Gram-negative organisms should always be considered.

2.5.6.2. Aspiration Pneumonia

For chemical pneumonitis, the use of corticosteroids and antibiotic agents is controversal. If steroids are given, they should be administered promptly (within 12 hr of aspiration) and continued for only a limited time (2 to 4 days).[126] Antimicrobial drugs are not indicated unless a subsequent bacterial infection develops.

For community-acquired cases of aspiration pneumonia, anaerobic bacteria are the major pathogens, and these strains are susceptible to penicillin G. The major exception is *Bacteroides fragilis* which has been recovered in 15 to 20% of patients.[117] Despite in vitro resistance, pulmonary infections involving *B. fragilis* generally respond satisfactorily to penicillin G.[117] Accordingly, penicillin G is considered the drug of choice for aspiration pneumonia acquired outside the hospital. Cases acquired within the hospital or an extended care facility frequently involve *S. aureus* and Gram-negative organisms in addition to anaerobes. Thus, an aminoglycoside, such as gentamicin, in combination with a semisynthetic penicillin or cephalosporin is appropriate.

For aspiration of large volumes of nontoxic fluids or particulate material, the obvious therapy is to clear the airways. Tracheal suctioning of fluids and extraction of solid particles by bronchoscopy is critical. Any infectious complications generally respond to penicillin providing the underlying lesion is removed.[126]

2.5.6.3. Atypical and the "New" Pneumonias

2.5.6.3a. Legionnaires' Disease. Erythromycin is the antibiotic of choice for patients suspected or diagnosed to have legionnaires' disease.[120,121] The suggested dose is 0.5 to 1.0 g every 6 hr. Other drugs, such as tetracycline and rifampin, have appeared to be less effective in test systems.

2.5.6.3b. Influenza. Amantadine is effective in the early treatment of influenza A cases if started within 24 to 48 hr of the onset of illness and should be continued for 4 to 5 days.[127] Prophylactic treatment with amantidine should be started as soon as possible after exposure to a patient infected with influenza A.

2.5.6.3c. The "New" Pneumonias. Because the diagnosis of these diseases require special microbiological studies, therapy is empiric. This type of pulmonary infection should be suspected when conventional culturing techniques fail to identify a specific organism, and the patient does not respond to antibiotics commonly used to treat pneumonia. Present data indicate that all organisms implicated in the "new" pneumonias are sensitive to erythromycin.[123] Thus, after appropriate procedures needed to recover the organism have been performed (culture of sputum, collection of blood for later serologic study, and possible biopsy of the lung), 1 g of erythromycin should be administered intravenously every 6 hr.[123]

2.5.7. Prophylactic Immunization

2.5.7.1. *S. pneumoniae* Pneumonia

Although infection due to *S. pneumoniae* represents less than 25% of all cases of pneumonia, it is estimated that as many as 500,000 cases of pneumococcal pneumonia occur annually in the United States.[128] The disease continues to have an overall case fatality rate of 5 to 10%. Mortality is highest in patients with bacteremia or meningitis, those with underlying medical conditions, and in older persons. In 1977, a pneumococcal polysaccharide vaccine was licensed for use; it contains purified capsular material of 14 types of *S. pneumoniae*. These 14 bacterial types are responsible for 68% of bacteremic pneumococcal disease in the United States.[128] The Advisory Committee for Immunization Practices of the Public Health Service has recommended that the pneumococcal vaccine should be given to adults with chronic lung and cardiovascular diseases, diabetes, renal disease, sickle cell disease, and immunocompromised conditions since they are at increased risk of developing pneumococcal infections as well as experiencing more severe pneumococcal illness.[129] Although the Advisory Committee did not recommend routine immunization for the general population,[129] it is common practice for physicians to prescribe the pneumococcal vaccine for elderly patients since the benefits appear to outweigh the minimal risks involved. At the present time, pneumococcal vaccine should be given only once to adults.[129]

2.5.7.2. Influenza Pneumonia

Influenza virus infections occur yearly in the United States, although incidence and geographic distribution vary considerably. Influenza vaccine contains antigens of influenza viruses expected to circulate in the population during the next influenza season. *Annual* vaccination is recommended for all high-risk persons, including those with chronic lung and cardiovascular diseases, diabetes, renal disease, chronic anemia such as sickle cell disease, conditions with compromised immune mechanisms including malignancies and immunosuppressive therapy, and those who are 65 years of age or more.[130]

References

1. Wynne, J. W., 1979, Pulmonary disease in the elderly, in: *Clinical Geriatrics* (I. Rossman, ed.), J. B. Lippincott Co., Philadelphia.
2. Hutchinson, J., 1946, On the capacity of the lungs and on respiratory functions, with a view of establishing a precise and easy method of detecting disease by the spirometer, *Med. Air Trans. (London)* 29:662–289.
3. Muiesan, G., Sorbini, C. A., and Grassi, V., 1971, Respiratory function in the aged, *Bull. Physiopath. Resp.* 7:973–1009.

4. Morris, J. F., Kolski, A., and Johnson, L. C., 1971, Spirometric standards for healthy nonsmoking adults, *Am. Rev. Respir. Dis.* 103:57-67.

5. Cotes, J. E., Rossiter, C. E., Higgins, I. T. T., and Gilson, J. C., 1966, Average normal values for the forced expiratory volume in white caucasian males, *Br. Med. Jr.* 1:1016-1019.

6. Kory, R. C., Callahan, K., Boren, H. G., and Syner, J. C., 1961, The Veterans Administration–Army cooperative in normal men, *Am. J. Med.* 30:243-258.

7. Knudson, R. J., 1981, How aging affects the normal adult lung, *J. Respir. Dis.* 2:74-84.

8. Knudson, R. J., Clark, D. F., Kennedy, T. C., and Knudson, D. E., 1977, Effect of aging alone on mechanical properties of the normal adult human lung, *J. Appl. Physiol.: Respirat. Environ. Exercise Physiol.* 43:1054-1062.

9. Turner, J. M., Mead, J., and Wohl, M. E., 1968, Elasticity of human lungs in relation to age, *J. Appl. Physiol.* 25:664-671.

10. Mellemgaard, K., 1966, Alveolar-arterial oxygen difference: Size and components in normal man. *Acta Physiol. Scand.* 67:10-20.

11. Sorbini, C. A., Grassi, V., Solinas, E., and Muiesan, G., 1968, Arterial oxygen tension in relation to age in healthy subjects, *Respiration,* 25:3-10.

12. Ricci, B., 1967, *Physiological Basis of Human Performance,* Lea and Febiger, Philadelphia.

13. Black, L. F. and Hyatt, R. E., 1969, Maximal respiratory pressures: Normal values and relationship to age and sex, *Am. Rev. Respir. Dis.* 99:696-702.

14. Kronenberg, R. S. and Drage, C. W., 1973, Attenuation of the ventilatory and heart rate responses to hypoxia and hypercapnia with aging in normal men, *J. Clin. Invest.* 52:1812-1819.

15. Peterson, D. D., Pack, A. I., Silage, D. A., and Fishman, A. P., 1981, Effects of aging on ventilatory and occlusion pressure responses to hypoxia and hypercapnia, *Am. Rev. Respir. Dis.* 124:387-391.

16. Gerrard, J. W., Cockcroft, D. W., Mink, J. T., Cotton, D. J., Poonawala, R., 1980, Increased nonspecific bronchial reactivity in cigarette smokers with normal lung function, *Am. Rev. Respir. Dis.* 122:557-581.

17. White, J. R. and Froeb, H. F., 1982, Small-airways dysfunction in nonsmokers chronically exposed to tobacco smoke, *N. Engl. J. Med.* 302:720-723.

18. Bossé, R., Sparrow, D., Rose, C. L., and Weiss, S. T., 1981, Longitudinal effect of age and smoking cessation on pulmonary function, *Am. Rev. Respir. Dis.* 123:378-381.

19. Buist, A. S., Nagy, J. M., and Sexton, G. J., 1979, The effect of smoking cessation on pulmonary function: A 30-month follow-up of two smoking cessation clinics, *Am. Rev. Respir. Dis.* 120:953-957.

20. Jones, N. L., Campbell, E. J. M., Edward, R. H. T., and Robertson, D. G., 1975, *Clinical Exercise Testing,* W. B. Saunders Co., Philadelphia.

21. Astrand, P-O., 1976, Quantification of exercise capability and evaluation of physical capacity in man, *Prog. Cardiovasc, Dis.* 19:51-67.

22. Astrand, P-O. and Rodahl, K., 1970, *Textbook of Work Physiology,* McGraw-Hill, New York.

23. Ouellet, Y., Poh, S. C., and Becklake, M. R., 1969, Circulatory factors limiting maximal aerobic exercise capacity, *J. Appl. Physiol.* 27:874-880.

24. Mahler, D. A. and Loke, J., 1981, Lung function after marathon running at warm and cold ambient temperatures, *Am. Rev. Respir. Dis.* 124:154–157.

25. Mahler, D. A. and Loke, J., 1981, Pulmonary dysfunction in ultramarathon runners, *Yale J. Biol. Med.* 54:243–248.

26. Loke, J., Mahler, D. A., and Virgulto, J., 1982, Respiratory muscle fatigue after marathon running, *J. Appl. Physiol: Respirat. Environ. Exercise Physiol.* 52:821–824.

27. Astrand, I., Astrand, P-O., Hallback, I., and Kilbom, A., 1973, Reduction in maximal oxygen uptake with age, *J. Appl. Physiol.* 35:649–654.

28. Dehn, M. M. and Bruce, R. A., 1972, Longitudinal variations in maximal oxygen intake with age and activity, *J. Appl. Physiol.* 33:805–807.

29. Robinson, S., Dill, D. B., Tzankoff, S. P., Wagner, J. A., and Robinson, R. D., 1975, Longitudinal studies of aging in 37 men, *J. Appl. Physiol.* 38:263–267.

30. Brandfonbrener, M., Landowne, M., and Shock, N. W., 1955, Changes in cardiac output with age, *Circulation* 12:557–566.

31. Becklake, M. R., Frank, H., Dagansis, G. R., Ostiguy, G. L., and Guzman, C. A., 1965, Influence of age and sex on exercise cardiac output, *J. Appl. Physiol.* 20:938–947.

32. Conway, J., Wheeler, R., and Sannerstedt, R., 1971, Sympathetic nervous activity during exercise in relation to age, *Cardiovasc. Res.* 5:577–581.

33. Julius, S., Antoon, A., Whitlock, L. S., and Conway, J., 1967, Influence of age on the hemodynamic response to exercise, *Circulation* 36:222–230.

34. Granath, A., Jonsson, B., and Strandell, T., 1964, Circulation in healthy old men studied by right heart catheterization at rest and during exercise in supine and sitting position, *Acta Med. Scand.* 176:425–446.

35. Lange-Anderson, K., Shephard, R. J., Denolin, H., Varnauskas, E., and Masironi, R., 1971, *Fundamentals of Exercise Testing,* World Health Organization, Geneva.

36. Port, S., Cobb, F. R., Coleman, E., and Jones, R. H., 1980, Effect of age on the response of the left ventricular ejection fraction to exercise, *N. Engl. J. Med.* 303:1133–1137.

37. Norris, A. H., Shock, N. W., and Yiengst, M. J., 1955, Age differences in ventilatory and gas exchange responses to graded exercise in males, *J. Gerontol.* 10:145–155.

38. Tzankoff, S. P., Robinson, S., Pyke, F. S., and Brown, C. A., 1972, Physiological adjustments to work in older men as affected by physical training, *J. Appl. Physiol.* 33:346–350.

39. Hanson, J. S., Tabakin, B. S., Levy, A. M., and Needle, W., 1968, Longterm physical training and cardiovascular dynamics in middle-aged men, *Circulation* 38:783–799.

40. Naughton, J. P. and Nagle, F., 1965, Peak oxygen intake during physical fitness program for middle-aged men, *JAMA* 191:899–901.

41. Barry, A. J., Daly, J. W., Pruett, E. D. R., Steinmetz, J. R., Page, H. F., Birkhead, N. D., and Rodahl, K., 1966, The effects of physical conditioning on older individuals. I. Work capacity, circulatory–respiratory functions, and work electrocardiogram, *J. Gerontol.* 21:182–191.

42. Holloszy, J. O., 1973, Biochemical adaptations to exercise: Aerobic metabolism,

in: *Exercise and Sport Sciences Reviews,* Volume 1 (J. H. Wilmore, ed.) Academic Press, New York, pp. 46-102.

43. Meneely, G. R. (Chairman), 1962, Definitions and classification of chronic bronchitis, asthma, and pulmonary emphysema, *Am. Rev. Respir. Dis.* 85:762-768.

44. Deal, E. C., McFadden, E. R., Jr., Ingram, R. H., Jr., Strauss, R. H., and Jaeger, J. J., 1979, Role of respiratory heat exchange in production of exercise-induced asthma, *J. Appl. Physiol.: Respirat. Environ. Exercise Physiol.* 46:467-475.

45. Dosman, J. F., Bode, F., Urbanetti, J., Martin, R., and Macklem, P. T., 1975, The use of helium-oxygen mixture during maximum expiratory flow to demonstrate obstruction in small airways in smokers, *J. Clin. Invest.* 55:1090-1099.

46. Snider, G. L., Kory, R. C., and Lyons, H. A., 1967, Grading of pulmonary function impairment by means of pulmonary function tests, *Chest* 52:270-271.

47. Burrows, B. and Earle, R. H., 1969, Course and prognosis of chronic obstructive lung disease: A prospective study of 200 patients, *N. Engl. J. Med.* 280:397-404.

48. Snider, G. L. (Chairman), 1974, Criteria for the assessment of reversibility in airways obstruction, *Chest* 65:552-553.

49. Dull, W. L., Alexander, M. R., and Kasik, J. E., 1981, Isoproterenol challenge during placebo and oral theophylline therapy in chronic obstructive pulmonary disease, *Am. Rev. Resp. Dis.* 123:340-342.

50. McFadden, F. R. and Lyons, H. A., 1968, Arterial-blood gas tensions in asthma, *N. Engl. J. Med.* 278:1027-1032.

51. Matthay, R. A., Schwarz, M. I., Ellis, J. H., Jr., Steele, P. P., Siebert, P. E., Durrance, J. R., and Levin, D. C., 1981, Pulmonary artery hypertension in chronic obstructive pulmonary disease: Chest radiographic assessment, *Invest. Radiol.* 16:95-100.

52. Stubbing, D. G., Pengelly, L. D., Morse, J. L. C., and Jones, N. L., 1980, Pulmonary mechanics during exercise in subjects with chronic airflow obstruction, *J. Appl. Physiol.: Respirat, Environ. Exercise Physiol.* 49:511-515.

53. Jones, N. L., Jones, G., and Edwards, R. H. T., 1971, Exercise tolerance in chronic airway obstruction, *Am. Rev. Respir. Dis.* 103:477-491.

54. Minh, V., Lee, H. M., Dolan, D. G., Light, R. W., Bell, J., and Vasquez, P., 1979, Hypoxemia during exercise in patients with chronic obstructive pulmonary disease, *Am. Rev. Respir. Dis.* 120:787-794.

55. Grassino, A., Gross, D., Macklem, P. T., Roussos, C., and Zagelbaum, G., 1979, Inspiratory muscle fatigue as a factor limiting exercise, *Bull. Europ. Physiopathol. Respir.* 15:105-111.

56. Delgado, H. R., Braun, S. R., Skatrud, J. B., Reddan, W. G., and Pegelow, D. F., 1982, Chest wall and abdominal motion during exercise in patients with chronic obstructive pulmonary disease, *Am. Rev. Respir. Dis.* 126:200-205.

57. Pardy, R. L., Rivington, R. N., Despas, P. J., and Macklem, P. T., 1981, The effects of inspiratory muscle training on exercise performance in chronic airflow limitation, *Am. Rev. Respir. Dis.* 123:426-433.

58. Khaja, F. and Parker, J. O., 1971, Right and left ventricular performance in chronic obstructive lung disease, *Am. Heart J.* 82:319-327.

59. Minh, V-D., Lee, H. M., Vasquez, P., Shepard, J. W., and Bell, J. W., 1979, Relation of $\dot{V}O_2$max to cardiopulmonary function in patients with chronic obstructive lung disease, *Bull. Europ. Physiopath. Respir.* 15:359-375.

60. Matthay, R. A., Berger, H. J., Davies, R. A., Loke, J., Mahler, D. A., Gottschalk, A., and Zaret, B. L., 1980, Right and left ventricular exercise performance in chronic obstructive pulmonary disease: Radionuclide assessment, *Ann. Int. Med.* 93:234–239.

61. Mahler, D. A., Matthay, R. A., Berger, H. J., Brent, B. N., Loke, J., and Zaret, B. L., 1982, Right ventricular exercise performance in severe obstructive airway disease: Combined hemodynamic and radionuclide assessment, *Am. Rev. Respir. Dis.* 125:80 (Abstract).

62. Mahler, D. A., Weinberg, D. H., Wells, C. K., and Feinstein, A. R., 1982, Measurement of dyspnea: Description of two new indexes, interobserver agreement, and physiologic correlations, *Am. Rev. Respir. Dis.* 125:138 (Abstract).

63. Wolfe, J. D., Tashkin, D. P., Calvarese, B. and Simmons, M., 1978, Bronchodilator effects of terbutaline and aminophylline alone and in combination in asthmatic patients, *N. Engl. J. Med.* 298:363–367.

64. Eaton, M. L., Green, B. A., Church, T. R., McGowan, T., and Niewoehner, D. E., 1980, Efficacy of theophylline in "irreversible" airflow obstruction, *Ann. Int. Med.* 92:758–761.

65. Emirgil, C., Sobol, B. J., Norman, J., Muskowitz, E., Goyal, P., and Wadhwani, B., 1969, A study of the long-term effect of therapy in chronic obstructive pulmonary disease, *Am. J. Med.* 47:367–377.

66. Rossing, T. H., Fanta, C. H., Goldstein, D. H., Snapper, J. R., and McFadden, Jr., E. R., 1980, Emergency therapy of asthma: Comparison of acute effects of parental and inhaled sympathomimetics and infused aminophylline, *Am. Rev. Respir. Dis.* 122:365–371.

67. Shim, C. and Williams, M. H., Jr., 1980, Bronchial response to oral vs. aerosol metaproterenol in asthma, *Ann. Int. Med.* 93:428–431.

68. Dulfano, M. and Glass, P., 1973, Evaluation of a new beta$_2$ adrenergic receptor stimulant, terbutaline, in bronchial asthma, II. Oral comparison with ephedrine, *Curr. Ther. Res.* 15:150–157.

69. Sly, R., Bodie, B., and Faciano, J., 1977, Comparison of subcutaneous terbutaline with epinephrine in the treatment of asthma in children, *J. Allergy Clin. Immunol.* 59:128–135.

70. Mitenko, P. A. and Ogilvie, R. I., 1973, Rational intravenous doses of theophylline, *N. Engl. J. Med.* 289:600–603, 1973.

71. Weinberger, M., Hendeles, L., and Ahrens, R., 1980, Pharmacologic management of reversible obstructive airways disease, *Med. Clin. North Am.* 65:579–613.

72. Aubier, M., Murciano, D., Viires, N., Lecocguic, Y., Fleury, B., and Pariente, R., 1982, Protective effects of aminophylline in diaphragmatic fatigue in acute respiratory failure, *Am. Rev. Respir. Dis.* 125:206 (Abstract).

73. Hendeles, L., Weinberger, M., and Bighley, L., 1977, Absolute bioavailability of oral theophylline, *Amer. J. Hosp. Pharm.* 34:525–527.

74. Jusko, W. J., Koup, J. R., Vance, J. W., Schentag, J. J., and Kuritzky, P., 1977, Intravenous theophylline therapy: Nomogram guidelines, *Ann. Int. Med.* 86:400–404.

75. Piafsky, K. M., Sitar, D. S., Rangno, R. E., and Ogilvie, R. I., 1977, Theophylline disposition in patients with hepatic cirrhosis, *N. Engl. J. Med.* 296:1495–1497.

76. Reitberg, D. P., Bernhard, H., and Schentag, J. J., 1981, Alteration of theophyl-

line clearance and half-life by cimetidine in normal volunteers, *Ann. Int. Med.* 95:582–585.

77. Arnaud, A., Vervloet, D., Dugue, P., Orehek, J., and Charpin, J., 1979, Treatment of acute asthma: Effect of intravenous corticosteroids and beta$_2$ adrenergic agonists, *Lung* 156:43–48.

78. Albert, R. K., Martin, T. R., and Lewis, S. W., 1980, Controlled clinical trial of methylprednisolone in patients with chronic bronchitis and acute respiratory insufficiency, *Ann. Int. Med.* 92:753–758.

79. Ackerman, G. L. and Nolan, C. M., 1968, Adrenocortical responsiveness after alternate-day corticosteroid therapy, *N. Engl. J. Med.* 278:405–409.

80. Ballin, J. C., 1976, Evaluation of a new aerosolized steriod for asthma therapy, *JAMA* 236:2891–2893.

81. Byyny, R. L., 1976, Withdrawal from glucocorticoid therapy, *N. Engl. J. Med.* 295:30–32.

82. Hodson, M. E., Batten, J. C., Clarke, S. W., and Gregg, I., 1974, Beclomethasone dipropionate aerosol in asthma, *Am. Rev. Respir. Dis.* 110:403–408.

83. Williams, M. H., 1981, Beclomethasone dipropionate, *Ann. Int. Med.* 95:464–467.

84. A controlled trial by the British Thoracic and Tuberculosis Association, 1975, Inhaled corticosteroids compared with oral prednisone inpatients starting long-term corticosteroid therapy for asthma, *Lancet* ii:469–473.

85. Nocturnal Oxygen Therapy Trial Group, 1980, Continuous or nocturnal oxygen therapy in hypoxemic chronic obstructive lung disease, *Ann. Int. Med.* 93:391–398.

86. Boysen, P. G., Block, A. J., Wynne, J. W., Hunt, L. A., and Flick, M. R., 1979, Nocturnal pulmonary hypertension in patients with chronic obstructive pulmonary disease, *Chest* 76:536–542.

87. Tirlapur, V. G. and Mir, M. A., 1982, Nocturnal hypoxemia and associated electrocardiographic changes in patients with chronic obstructive airways disease, *N. Engl. J. Med.* 306:125–130.

88. Report of the Medical Research Council Working Party, 1981, Long term domiciliary oxygen therapy in chronic hypoxic cor pulmonale complicating chronic bronchitis and emphysema, *Lancet* i:681–686.

89. Block, A. J., 1982, Dangerous sleep: Oxygen therapy for nocturnal hypoxemia. *N. Engl. J. Med.* 306:166–167.

90. Belman, M. J. and Wasserman, K., 1981, Exercise training and testing in patients with chronic obstructive pulmonary disease, *Basics RD* 10:1–6.

91. Grassino, A., Gross, D., Macklem, P. T., Roussos, Ch., and Zagelbaum, G., 1979, Inspiratory muscle fatigue as a factor limiting exercise. *Bull. Eur. Physiopathol. Respir.* 15:105–111.

92. Belman, M. J. and Mittman, C., 1980, Ventilatory muscle training improves exercise capacity in chronic obstructive pulmonary disease patients, *Am. Rev. Respir. Dis.* 121:273–280.

93. Franciosa, J. A. and Fischer, H. A., 1981, Right ventricular unloading: Lessons from the left, *Ann. Int. Med.* 95:647–648.

94. Rubin, L. J. and Peter, R. H., 1981, Hemodynamics at rest and during exercise after oral hydralazine in patients with cor pulmonale, *Am. J. Cardiol.* 47:116–122.

95. Simonneau, G., Eacourrou, P., Duroux, P., and Lockhart, A., 1981, Inhibition of hypoxic pulmonary vasoconstriction by nifedipine, *N. Engl. J. Med.* 304:1582–1585.

96. Muramoto, A., Caldwell, J., Lakshinarayan, S., Albert, R. K., and Butler, J., 1981, Nifedipine reduces pulmonary artery pressure at a comparable cardiac output in patients with chronic obstructive pulmonary disease, *Circulation* 64(Suppl. IV):179 (Abstract).

97. Matthay, R. A. and Berger, H. J., 1981, Cardiovascular performance in chronic obstructive pulmonary disease, *Med. Clin. North Am.* 65:489–524.

98. Abraham, A. S., Cole, R. B., and Bishop, J. M., 1968, Reversal of pulmonary hypertension by prolonged oxygen administration in patients with chronic bronchitis, *Circ. Res.* 23:147–157.

99. Olvey, S. K., Reduto, L. A., Stevens, P. M., Deaton, W. J., and Miller, R. R., 1980, First-pass radionuclide assessment of right and left ventricular ejection fraction in chronic pulmonary disease: Effect of oxygen upon exercise response, *Chest* 78:4–9.

100. Gertz, I., Hedensteirna, G., and Wester, P. O., 1979, Improvement in pulmonary function with diuretic therapy in the hypervolemic and polycytemic patient with chronic obstructive pulmonary disease, *Chest* 75:146–151.

101. Green, L. H. and Smith, T. W., 1977, The use of digitalis in patients with pulmonary disease, *Ann. Int. Med.* 87:459–465.

102. Mathur, P. N., Powles, A. C. P., Pugsley, S. O., McEwan, M. P., and Campbell, E. J. M., 1981, Effect of digoxin on right ventricular function in severe chronic airflow obstruction, *Ann. Int. Med.* 95:283–288.

103. Center for Disease Control, 1980, Annual Summary 1979, *Morbid. Mortal. Weekly Rep.* 28:54–55.

104. Siegel, J. S., 1982,Some demographic aspects of aging in the United States, in: *The Epidemiology of Aging* (A. M. Ostfeld and D. C. Gibson, eds.), DHEW, Publication No. (NIH) 77–711, Bethesda, Md.

105. Sullivan, R. J., Dowdle, W. R., Marine, W. M., 1972, Adult pneumonia in a general hospital: Etiology and host risk factors, *Arch. Int. Med.* 129:935–942.

106. Phair, J. P., Kauffman, C. A., Bjornson, A., 1978, Host defenses in the aged: Evaluation of components of the inflammatory and immune responses, *J. Infect. Dis.* 138:67–73.

107. Buckley, C. E. and Dorsey, F. C., 1970, The effect of aging on human serum immunoglobulin concentrations, *J. Immunol.* 105:964–972.

108. Weksler, M. E. and Hutteroth, T. H., 1974, Impaired lymphocyte function in aged humans, *J. Clin. Invest.* 53:99–104.

109. Elright, J. R. and Rytel, M. W., 1980, Bacterial pneumonia in the elderly, *J. Am. Geriatr. Soc.* 28:220–223.

110. Garb, J. L., Brown, R. B., Garb, J. R., and Tuthill, R. W., 1978, Differences in etiology of pneumonias in nursing home and community patients, *JAMA* 240:2169–2172.

111. Valenti, W. M., Trudell, R. G., and Bentley, D. W., 1978, Factors predisposing to oropharyngeal colonization with gram-negative bacilli in the aged, *N. Engl. J. Med.* 298:1108–1111.

112. Stamm, W. E., 1979, Gram-negative pneumonias: Diagnosis and management, *Drug Ther.* 9:69–80.
113. Wanner, A., 1979, The role of mucociliary dysfunction in bronchial asthma, *Am. J. Med.* 67:477–485.
114. Frame, P. T., 1982, Acute infectious pneumonia in the adult, *Basics RD* 10:1–8.
115. Robbins, S. L. and Cotran, R. S., 1979, Pneumonia, in: *Pathologic Basis of Disease,* W. B. Saunders Co., Philadelphia.
116. Oswald, N. C., Simon, G., and Shooter, R. A., 1961, Pneumonia in hospital practice, *Br. J. Dis. Chest* 55:109–118.
117. Bartlett, J. G. and Gorbach, S. L., 1975, The triple threat of aspiration pneumonia, *Chest* 68:560–566.
118. Mendelson, C. L., 1946, The aspiration of stomach contents into the lungs during obstetric anesthesia, *Am. J. Obstet, Gynecol.* 52:191–205.
119. Greenfield, L. J., Singleton, R. P., McCaffree, D. R., 1969, Pulmonary effects of experimental graded aspiration of hydrochloric acid, *Ann. Surg.* 170:74–86.
120. Center for Disease Control, 1978, Legionnaires' disease: Diagnosis and management, *Ann. Int. Med.* 88:363–365.
121. Kirby, B. D., Snyder, K. M., Meyer, R. D., and Finegold, S. M., 1978, Legionnaires' disease: Clinical features of 24 cases, *Ann. Int. Med.* 89:297–309.
122. Douglas, R. G., Jr., 1976, Influenza: The disease and its complications, *Hosp. Practice* (Dec):43–50.
123. Weinstein, L., 1980, The "new" pneumonias: The doctor's dilemma, *Ann. Int. Med.* 92:559–561.
124. Edelstein, P. H., Meyer, R. D., and Finegold, S. M., 1980, Laboratory diagnosis of Legionnaires' disease, *Am. Rev. Respir. Dis.* 121:317–327.
125. Hébert, G. A., Thomason, B. M., Harris, P. P., Hicklin, M. D., and McKinney, R. M., 1980, "Pittsburgh Pneumonia Agent": A bacterium phenotypically similar to Legionella pneumophila and identical to the TATLOCK bacterium, *Ann. Int. Med.* 92:53–54.
125a. Roberts, R. B., 1982, Antimicrobial therapy, in: *Cecil Textbook of Medicine* (J. B. Wyngaarden and L. H. Smith, Jr. eds.), W. B. Saunders, Philadelphia, pp. 71–83.
125b. Kirby, W. M. M., Chemotherapy of infection, in: *Harrison's Principles of Internal Medicine* (K. J. Isselbacher, R. D. Adams, E. Breunwald, R. G. Petersdorf, and J. D. Wilson, eds.), McGraw-Hill, New York, pp. 573–586.
126. Bartlett, J. G., 1980, Aspiration pneumonia, *Clin. Notes Respir. Dis.* 18:(4):3–8.
127. Position paper of the ATS ad hoc advisory committee on influenza, 1981, Prevention of influenza and pneumonia, *Am. Thoracic Soc. News,* p. 41.
128. Broome, C. V. and Facklam, R. R., 1981, Epidemiology of clinically significant isolates of *Streptococcus pneumoniae* in the United States, *Rev. Infect. Dis.* 3:277–280.
129. Recommendation of the Immunization Practices Advisory Committee, 1981, Pneumococcal polysaccharide vaccine, *Morbid. Mortal. Weekly Rep.* 30:410–419.
130. Recommendation of the Public Health Service Immunization Practices Advisory Committee, 1981, Influenza vaccine 1981-82, *Morbid. Mortal. Weekly Rep.* 30:279–288.

Gastroenterology and the Elderly

Thomas W. Sheehy

3.1. Esophagus

3.1.1. Dysphagia

Esophageal disorders, such as esophageal motility disorders, infections, tumors, and other diseases, are common in the elderly. In the elderly, dysphagia usually implies organic disease. There are two types: (1) pre-esophageal and (2) esophageal. Both are further subdivided into motor (neuromuscular) or structural (intrinsic and extrinsic) lesions.[1]

3.1.2. Pre-esophageal Dysphagia

Pre-esophageal dysphagia (PED) usually implies neuromuscular disease and may be caused by pseudobular palsy, multiple sclerosis, amytrophic lateral sclerosis, Parkinson's disease, bulbar poliomyelitis, lesions of the glossopharyngeal nerve, myasthenia gravis, and muscular dystrophies. Since PED is due to inability to initiate the swallowing mechanism, food cannot escape from the oropharynx into the esophagus. Such patients usually have more difficulty swallowing liquid

THOMAS W. SHEEHY • The University of Alabama in Birmingham, School of Medicine, Department of Medicine; and Medical Services, Veterans Administration Medical Center, Birmingham, Alabama 35233.

than solids. They sputter or cough during attempts to swallow and often have nasal regurgitation or aspiration of food.

3.1.3. Dysfunction of the Cricopharyngeus Muscle

In the elderly, this is one of the more common forms of PED.[2] These patients have the sensation of an obstruction in their throat when they attempt to swallow. This is due to incoordination of the cricopharyngeus muscle. When this muscle fails to relax quickly enough during swallowing, food cannot pass freely into the esophagus. If the muscle relaxes promptly but closes too quickly, food is trapped as it attempts to enter the esophagus. Usually, solids can be swallowed more easily than liquids.

Cricopharyngeal dysphagia is attributed to failure of vagal control. In an attempt to see if the condition is more frequent with age, Paiget and Fouillet studied 100 symptomless individuals over age 65 years.[3] Thirty-eight percent of the men and 15% of the women had neurological dysfunction of their hypopharynx.

3.1.3.1. Diagnosis

Diagnosis is based on the history of inability to drink fluids readily (85%), excessive expectoration of saliva (30%), weight loss (50%), and heartburn (50%) due to gastroesophageal reflux. It is confirmed by cineroentgenography. Failure of the cricopharyngeal muscle to relax leads to puddling of contrast material in the valleculae and pyriform sinuses. Hypopharyngoscopy and esophagoscopy are necessary to exclude other diseases.

3.1.3.2. Complications

Complications include chronic irritation of the larynx, aspiration, and the development of a Zenker's diverticulum. Eventually, many patients develop chronic bronchitis or bronchiectasis as the result of repeated aspiration.

3.1.3.3. Treatment

Treatment consists of cricopharyngeal myotomy. Usually this procedure results in prompt relief whereas bouginage is seldom helpful. Myotomy is also effective for patients with cricopharyngeal dysphagia, and gastroesophageal reflux secondary to motor neuron disease.[4-8]

Formerly, a Zenker's diverticulum had to be removed surgically. This is no longer necessary because even those older patients with a severe obstruction in the advanced stage of the disorder responded successfully to myotomy alone. Once the obstruction is relieved, the diverticulum begins to involute.[6] The advantages of this approach are: (1) a shorter operating time, (2) ability to resume oral feedings promptly, (3) elimination of the need for a Levine tube, (4) a decreased risk of suture line leakage and stricture formation, and (5) no need for antibiotics.[6]

3.1.3.4. Esophageal Dysphagia

Esophageal dysphagia too is classified according to motor dysfunction or structural abnormalities.[1] Motor disorders usually cause a greater dysphagia for liquids than solids, whereas structural lesions are associated with more difficulty in swallowing solids. Motor abnormalities leading to dysphagia include achalasia, diffuse esophageal spasm, and neuropathy secondary to diabetes or alcoholism.

3.1.4. Achalasia of the Lower Esophagus

In this disorder, the muscular wall of the distal esophagus is narrow while the proximal esophagus is dilated and tortuous. Achalasia has been attributed to degeneration of neural elements within the essophagus, the vagus, and the dorsal motor nucleus in the brain stem.[9] Only a few ganglion cells are found in the esophageal wall and there is a degeneration of Auerbach's plexus. Electron microscopic studies have shown varying degrees of degeneration within the branches of the vagal nerve. Whatever the basic lesion, the results are an increase in lower esophageal sphractel (LES) pressure; incomplete relaxation of the sphincter during swallowing, and an absence of effective esophageal peristalsis during the swallowing act. Stasis results, leading to inflammation or ulceration of the mucosal lining.

3.1.4.1. Clinical Findings

Achalasia occurs in 1 per 100,000 population per year. Afflicted patients complain of difficulty in swallowing. Early in the affliction, they have more difficulty swallowing liquids than solids. Later, as the disorder progresses, undigested foods are often regurgitated. Since bile is absent, regurgitated food does not taste bitter. Nocturnal aspiration results in spasms of nocturnal coughing and often to pulmonary complications. Odynophagia occurs with ingestion of hot or cold food or beverages. This pain is substernal and radiates to the shoulders or back and even down the arms, mimicking angina.[10,11]

Eventually, the esophagus dilates and loses its capability to propel food into the stomach. Manometric studies show an elevated LES pressure. This prevents the sphincter from relaxing normally on swallowing and eliminates esophageal peristalsis.

3.1.4.2. Diagnosis

Mecholyl (acetyl-β-methylcholine-chloride) is a valuable aid to diagnosis. Five to 10 mg given subcutaneously increases the baseline LES pressure in 80%

of patients with achalasia and keeps it elevated for 5 to 10 min.[12] Normally, mecholyl does not increase baseline esophageal pressure. If mecholyl induces severe chest pain, the administration of atropine sulfate usually relieves it.

3.1.4.3. Treatment

Treatment is directed toward reducing the elevated resting pressure of the LES. This can be accomplished by forceful pneumatic dilatation or by surgical myotomy. Symptomatic improvement occurs with either procedure, if it succeeds in reducing the LES resting pressure. Unfortunately, neither treatment leads to a return of normal esophageal peristalsis. At present, most gastroenterologists favor pneumatic dilatation as the primary method of treatment.[13,14]

3.1.5. Diffuse Esophageal Spasm

Diffuse esophageal spasm (DES), too, arises from neuromuscular abnormality. As a result of the spasm, the radiologic appearance of the esophagus is distorted during contrast study, yielding the "corkscrew," "curling," or "rosary-bead" esophagus.

Dysphagia occurs after swallowing hot or cold beverages and on attempting to swallow both liquids and solids. Often, the pain is so severe, it awakens patients from their sleep. The pain's radiation pattern, too, can mimic angina pectoris and it is often relieved by nitroglycerin.

The pathologic lesion is similar to that observed in achalasia, i.e., abnormalities of Auerbach's plexus and Wallerian degeneration of the vagal nerve branches.

3.1.5.1. Diagnosis

Diagnosis requires both manometric and radiologic studies. Manometric studies reveal abnormally high esophageal waves, i.e., with an amplitude greater than 35 mm Hg. In contrast to achalasia, however, LES pressure is normal despite diffuse spasm. The sphincter relaxes completely upon swallowing.[15]

Secondary esophageal spasm often developes in patients with alcoholic or other forms of neuropathy.

3.1.5.2. Presbyesophagus

Originally, presbyesophagus was touted as a common condition among the elderly.[16] Actually, most of the patients studied originally had diabetes mellitus, senile dementia, or peripheral neuropathy that accounted for their abnormal motility. Recent studies have shown no evidence of impaired peristalsis in healthy older patients.[17]

3.1.5.3. Treatment for DES

Three forms of treatment are available: (1) medical, (2) dilatation, and (3) surgical.[18] Medical therapy is beneficial in 50% of the patients when there is gastric reflux. Sublingual nitroglycerin 1/200 grain is given 15 to 20 min before meals. If this is successful, long-acting nitrates, such as isosorbide dinitrate, are substituted for more prolonged relief.[19] In the absence of gastric reflux, anticholenergic agents are often helpful.

Bouginage, with a 40 French dilator is reserved for extremely symptomatic patients. Pneumatic dilatation of the LES is reserved for patients with associated achalasia and elevated LES pressures. Esophageal myotomy is used when symptoms are severe or incapacitating.[20] In the Mayo Clinic series, two-thirds of the patients treated surgically had good results.[21]

3.1.6. Structural Lesions

Other causes of dysphagia must also be considered. These include esophageal carcinoma, peptic or caustic esophageal strictures, an enlarged left atrium, an aortic arch aneurysm, an aberrant subclavian artery, dysphagia lusoria, metastatic carcinoma, and benign esophageal tumors.

3.1.7. Esophagitis

Esophagitis may develop secondary to infections, tumors, corrosives, or from the reflux of acid or bile.

3.1.7.1. Infectious Esophagitis

Formerly, diphtheria, scarlet fever, and tuberculosis were common causes of esophagitis. Today, infectious esophagitis is usually due to invasion by herpes simplex or *Candida albicans*. Even these entities are relatively rare.[23,24]

3.1.7.2. Reflux Esophagitis

This is defined as esophageal inflammation caused by reflux of acid or bile. Several recent reviews have covered the diagnostic, therapeutic, and clinical aspects of this disorder.[24-26]

3.1.7.3. Pathogenesis

Reflux esophagitis is a multifactorial disease wherein the antireflux mechanism, i.e., the LES, the volume of gastric fluid; the potency of the refluxed material; the efficiency of esophageal clearance; and tissue resistance are all involved.[27]

The intrinsic tone of the LES is a major factor in preventing gastroesophageal reflux. It is maintained by neural, hormonal, and myogenic factors.[28,29] When the LES pressure falls to 10 mm Hg or less, sphincteric action is probably impaired sufficiently to allow reflux. Patients with severe esophagitis usually have lower LES pressures than patients with mild reflux esophagitis.[30] Patients with normal LES pressures and esophagitis may not have sample pressures that are truly representative. The resting LES pressure does exhibit considerable temporal variation and it may fall significantly after eating fat or chocolate, or drinking alcohol.[27,31,32] A large gastric volume probably increases both the chance for and the amount of reflux.[4,10] Gastric volume is determined by the quantity of ingested food, the rates of gastric secretion and gastric emptying, and the frequency of reflux. Abnormalities of any of these factors can lead to an excessive gastric volume that favors reflux and development of esophagitis.

The composition of the refluxing material is related to tissue injury. Even a small amount of pepsin in an acid milieu (i.e., pH 2 or less) may induce severe esophagitis.[33]

Biliary or alkaline esophagitis results from the corrosive effect of bile and pancreatic secretion.[22] Conjugated bile salts damage the esophageal mucosa at an acid pH; deconjugated bile salts and trypsin are more injurious at a neutral pH.[35] Bile acids also increase the permeability of the esophageal mucosa to hydrogen ions.[24]

Esophageal clearance is enhanced by gravity, persistalsis, and saliva. Persistalsis is the primary force behind esophageal clearance while saliva is important in maintaining the lumenal pH above 3. Patients with reflux esophagitis are more apt to have noctural symptoms because the effect of gravity is lost in the recumbent position and salivation ceases at night.[27] Swallowing frequency, normally once per minute, also decreases at night. Tissue resistance is also decreased in patients with reflux esophagitis.

3.1.7.4. Clinical Findings

Patients complain either of "heartburn" or chest pain. The former may be worsened by eating, by hot drinks, or sleep. Chest pain may simulate angina and is characterized as a squeezing, crushing, or burning sensation.

3.1.7.5. Diagnosis

An esophagram should be obtained to rule out neoplasms and other lesions. Double contrast radiography is extremely accurate for diagnosing reflux esophagitis, 80 to 90% positive. A new isotopic method for evaluating reflux appears to be relatively sensitive and specific.[36] Recently the sensitivity and reliability of the acid perfusion (Bernstein) test has been improved, by the addition of ataurine bile salt conjugate to 0.1N HCl.[37]

Endoscopy allows identification of mucosal lesions and permits mucosal biopsy. At endoscopy, the mucosa often is discolored and ulcers, exudates, and lumenal narrowing may be observed. Histologically, the mucosa is infiltrated with polymorphonuclear or mixed polynuclear round cells and there is usually evidence of erosion or ulceration. These histologic findings are necessary for diagnosis. Occasionally, at endoscopy, there is no visible evidence of esophagitis. In these patients, microscopic examination of the biopsy reveals the characteristic inflammation.

3.1.7.6. Treatment

Symptomatic therapy consists of the use of antacids, 30 ml 1 hr after meals and at bedtime, along with elevation of the head of the bed on 4-inch blocks. Patients should avoid materials that reduce esophageal sphincter pressure, such as caffeine, alcohol, chocolate, and peppermint. They should also refrain from eating before bedtime. Overweight individuals are helped by losing weight since obesity is associated with increased reflux. Bethanechol, 10 to 15 mg 3 times daily and at bedtime, is often helpful. For those who develop scarring or cicatricial lesions, dilitation is required. If medical therapy fails, antireflux surgery may be necessary.

3.2. Stomach

3.2.1. Upper Gastrointestinal Bleeding

The major causes of upper gastrointestinal bleeding (UGIB) have not changed significantly over the past 25 years. Table I lists the etiology and the mortality observed in 633 patients with UGIB over a 5-year period (1975 to 1980) (T. W. Sheehy, personal observations). The results are comparable to those observed in other large studies (Table II).[38-40] Patients with UGIB tend to be elderly. Forty-eight percent of Allen's patients with UGIB were over age 60, although 40% of the men and 60% of the women in Schiller's series were 68 years of age or greater.[41] In the national survey conducted in the American Society of Gastroenterology study, the average age of patients with UGIB was 57 years $\pm$ 17.5 years.[41] Yet, few studies of UGIB in the elderly are available. Chang and his associates studied 66 patients over age 65 with massive UGIB. Thirty had duodenal ulcers, 17 gastric ulcers, 7 gastritis, 7 esophageal varices, 2 marginal ulcers, and 3 had an undetermined bleeding site. Seventy percent experienced hypovolemic shock, yet with early endoscopic diagnosis and appropriate surgery, the mor-

Table I.   Etiology and Mortality of Upper Gastrointestinal Tract Hemorrhage in 633 Patients[a,b]

	No. (%)	Deaths	Alcoholic liver disease (%)
Duodenal ulcer	122 (19.3)	4	18.1
Gastritis	107 (16.9)	4	23.6
Esophageal varices	72 (11.4)	14	98.6
Mallory–Weiss tear	53 (8.4)	6	96.2
Gastric ulcer	45 (7.1)	4	15.7
Esophagitis	25 (3.9)	—	19.3
Duodenitis	21 (3.3)	—	30.3
Gastric carcinoma	10 (1.6)	—	10.0
Stomal ulcer	10 (1.6)	—	20.0
Warfarin	24 (3.8)	—	13.0
Unknown	26 (4.1)	5	19.2
Multiple lesions	118 (18.6)	14	57.5
Total	633	51	

[a]Study by T. W. Sheehy and R. Navarre, *Ala. J. Med. Sci.,* 1983, in press.
[b]All patients had endoscopy, UGI series, or both studies within the initial 36 hr of admission.

Table II.   Causes of Upper GI Bleeding

	ASGE (1981)[41] % (No.)	Palmer (1970)[100a] % (No.)	Thomas-Rees (1954)[100b] % (No.)	Sheehy (1981)[a] % (No.)
Duodenal ulcer	24.3 (541)	27.1 (406)	32.6 (157)	19.3 (122)
Gastric erosions	23.4 (521)	12.8 (193)		16.9 (107)
Gastric ulcer	21.3 (474)	12.4 (186)	17.3 (84)	7.1 (45)
Varices	10.3 (229)	19.6 (295)	3.5 (17)	11.4 (72)
Mallory–Weiss tear	7.2 (160)	4.8 (77)		8.4 (53)
Esophagitis	6.3 (141)	7.2 (109)		3.9 (25)
Erosive duodenitis	5.8 (128)			3.3 (21)
Neoplasm	2.9 (64)	0.5 (7 Esophagus) 1.4 (21 Gastric)	5.1 (25)	1.6 (10)
Stomal ulcer	1.8 (41)	3.1 (47)	2.9 (14)	1.6 (10)
Esophageal ulcer	1.7 (37)	0.7 (10)		
Osler's disease	0.5 (11)	0.5 (8)		(3)
Warfarin				3.8 (24)
Other	6.3 (139)	6.9 (141)	38.4 (186)	4.1 (26)
Multiple lesions[b]	32.2 (696)[b]	38.6 (530)		18.6 (118)
Total	2486	1500	483	633

[a]Unpublished observations.
[b]These patients had one or more potential bleeding lesions in addition to the actual bleeding lesions recognized at endoscopy. In the ASGE study, there were two lesions in 532 patients, three lesions in 126 patients, and four lesions in 38 patients.

tality among the 39 surgically treated patients was only 5%. Surgical morbidity was high, however, because of associated diseases, such as diabetes, pulmonary disease, hypertension, and atherosclerosis.[42]

3.2.1.1. Early Endoscopy—Pro and Con

3.2.1.1a. Early Endoscopy—Con. A detailed review of the causes of UGIB is not possible within the limitations of this treatise. Nonetheless, there are certain points relating to UGIB that need to be reviewed. There is general agreement that gastroendoscopy (GE) provides a much higher diagnostic yield (50 to 95%) than upper gastrointestinal radiological studies (50 to 70%), even with double contrast examinations (65 to 80%).[38–43] There is disagreement, however, on the need for early endoscopy in patients with UGIB, i.e., within the first 12 to 24 hr of bleeding. Several studies have suggested that early endoscopy does not decrease mortality or shorten a hospital stay and, therefore is not necessary.[34–40,44,45] These investigators suggested that barium radiologic studies or endoscopy can be done later because 75 to 80% of patients with UGIB stop bleeding spontaneously within 24 to 48 hr. Some even question the need to treat alcoholic cirrhotics who are bleeding, because of the cost and lack of patient compliance.[46] This approach is not universally accepted for several reasons. If the patients do not stop bleeding, they will probably have to undergo endoscopy. This occurred in the study of Peterson et al. wherein the need for early endoscopy was evaluated randomly in 202 patients with UGIB.[44] Even though randomization was carried out after the patients stopped bleeding, 32 of the 102 nonendoscoped patients rebled. They had to be endoscoped later to establish a diagnosis so that definitive treatment could be undertaken.

3.2.1.1b. Early Endoscopy—Pro. Proponents of early endoscopy believe it ensures a more accurate diagnosis; leads to early, appropriate therapy; and permits selection of patients with a high rebleeding risk. Bleeding that recurs after hospitalization for an acute bleeding ulcer can result in a twelvefold increase in mortality.[47] The presence at endoscopy of certain stigmata such as the "visible vessel," or slough in an ulcer will identify 55 to 90% of ulcer patients who are likely to rebleed and therefore are at greater risk of death.[47–50] Early endoscopy also identifies the highly lethal lesions that are more often missed by upper gastrointestinal barium studies, namely esophageal varices, Mallory–Weiss tears, and multiple lesions. It can also be carried out effectively on patients too ill to be moved to a radiologic suite.

According to one recent study, early endoscopy and appropriate treatment lowered mortality from UGIB from 9% to 2.4% over a 6-year period.[51] A major cause of death in any group of patients with UGIB is bleeding esophageal varices. The finding that propranolol reduces portal hypertension in cirrhotics and decreases variceal rebleeding may be a real breakthrough in the care of this lethal condition.[52] If verified, such treatment would substantially reduce mortality due to UGIB.

3.2.1.2. Therapeutic Endoscopy

Therapeutic endoscopy is in its infancy, but, to date, the treatment of active bleeding sites with laser therapy and the use of sclerosing solutions for bleeding varices has not proven highly successful. Sclerosing therapy reduces the immediate risk of rebleeding from esophageal varices, and may decrease later risks of rebleeding. However, over all survival from bleeding varices is not improved, and many patients develop esophageal ulcers as the result of treatment.

At present, patients with massive UGIB and characteristic orthostatic changes should be placed in an intensive care unit and undergo early endoscopy. This and supportive treatment and/or surgery will optimize the chances of the elderly bleeder for survival.

3.2.2. Peptic Ulcer Disease

Age does not decrease the incidence or dim the suffering caused by ulcer disease. Many patients experience the disease for the first time after age 60.[53] Among older patients, the disease is more serious and complications are more frequent. Gastric ulcers and duodenal ulcers are referred to, herein, as peptic ulcer disease (PUD). However, each has its own clinical and pathophysiologic characteristics.

3.2.2.1. Incidence

PUD is prevalent among the elderly. Between 1970 and 1978, the percentage of persons over age 60 in the United States increased from 14 to 15%, although

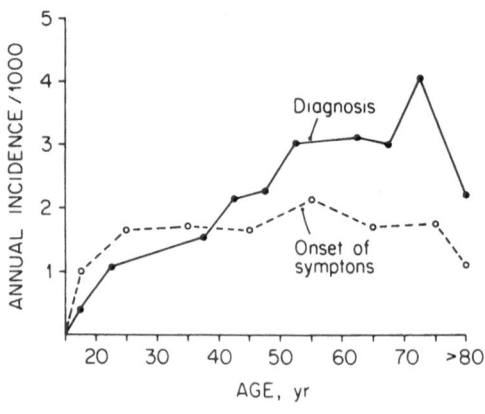

Figure 1. Incidences of new cases of duodenal ulcer (DU) in men according to age of onset of symptoms and age at time of diagnosis. Incidence by onset of symptoms reaches plateau at age 25, but incidence by time of diagnosis keeps increasing to age 75. Adapted from: Grossman, M. I., 1981, *Peptic Ulcer: A Guide for the Practicing Physician*, 1st ed., Yearbook Publishers, Inc., Chicago.

the number of people this age who are hospitalized for duodenal ulcers (DU) rose from 27 to 36% and for gastric ulcer from 40 to 48%,[54-57] Fig. 1 shows the incidence of DU by onset of symptoms and diagnosis. Incidence of symptoms reaches a plateau by age 25 years, whereas the incidence by diagnosis increases steadily to age 75.

The incidence for gastric ulcer also increases between 40 and 65 years.[55] Although PUD does not affect life expectancy, unless complications occur, the death rate due to PUD increased with age. In 1977, in the United States, it rose from 1 per 100,000 at age 45 to 48 per 100,000 at age 85.[55]

3.2.2.2. Etiology

Hydrochloric acid and pepsin are essential to the development of duodenal ulcer, but not necessarily to the evolution of a gastric ulcer. Heredity plays a role. One-half of all patients with DU have hyperpepsinogenemia I as the result of an autosomal dominant trait.[58] DU is more common in "individuals with blood group O and in 'secretors,' i.e., individuals who secrete blood group substances into their saliva and gastric juice." (p. 21)[55] Since ulcer disease is not explained by simple Mendelian genetics, two theories, the "polygenic" and the "heterogeneity" concept have been proposed as explanations.[59-65]

Smoking is associated with an increased incidence for peptic ulcer disease and with delayed ulcer healing. Excessive aspirin ingestion doubles one's chance for acquiring a gastric but not a doudenal ulcer. Contrary to popular opinion, stress, occupation, and personality type are no longer considered risks for ulcer disease.[61]

Patients with duodenal ulcers have the capacity to produce more gastric acid and pepsin then normal individuals. Their parietal cell mass is greater; the response of these cells to pentagastrin, gastrin, and to histamine is increased and gastrin release is thought to be greater than normal following ingestion of food. Duodenal ulcer patients often have elevated plasma levels of pepsin I presumably as the result of a greater number of pepsinogen-I-producing cells. Because of heterogeneity, however, not all these changes are found in every ulcer patient.

3.2.2.3. Diagnosis

One feature unique to PUD is the unreliability of the history. Less than 50% of patients with a history suggestive of PUD have endoscopic evidence for ulcer.[66] In the elderly, epigastric ulcer pain is less common and often bears no temporal relation to meals. Eating may actually make the pain worse. Symptoms are apt to be vague with no pattern of pain relief following eating. Often, there is a substantial loss of weight and a loss of appetite. Ninety percent have nocturnal pain, but such pain is common to other chronic abdominal disorders in the aged, as is relief by antacids.[48]

Despite the unreliability of the history and a paucity of physical findings, in ulcer disease, both are essential to determine the elderly patient's health status. It is important to know if the patient has an ulcer history, is taking medications that can induce a gastric ulcer, and has other diseases, e.g., cardiovascular, renal, or pulmonary disease. The best way to make the diagnosis is by upper gastrointestinal radiologic study or endoscopy. Endoscopy is the more accurate but it is more expensive.[48] In older patients with gastric ulcers, endoscopy is essential to rule out malignancy. Six to 8 biopsies are taken from the ulcer side and 1 or 2 are taken from the ulcer base at the time of endoscopy. Brush cytology of the ulcer is also mandatory before initiating treatment for gastric ulcer.

3.2.2.4. Clinical Course

More than one-half of the patients over 60 years with ulcer disease experience the disease for the first time. The elderly ulcer patient suffers a disproportionate number of serious complications, and their ulcer disease is often masked by the presence of other serious illnesses. Diagnosis is often delayed by the belief that ulcer is uncommon among the aged.[63,64]

The aged with symptomatic ulcer disease usually have a serious course. Only 1 in 4 can be expected to become asymptomatic. About one-half develop major complciations as the first sign of their ulcer. Twenty percent will be hospitalized with a bleeding complication sometimes in the course of their disease.[63,64] Many obtain relief only with surgery. Although patients over age 60 constitute only 15% of the ulcer population, they account for 80% of all ulcer deaths.[66]

3.2.2.5. Treatment of Ulcer Disease

Cimetidine and antacids are effective in promoting healing of duodenal ulcers. Cimetidine (200 to 300 mg) taken with meals and at bedtime (300 to 400 mg) leads to healing of 85% of duodenal and 65% of gastric ulcers within 4 to 6 weeks.[48,67] Cimetidine is even effective in healing ulcers in patients with the Zollinger–Ellison syndrome.[68] Pain relief occurs earlier and more frequently than healing with both cimetidine and antacids, a fact revealed by serial endoscopic examinations.[67–69] In one of these studies, 75% of duodenal ulcer patients were asymptomatic by the fourth week of treatment, but only 70% of those without symptoms had endoscopic evidence of healing. Many developed asymptomatic recurrences.

In contrast, cimetidine is no better than placebo for treatment of gastric ulcers. Placebo led to pain relief in 67% of patients while cimetidine relieved pain in 80% at the end of 4 weeks. Endoscopically, ulcer healing was not significantly different.[70]

Sucralfate, a newly introduced sulfate disaccharide, (1 g before each meal and at bedtime) is as effective as cimetidine in the short-term healing of duodenal ulcer.[71]

3.2.2.6. Long-Term Therapy with Cimetidine

Long-term cimetidine therapy prevents duodenal ulcer recurrence. Eighty percent of duodenal ulcer patients relapse within 1 year without maintenance therapy. With maintenance therapy, the relapse rate is reduced to 20%.[72]

3.2.2.7. Side Effects

Sucralfate is practically nonabsorbable. It is believed to act locally at the ulcer site to block the erosive effects of acid, pepsin, and bile.[71] The only notable side effect reported to date is constipation. Side effects due to cimetidine include gynecomastia, agranulocytosis, and mental confusion. Confusion occurs more commonly in the elderly; particularly in those with hepatic or renal disease and higher than normal blood levels. Somnolence is common in the old, and drugs like Librium® and Valium® increase it. Cimetidine inhibits the hepatic microsomal enzyme metabolism of chlordiozepoxide (Librium) and diazepam (Valium), but not oxazepam (Serax®) or lorazepam (Ativan®).[73,74] It also slows the metabolism of theophylline and propanolol hydrochloride (Inderal®) and potentiates the hypoprothrombinemic effect of warfarin.[75-77] It may lead to elevation of serum transaminase (SGOT, SGPT) levels, but rarely causes clinical hepatitis. In general, reactions are relatively rare and usually are short-term.

3.2.2.8. Antacids

Thirty milliliters of a potent antacid, given 1 and 3 hr after meals and at bedtime, promotes healing within 4 to 8 weeks.[78,79] Hypersecretors require about 80 meq/hr of neutralizing capacity. Fortunately, high potency antacids, like Mylanta II®, Gelusil II®, and Maalox Therapeutic Concentrate® provide about 120 meq/30 ml. Less potent antacids have to be given, in greater amounts, to hypersecretors, i.e., 60 (Maalox®) to 100 ml (Amphogel®), 7 times daily.

3.2.2.9. Side Effects of Antacids

Diarrhea is common with antacids containing magnesium hydroxide. Aluminum hydroxide preparations tend to cause constipation. Older patients with hypertension or borderline cardiac failure should be given a low sodium antacid, e.g., Riopan®. Commercial antacid preparations containing calcium, e.g., Tums®, Rolaids® are dangerous to the elderly, particularly those with renal dysfunction. These agents can induce the milk–alkali syndrome (MAS) or cause acid rebound.[80]

3.2.3. New Drugs

Several new histamine$_2$ (H$_2$) receptors antagonists are now under evaluation for ulcer treatment. Rantidine is a more potent acid inhibitor than cimetidine and only needs to be given twice daily for effective healing.[81] Trithiozine, an alkoxy-thiobenzamide, has been used extensively and successfully for ulcer therapy in Italy.[81] It has antiscretory and tranquilizing properties but is without antichole-nergic, antihistamenic, or ganglion-blocking effects.

Prostaglandin E_2 (PGE_2) is present in lower than normal concentrations in gastric mucosa of ulcer patients. Experimentally, it exhibits gastric secretion and prevents ulceration. Synthetic analogs of PGE_2 are known to increase the healing rate.[79] Undoubtedly, some of the new agents will play an important role in future therapy.

3.2.3.1. Predicators of Ulcer Healing

Five factors are known to affect ulcer healing. In order of importance, they are as follows: (1) sex (women heal more rapidly than men), (2) alcohol [small doses (20 mg/day) may actually improve healing], (3) smoking (impairs healing), (4) age (the elderly heal more slowly), and (5) cimetidine and antacids (potentiate healing).[72]

3.2.3.2. Complications

Major complications of duodenal ulcer in the elderly are similar to those found in the young, namely, bleedings, perforation, obstruction, and intractibility.

3.2.3.3. Bleeding

Bleeding, the most common complication, accounts for over one-half of all fatal ulcer cases. One-half of all patients with bleeding ulcers are over age 50 years and their chances for bleeding are twice that of younger ulcer patients. If bleeding is the first sign of ulcer disease, the risk of rebleeding is doubled in both young and old. After age 70, the risk of bleeding in a duodenal ulcer patient increases 7% yearly.[64] At this age, massive bleeding is common and, in Brooks' study, it was the first sign of disease in 80% of fatal cases.[82] When older patients require surgery for uncontrolled bleeding, the mortality approaches 50%.

3.2.3.4. Factors Predisposing to Rebleeding

Since the death rate increases considerably with rebleeding, factors predis-posing to recurrent hemorrhage should be looked for carefully. These include age, hypertension, massive bleeding, increased transfusion requirements, and certain endoscopic observations. Table II shows the incidence of bleeding ulcers in several large series of patients with UGIB. Ulcer disease is still the most common cause of UGIB.

3.2.3.5. Diagnosis of Bleeding Ulcers

Nasogastric aspiration for blood or heme-positive material is a simple and accurate means of localizing UGIB. Less than 1% of patients with UGIB have negative nasogastric aspirations. A linear correlation also exists between the color of the nasogastric aspirate (NGA) and active UGIB.[48] Forty-eight percent of patients with a bloody NGA have active bleeding or at least oozing lesions at endoscopy.[48]

The color of the NGA and stools are also related to mortality. Bleeding patients with a clear NGA and brown stool have a mortality of 7.9%. When both are bloody, mortality is about 28%.[43,48] Red or maroon stools in ulcer patients are associated with increased mortality, transfusion requirements, complications, and the need for surgery.

3.2.3.6. Endoscopy versus Barium Radiologic Studies

Barium studies of the upper GI tract miss or lead to misdiagnosis of duodenal ulcers in 20 to 40% of bleeding patients. In contrast, endoscopy reveals up to 95% of the lesions responsible for UGIB.[48] Although double contrast barium studies are superior diagnostically to routine barium studies in patients with UGIB, few hospitals provide this service. All agree that endoscopy is the best method to make the diagnosis of bleeding ulcers. However, not all agree that it should be done immediately for UGIB.[83-86]

3.2.3.7. Rebleeding

Rebleeding after hospitalization is extremely lethal, particularly for the aged. Twenty to 30% of patients with UGIB rebleed and one of every three patients with bleeding gastric ulcers rebleed.[84] Patients who rebleed require emergency surgery.[83] Under these circumstances, mortality following surgery often exceeds 50%. Endoscopy is extremely valuable for detecting patients who will rebleed. Foster, Griffiths and Swain found the presence of "visible" vessel highly prognostic.[49,50,84,85]

3.2.3.8. Treatment of Bleeding Ulcers

Resuscitative and supportive measures constitute the initial therapeutic steps in management of UGIB. Four double-blinded control studies have shown that neither oral or parenteral cimetidine or antacids stop ulcer bleeding or prevent rebleeding. Even so, most physicians will administer these agents after diagnosis.[86-89]

Somatostatin is a potent inhibitor of pentagastrin-stimulated hydrochloric acid and pepsin secretion by the stomach as well as gastrin release. Recently, it was found helpful in bleeding ulcer patients. In this randomized study, eight of ten bleeding patients responded to an intravenous somatostatin bolus of 250 µg followed by 250 µg every hour for 48 to 120 hr. In contrast, cimetidine was ineffective in these patients.[89]

3.2.3.9. Prognosis

High risk factors associated with UGIB include: Age ($>$ 60 years); six or more blood transfusions; absence of a preoperative diagnosis; over 60 years old with systolic blood pressure of under 100 mm Hg; and a history of cardiac, respiratory, renal, or hepatic disease, or the presence of congestive heart failure.[90]

3.2.3.9a. Perforation and Penetration. These complications occur in 5 to 10% of patients with PUD. The risk of perforation doubles after age 50 years.[90] Perforation is the first manifestation of disease in 20% of older patients with duodenal ulcer and in 11% of those with gastric ulcer. About one to ten ulcer patients with perforations will bleed from their ulcer. Perforation accounts for 25% of all ulcer-related deaths, the mortality rate increasing sharply with age.[63,66,91,92,]

Factors affecting the outcome of perforation and associated with increased morbidity and mortality include: (1) age, (2) delay in diagnosis and surgical treatment, (3) recent onset of ulcer symptoms before perforation, and (4) presentation with gastrointestinal bleeding.[91,92]

Surgery is essential to treatment. Simple closure of the perforation is still effective and preferred by some surgeons. Others prefer proximal gastric vagotomy.[93,94]

3.2.4. Giant Duodenal Ulcer

Giant duodenal ulcer is, in effect, a posterior penetrating lesion, 3 to 6 cm in size. These ulcers are more common in the elderly and are associated with a high complication rate. Usually the diagnosis is delayed, e.g., only 11 of the 34 cases reported by Lumsten et al. were diagnosed radiologically because the entire duodenal bulb was erroded.[95] Similar erosion was found in 18 of 26 patients studied by Eisenberg and his co-workers.[96] Due to the propensity of giant ulcers to penetrate posteriorly, their base is often composed of necrotic pancreatic tissue. Perforation is much less common than bleeding, which occurs in 50% of patients with giant ulcers. Since mortality is high (40 to 50%), surgery is essential for cure. Recently, however, treatment with cimeditine was shown to be effective in one-half of 26 patients with giant ulcers.[97] Only two died. The combination of UGIB and posterior penetration should always raise the possibility of giant duodenal ulcer.

3.2.4.1. Obstruction

Overall, the incidence of obstruction is 4%, but it rises to 10% in the elderly.[55,82] Patients with obstructions usually have a history of long-standing ulcer disease. Edema and spasm of the bulb secondary to ulcer disease are usually responsible for the blockage. Neurogastric suction in conjunction with fasting and parenteral fluid support usually provide temporary relief. Symptoms are similar to those found in the young, but weight loss can be marked and, in older patients, suggests the possibility of cancer.[56]

3.2.4.2. Surgery

Surgery for ulcer disease in the elderly carries a significant risk and considerable morbidity. In the Nottingham Study, surgical mortality was 10% for patients under 60 with bleeding duodenal ulcers but was 25% for those over 60 years of age.[98] Since the course of ulcer disease is unpredictable, most patients are treated medically at onset and then followed. Surgery is considered for patients with the ulcer complications noted previously.

About 20% of Americans with duodenal ulcers require surgery. A significant number (5%) are incapacitated by surgery and even more (10 to 40%) develop chronic ill effects.[56,98] Hence, the decision to operate should not be taken lightly. Surprisingly, the bulk of operations are carried out for intractable disease upon patients who have not rebled, perforated, or obstructed. Not surprisingly, these patients have a higher risk of postoperative complications than patients who have bled or perforated.

The indications for surgery are: recurrent bleeding, obstruction, intractibility, and perforation. About 30% of patients with a bleeding ulcer have a second hemorrhage within 5 years. Chances for rebleeding a third time approach 60%. Each episode carries a 7% chance of death. Early surgery has decreased the mortality rate for patients with bleeding gastric ulcers that also have a high rate of rebleeding.[56,82,98]

Recent studies have shown that definitive surgery is required within 10 years in over one-half of patients who have had a simple closure of their perforations. For this reason, many surgeons now carry out definitive surgery at the time of perforation in patients with a long history of ulcer disease.[56,91,94]

At present, proximal truncal (parietal cell) vagotomy is the operation of choice for severe or intractable duodenal ulcer disease.[99-101] Among 233 patients subjected to this operation at the Mayo Clinic,[101] there was no mortality. Postoperative symptoms such as nausea and diarrhea were seen in less than 3%, but recurrence rate was 4.9%. The recurrence rate was 12.3% among 154 duodenal ulcer patients treated with vagotomy and pyloroplasty at the same institution. Diarrhea occurred in 16.2% and dumping in 7.8% of these patients.[101] The appropriate surgical procedure for complications of gastric ulcer disease remains a matter of individual choice. The end results of gastric resection with vagotomy versus oversewing the bleeding point of the gastric ulcer together with a vagotomy plus a drainage procedure do not appear to differ significantly.

3.2.5. Gastritis

Acute gastritis (AG) and chronic gastritis (CG) are common afflictions of the elderly. Achlorhydria in the elderly is usually due to CG. The frequency of achlorhydria rises steadily with age. About 30% are afflicted by the age of 70 years.[102]

3.2.5.1. Etiology

AG is usually associated with viral enteritis, food poisoning, and bacterial toxins and has a rapid onset. Tobacco, alcohol, and salicylates, hot drinks, iron deficiency, pernicious anemia, bile reflux, and allergy have all been associated with CG.[103-104] Atrophic gastritis develops in the wake of superficial gastritis. The mean transition time is about 17 years.[105] Atrophic gastritis is common in the sixth and seventh decades.

3.2.5.2. Clinical Findings

In AG, symptoms vary considerably due to differing causes. They include anorexia, nausea, vomiting, epigastric fullness, and pain. If infection is the cause, then fever, headache, diarrhea, and flulike symptoms usually develop. Dehydration and prerenal azotemia are common in the aged if vomiting or diarrhea are severe.

In chronic gastritis, symptoms are usually vague and nondescript and may consist of epigastric tenderness or flatulence. Clinical findings are usually unremarkable unless other diseases, e.g., gastric ulcer or carcinoma, are present. Chronic gastritis is never diagnosed until other possibilities are eliminated.

3.2.5.3. Diagnosis

Diagnosis of both AG and CG requires invasive procedures. In CG, radiographic studies may show thinning of the gastric folds. Endoscopically, the mucosa appears thin. Visible mucosal capillaries and superficial erosions may be seen.[104] Biopsy is confirmatory, revealing glandular atrophy and infiltration of the lamina propria with lymphocytes and plasma cells. Hypochlorhydria in CG is associated with a raised fasting serum gastrin level and gastrin cell hyperplasia.[102]

3.2.5.4. Treatment

This is supportive for AG. It consists of replenishing fluid, maintaining electrolyte balance and refraining from solid food during the acute episode.

There is no specific treatment for CG. Removal of aggravating factors such as alcohol, salicylates, nonsteroidal antiinflammatory drugs, and caffeine helps early in the course of the disease. Once atrophic gastritis develops, however, the lesion is usually irreversible. Vitamin B_{12} improves the chronic gastritis associated with pernicious anemia. Regeneration of chief and parietal cells occurs to a considerable extent.[105]

3.3. Hepatobiliary Disease

By age 65, liver mass has decreased from 2.5 to 1.5% of total body mass while hepatic blood has decreased by 40%. Even so, there is sufficient liver mass to allow normal liver function and bile salt production. The hepatobiliary system of the geriatric patient is subject to the same diseases as the young. In this brief treatise, we can only mention a few of these.

3.3.1. Cirrhosis

Few advances have been made in the diagnosis and treatment of cirrhosis. However, the morphological classification has been changed so that cirrhosis is now classified as micronodular ($<$ 1 mm nodules) or macronodular ($>$ 1 mm nodules).

3.3.1.1. Etiology

Drugs, notably alcohol, and viral infections are the primary causes of cirrhosis.[106-110] In this country, the incidence of cirrhosis peaks when the patient is between 55 and 75 years, and the disease declines thereafter. Alcoholism, a prime factor in cirrhosis, is common in the elderly, the incidence ranging from 7 to 17%.[111,112] *Senile cirrhosis* is a term often used to describe cirrhosis in the octogenerian.

3.3.1.2. Clinical Findings

Clinical findings are essentially those seen in the young, except they may be compounded by systemic diseases.

3.3.1.3. Treatment

Treatments for ascites, portal encephalopathy, and fulminant hepatic failure have not changed significantly.[106–112,116]

3.3.2. Viral Hepatitis

All three forms of viral hepatitis (A, B, and nonA–nonB) occur in the elderly, but none occurs with the frequency seen in youth. Clinical manifestations, laboratory abnormalities, and other features of the disease are essentially the same. However, morbidity and mortality are greater in the aged.

3.3.3. Chronic Active Hepatitis

Chronic active hepatitis (CAH), too, occurs with less frequency in the aged.

3.3.3.1. Etiology

CAH is believed to be the result of an altered immune response to viral hepatitis or drugs such as methyl-DOPA, isoniazid, oxyphenasiten, and nitrofurantoin.[113] Accordingly, the etiologic agent alters the hepatocyte membrane in such a manner that the immune system does not recognize it as self and produces antibodies to its own liver cells.[114]

Ten to 50% of all cases of CAH result from infectious hepatitis B. High titers of hepatitis B core antibody correlate with continued viral reproduction within the liver. They are indicative of persistent infection, even in the absence of a positive serum hepatitis B surface antigen. NonA–nonB hepatitis virus is responsible for 20% of CHA.[115,116]

3.3.3.2. Clinical Findings

The patient is often symptom-free, the only evidence of disease being abnormal liver function studies. Symptomatic patients usually complain of fatigue, anorexia, weakness, and malaise. With progression, the manifestations of cirrhosis and its complications may evolve.

3.3.3.3. Diagnosis

Diagnosis requires biochemical and histologic evidence of liver disease 6 months after a bout of acute viral or drug-induced hepatitis. Histological evidence consists of infiltration of the parenchyma and portal zones by plasma cells and lymphocytes, piecemeal necrosis, and formation of intralobular septa.

3.3.3.4. Treatment

For patients with CAH who are HBsAg-negative, steroids and azathioprine are the mainstays of therapy. Prednisone, 30 mg daily, is given to patients with symptomatic disease who have morphologically severe lesions.[117,118] With improvement, the dosage is reduced to a maintenance level that controls symptomatology and leads to improvement in liver chemistries. Insufficient data are available to determine the need for treating HBsAg-positive patients. Indeed, Lam and his associates claim prednisone hastens relapse and increases complications in these patients.[119] There is suggestive evidence, too, that azothiaprine therapy is harmful in CAH–HBsAg-positive patients. Among the newer modes of therapy, transfer factor and levamisole have not proven efficacious. Available data for antiviral chemotherapy with interferon and vidabrine are also insufficient to determine if these agents will be therapeutically beneficial.

3.3.3.5. Prognosis

The natural history of CAH has not yet been established and its course varies considerably. For patients who fail to improve with treatment, the course is one of progressive deterioration. About two-thirds of these patients die within 5 years of onset of symptoms.

3.4. Cholelithiasis

3.4.1. Incidence

The true incidence of cholelithiasis is unknown. It varies among nations and races. The highest incidence is found in Sweden and the lowest among the Masai of Africa. In Sweden, 70% of women over age 70 and 50% of men in their 90s have gallstones.[120] About 20,000,000 Americans have gallstones, and each year, 500,000 undergo a cholecystectomy.[121] In the Framingham study, the incidence was 8% over a 10-year period.[120] Gallstones are more common in women than in men in this country. They occur more frequently in multiparous women. Most Americans (80%) have cholesterol stones, 10% have mixed stones containing cholesterol and pigment, and 10% have pure pigmented stones.[120a]

3.4.1.1. Etiology

The high prevalence rate in Western countries has been attributed to a high consumption of refined carbohydrates which induce lithogenic bile formation.[120] Other factors associated with increased prevalence are obesity, cirrhosis, and

Crohn's disease. The incidence is doubled in cirrhosis and increased two- to five-fold in Crohn's disease. Hemolysis is responsible in cirrhosis and impaired absorption of bile salts in ileitis. Age and drugs (e.g., oral contraceptives and clofibrinate) are other factors.[122,123] Cholesterol stones develop if bile salt production is altered due to (1) defective bile synthesis, (2) a decrease in the enzyme necessary for bile synthesis (cholesterol-6-α-hydroxalase) or (3) an increase in cholesterol production secondary to an increase in the hepatic enzyme (hydroxymethyl-glutaryl-coenzyme-A-reductase) necessary for cholesterol synthesis.[124,125] The kinetics of biliary lipid secretion and gallbladder storage of bile have been reviewed recently by Mok, Von Bergmann, and Grundy.[126] Pigmented stones are usually associated with hemolysis, alcoholic liver disease, biliary tract infection, and advanced age.

3.4.1.2. Prognosis

Patients with gallstones are grouped into four categories: (1) the asymptomatic (50%), (2) the symptomatic (30%), (3) the dyspeptic (15%), and (4) the surgical (5%).[127] Fifty percent of symptomatic patients undergo cholecystectomy within 5 years due to recurrent symptoms, ductal obstruction, or pancreatitis. Over the same period, a similar percentage of asymptomatic patients become symptomatic. Twenty percent of the dyspeptics develop cholecystitis or biliary colic within a decade.

3.4.1.3. Treatment

Many surgeons consider the presence of gallstones a mandate for cholecystectomy. Their reasoning is based on two observatons, namely: (1) 50% of patients become symptomatic with age and (2) the elderly tolerate surgery less readily. The elderly account for 70% of the deaths associated with acute cholecystitis.[121] Cholecystectomy is also advocated for patients with diabetes mellitus, stable angina pectoris, and gallstones. These conditions increase complications and the surgical risk. Most physicians prefer to treat asymptomatic patients over 65 years of age conservatively, particularly those with renal or liver disease.[121]

3.4.1.4. Gallstone Dissolution

Advances in gallstone dissolution may eventually change therapy for the aged with gallstones. In the National Cooperative Gallstone Study, 900 patients with gallstones were treated with chenodeoxycholic acid (CA). The drug proved to be safe and effective, but it only dissolved stones in 13.5% of those taking 750 mg daily and in 5.2% of those taking 375 mg daily.[128] This dosage was probably inadequate.[129] The optimal oral dose recommended is 15 mg/kg per day for 2 years for radiolucent stones; larger stones may require even longer treatment. Slim patients achieve better results and women respond to treatment better than men.

Another oral preparation, ursodeoxycholic acid, is even more effective for stone dissolution.[129] The major side effects of CA are nausea, vomiting, diarrhea, and transient elevation of serum transaminase and cholesterol levels. Ursodeoxycholic acid does not increase serum transaminase levels or cause diarrhea as frequently. It will probably replace CA.

Monooctanoin, a digestive product of medium-chain triglycerides, is the most effective agent for direct contact dissolution of cholesterol stones. In vitro, it dissolved mixed cholesterol stones twice as fast as sodium cholate solutions. It can be infused into postcholecystectomy patients with retained bile duct stones via a T-tube or by percutaneous catheter at a rate of 3 to 10 mg/hr using a constant infusion pump. Such treatment leads to stone dissolution in 90% of patients after 4 to 21 days of therapy.[130,131]

3.4.2. Acute Cholecystitis

The major complication of cholelithiasis is acute cholecystitis. Among the elderly, this is a serious and often fatal illness and the number of affected patients is increasing.[121] Emergency cholecystectomy for the elderly carries a higher mortality (11 to 17%) than for the young (1 to 3%). Seventy percent of deaths from acute cholecystitis occur in the elderly.[121]

3.4.2.1. Etiology

Gallstones are the major cause of acute cholecystitis. With cystic duct blockage, bile accumulates leading to a chemical irritation of the mucosal lining and to inflammation of the gallbladder wall. With continued obstruction, bacterial invasion occurs via the lymphatics. *Escherichia coli* and *Enterococci* are the most common aerobic bacteria associated with acute cholecystitis. *Clostridium perfringens* and *Bacteroides fragilis* are the most commonly encountered anaerobic bacteria.[132] Emphysematous cholecystitis is usually due to infection with *Clostridia* and certain types of *E. coli*. This entity usually occurs in patients with diabetes mellitus.

Acalculous cholecystitis refers to acute cholecystitis in the absence of gallstones. Usually, it results from the bacteremia associated with extensive wounds or severe burns.[133]

3.4.2.2. Clinical Findings

The study of 88 elderly patients with acute cholecystitis by Morrow, Thomason, and Wilson exemplifies the problem in the aged.[134] All but one experienced some type of abdominal pain but only 34 had a temperature elevation above 37.8°C. Patients were divided into two groups. Group 1 consisted of 39 patients who required emergency surgery; 20 of whom had abdominal tenderness (74%). Less than one-half had peritoneal signs. Sixteen (41%) had peritonitis and 11

(28%) had jaundice. A mass was palpated in 7 (18%). Absence of overt right upper quadrant peritonitis led to a delay in diagnosis of longer than 24 hr in one-third. The 49 patients in Group 2 had elective surgery.

Leukocytosis occurred in 65% of acutely ill patients; total bilirubin and alkaline phosphatase levels were increased in 60%, SGOT and SGPT levels were elevated in 62%. Bactobilia was present in 70% of Group 1 patients and in 38% of Group 2 patients. Among Group 1 patients, 17 had acute cholecystitis, 9 empyema, 3 gangrenous cholecystitis, 4 perforated gallbladder, 6 subphrenic abscess, and 6 common bile duct stones. Among Group 2, 4 patients had acute cholecystitis, 2 empyema, 1 gangrenous cholecystitis, 1 perforated gallbladder, and 7 common duct stones. None of the patients who had elective surgery developed a subphrenic abscess.

In many older patients, emergency surgery was necessary because the diagnosis was obscured by a deceptively benign presentation. Associated diseases such as coronary artery disease (30%), severe pulmonary disease (25%), hypertension (15%), and diabetes mellitus (13%) further obscured the diagnosis.

3.4.2.3. Diagnosis

A plain film of the abdomen may reveal gallstones and a dilated or emphysematous gallbladder. Oral cholangiography and intravenous cholangiography are helpful in nonjaundiced patients. Ultrasonography is the most useful examination. This test has a specificity of 97% and a sensitivity of 88% in patients with acute biliary tract disease.[135]

3.4.2.4. Treatment

Initial therapy consists of bedrest, nasogastric suction to decompress the stomach, and intravenous fluid replacement. Pain can be relieved by meperidine hydrochloride or by intravenous indomethacin.[136] Indomethacin inhibits prostaglandin synthesis, thereby reducing intralumenal pressure and relieving biliary pain.[136] Antibiotics may be useful. Kefzolin 1 g intravenously every 6 hr and Ampicillin 500 mg intravenously or intramuscularly every 6 hr are usually preferred. This approach successfully relieves symptoms in 90% of patients within 72 to 96 hr.

In the past, a "cooling-off" period was often allowed so that surgery could be performed safely at a later time. Now, cholecystectomy is advocated within 24 to 72 hr of hospitalization.[137,138] Few surgeons perform cholecystostomy. In the acutely ill patient, cholecystostomy is associated with a much higher mortality than cholecystectomy (27% versus 2%).[121,139]

Medical therapy is employed for patients with severe complications such as acute pancreatitis, mycardial infarction, congestive heart failure, or severe respiratory disease in the hope of ameliorating the biliary condition temporarily. If successful, these patients are followed until elective cholecystectomy is feasible.

3.4.3. Choledocholithiasis

Fifteen percent of patients undergoing cholecystectomy have bile duct stones. Ultrasonography or computerized tomography readily reveal impacted stones or the presence of dilated bile ducts which suggests their presence. Percutaneous transhepatic cholangiography is also effective for localizing obstructing stones. This test should be done on the day of operation even though the Chiba (skinny) needle decreases bile leakage from the liver.[140] Operative cholangiography is another important advance. Like cholecystoscopy with a Stor–Hopkins choledoscope, it allows visualization of the entire biliary tree.

3.5. Acute Pancreatitis

3.5.1. Incidence

The incidence of acute pancreatitis (AP) increases with age. AP is the most important nonsurgical cause of the acute abdomen in the elderly. Although there are many causes of AP (Table III), 75 to 80% of patients have either gallstone

Table III.   Etiology of Pancreatitis

	Mortality (percent)
Alcohol	31[a]
Gallstones	13
Drugs—Thiazides	
Steroids	
Other—Hereditary	
Traumatic—Postsurgical	27
Posttraumatic	
Infection —Viral	
Metabolic—Hyperparathyroidism	
Hyperlipemia	
Hypercalcemia	
Hemochromatosis	
Diabetes	
Pregnancy	
Porphyria	
Uremia	
Idiopathic	17
Odd —Scorpion venom	
Vascular disease	
Peptic ulcer	
Liver disease	
Cirrhosis	
Small bowel disease	

[a] Adapted from Ranson, J. H. C., *Surg. Clin. North Am.* 61:55–70, 1981.

(GSP) or alcoholic pancreatitis (AAP).[141] Four kinds of pancreatitis have been recognized: acute pancreatitis, recurrent acute pancreatitis, recurrent chronic pancreatitis, and chronic pancreatitis.[142] AAP and GSP are the types of pancreatitis most often found in the elderly.

3.5.2. Alcoholic Pancreatitis

Alcoholism and AAP are common among the elderly. Fifty-two of our 200 patients with AAP were over age 55. AAP evolved after 6 to 19 years of heavy drinking. Secretory and eventually structural changes occur within the pancreas. Alcohol increases the protein content of pancreatic juice five- to sixfold, leads to its precipitation in intracalated ducts, and induces formation of "lactoferrin."[143] The risk of AAP increases linearly as a function of the quantity of alcohol and protein consumed. For every additional 20-g intake of alcohol, the risk is multiplied by a factor of 1.4. Fat consumption correlates quadratically with risk. It is increased by ingestion of both a low lipid diet (< 85 g/day) and a high lipid diet (> 110 g/day).[144,145]

3.5.3. Gallstone Pancreatitis

In contrast to AAP which involves the ductules, GSP involves the large pancreatic ducts. Eighty-five to 90% of patients with GSP have gallstones in their stools.[146,147] GSP may arise as result of a common channel with bile reflux, an obstructed or compressed duct, or edema and inflammation from passage of a stone through the ampulla of Vater.

3.5.4. Diagnosis

The clinical presentation of AP varies in the elderly. Often, the history is noncontributory, while physical findings, with the exception of tachycardia, upper abdominal pain and guarding, are nonspecific.[145] Clinically, the most important factor is to differentiate AP from other causes of an acute abdomen. An elevated serum amylase is found in 95% of older patients with AP and in 5% of the elderly with other causes of an acute abdomen.[148,149] Sixty percent of patients with GSP and 10 to 30% with AAP have jaundice. Serum bilirubin and serum transamylase levels are increased two- to threefold. Hypocalcemia is common with acute hemorrhagic pancreatitis. The amylase/creatinine ratio is not specific as intially anticipated. Lactoferrin is increased in the duodenal and pancreatic juices of patients with alcoholic, idiopathic, hereditary, and chronic pancreatitis and in a small number of normal individuals. This protein may prove to be a diagnostic aid for AP.[150]

Other diagnostic tests include a flat plate of the abdomen to determine if pancreatic calcification is present. If the patient is not jaundiced, intravenous cholangiography may help to identify the presence or absence of biliary tract disease.

Ultrasonography helps to assess the presence of cholelithiasis in jaundiced individuals. It is useless when the bowel is distended with gas or the patient is markedly obese. Sequential studies may detect liquification and pseudocyst formation in AAP. Computerized tomography is of little help in identifying gallstones, but it may reveal intrahepatic and common duct dilitation as well as changes in pancreatic and peripancreatic tissues.[140] Chiba-needle cholangiography is extremely helpful in jaundiced patients. It allows differentiation of acute pancreatitis from acute biliary disease with hyperamylasemia. Endoscopic retrograde cholangiography is an excellent way to visualize the pancreatic ducts, but it may induce pain identical to that experienced during an attack of pancreatitis.

3.5.5. Prognosis

Fortunately, acute pancreatitis is self-limiting in 95% of patients and acute necrotizing pancreatitis only develops in 5%, but 40 to 80% of these patients die.[151] Early diagnosis is imperative for survival with this entity. The greater the necrosis, the higher the mortality (28% for hemorrhagic versus 7% for edematous pancreatitis).[151] The unpredictability of acute necrotizing pancreatitis led Ranson et al. to look for prognostic signs.[152] Eleven signs were found to be helpful (Table IV). Patients with less than three have a low risk. Those with three or more positive signs have a high risk of death from major complications.

3.5.6. Treatment

3.5.6.1. Medical

The mild attack requires little more than fluid replacement. However, for acute nectorizing pancreatitis, patients require nasogastric suction, intravenous

Table IV. Early Prognostic Signs in Acute Pancreatitis That Correlate with Serious Illness or Death[a]

Admission
  Age: Over 55 years
  WBC: Over 16,000
  Glucose: Over 200 mg%
  LDH: Over 350 units
  SGOT: Over 250 SF
During first 48 hr
  Hct: Decrease of 10%
  BUN: Rise over 5 mg%
  Ca^{2+}: Below 8 mg%
  PaO_2: Below 60 mm Hg
  Base deficit over 4 meq/liter
  Estimated fluid sequestration over 6 liters

[a]Adapted from: Ranson, J. H. C., et al., *Surg. Gynec. Obstet.* 139:69–81, 1974.

fluid replacement, analgesic support, monitoring of their pulmonary artery and capillary wedge pressures, electrolytes, and fluid intake and output. Hyperalimentation and calcium and magnesium administration may be necessary. Peritoneal lavage is used for patients with three or more positive prognostic signs. In some, it produces a striking clinical improvement and it is often helpful in patients with cardiovascular and respiratory complications,[145,153] so monitoring of pulmonary function and arterial blood gases is important. This technique may also injure abdominal viscera and worsen ventilation.

3.5.6.2. Surgical

Early operative intervention for AAP is dangerous. Intraabdominal sepsis, pancreatic abscess, and the severity of respiratory complications are markedly increased.[154]

Early operative intervention for GSP carries a mortality of 7 to 8%; nonoperative mortality is higher.[155] Acosta and Ledesma advocate operative intervention for GSP within 24 to 48 hr of onset of symptoms.[146] Presumably, early decompression decreases the chance of edematous pancreatitis progressing to hemorrhagic pancreatitis. Ranson advocates supportive treatment of GSP until the symptoms have subsided before operating on these patients.[156] All agree that biliary tract pathology must be eliminated. Otherwise, 10 to 50% of these patients sustain repeated bouts of pancreatitis.[155,156]

Patients with GSP survive the fluid loss of hemorrhagic pancreatitis better than those with AAP. Hence, more survive to develop pancreatic abscesses and pancreaticoenteric fistulae.[157] Pseudocysts, pancreatic ascites, portal vein thrombosis, and chronic pancreatitis are more likely to be associated with alcoholic pancreatic pancreatitis.[158]

3.5.7. Complications

Hyperglycemia occurs in 50% of patients with AAP. Parathyroid hormone inactivation or a parahormone deficiency is thought to be responsible for hypocalcemia.[159] Hyperlipemia often occurs in alcoholics with Type I and IV, V hyperlipoproteinemia. Respiratory insufficiency results from pleural effusion, fluid overload, pneumonitis, and pulmonary infarction. Mild to moderate hypoxia occurs in 60% during the first 48 hr. Nonspecific factors contributing to pulmonary distress include pulmonary capillary damage, surfactant impairment, and altered respiratory muscle coordination. Respiratory distress usually develops after 4 to 5 days of illness.[160,161] Arterial blood gases are more predictive of an evolving acute respiratory distress syndrome (ARDS) than the chest X ray.

Pseudocysts occur in about 5% of patients. Overall mortality associated with their surgical drainage is 6 to 8%. Ten to 15% reoccur following surgery and 5% rupture.[162] Pseudocyst growth depends upon the continued existence of a fistula linking the cyst with the pancreatic duct.[163] If the inflammatory resection fails to seal off the retroperitoneal space, fluid drains anteriorly causing pancreatic ascites. If the inflammation process directs the leak posteriorly, fluid seeps upward into the pleural cavity yielding massive pleural effusions.[163,164] This is not to be confused with the small pleural effusions seen early in an acute attack.

3.6. The Colon

3.6.1. Diverticulosis

3.6.1.1. Incidence

It was not until the advent of contrast radiology that the frequency of diverticulosis was appreciated. The incidence increases from 5% at age 40 to 50% in the ninth decade (Table V).[165,166,166a-e,172]

3.6.1.2. Etiology

Until recently, it was believed that diverticuli resulted from either continued ingestion of a low fiber diet or from an abnormality of colonic motility.[167] A lack of dietary bulk was thought to cause partitioning of the colon into partially obstructed compartments with high intralumenal pressure. The latter presumably caused the mucosal lining to herniate along vascular channels through the bowel wall. However, high intralumenal pressures have also been observed in patients with the irritable bowel syndrome and may be invoked by food ingestion, morphine, and parasympathomimetic drugs.[167-169] Early enthusiasm for the high-fiber diets has waned as reports appeared claiming this type of diet fails to alleviate symptoms and merely acts as a stool softener.[169]

The abnormal motility concept evolved in 1926 after Barling reported that spasm of the colon observed at laparotomy produced tiny saccules along the longitudinal muscle bands.[170] These saccules disappeared when the spasm passed.

Table V. Incidence of Diverticuli

Year	Authors	Percent	Patients	Number examined
1930	Mayo, W. J.[165]	5.7	1,819	31,838
1930	Rankin, S. W., Brown, P. E.[166a]	5.6	1,398	24,620
1935	Oschner, H. C., Bargen, G. A.[166b]	7.0	Not given	2,747
1936	Willard, J. H., Bockus, H.[166c]	8.2	38	463
1953	Allen, A. W.[166d]	30	Not given	2,000
1939	Smith, C. C., Christensen, W. R.[166e]	22	Not given	1,016

Since then it has been learned that patients with asymptomatic diverticulosis and an irritable bowel syndrome have normal colonic motility whereas symptomatic patients with these diseases have abnormal motility indexes.[171-173]

3.6.1.3. Clinical Findings

Most patients with diverticulosis have few symptoms. Some complain of constipation, others of abdominal distension, and some of severe cramping pain. Constipation is more common than diarrhea and may alternate with it. The physical examination is not characteristic. Laboratory studies are also nonspecific except for the barium enema which is diagnostic. In some patients with lower quadrant pain, only muscular thickening and lumenal narrowing of the sigmoid is found on barium contrast study.

3.6.1.4. Diagnosis

Barium enema examination is essential for diagnosis. In 90% of patients, the disease involves the sigmoid colon. In 45 to 60%, it is the only area involved.

3.6.1.5. Prognosis

At one time, it was thought that the greater the number of diverticulae, the greater the chance for complications. This concept has never been proven. In two-thirds of patients, the disease remains relatively quiescent.[171] Of those treated medically, one-third have a recurrence of diverticulitis within 5 years.[174]

3.6.2. Diverticulitis

3.6.2.1. Etiology

Diverticulitis results from micro- or macro-perforation of the diverticulum. With rupture of the mucosa, bacteria escape into the limiting serosa yielding peridiverticular infection. With rupture through the serosa, bacteria escape into the peritoneum, yielding peritonitis. Usually both occur on the left side of the colon and lead to localizing or generalized peritonitis.

3.6.2.2. Diagnosis

Diverticulitis is characterized by pain in the left lower quadrant and a change in bowel habits. Fever is usually present, its degree depending upon the severity and extent of the inflammation. Involvement of surrounding organs such as the bladder or ureter may give rise to dysuria.

3.6.2.3. Clinical Findings

Usually tenderness to deep palpation is found in the left lower quadrant. Occasionally, there is rebound tenderness. About one-fourth of patients have a tender palpable mass in the left lower quadrant. If septicemia ensues, chills and fever become prominent. In the elderly, leukocytosis is often absent and the only indication of infection may be an increase in the number of immature neutrophils. Sigmoidoscopy may disclose an edematous reddened mucosa proximal to the rectosigmoid area. With perforation, upright films may reveal air under the diaphragm or dilitation of the colon suggesting possible obstruction. Barium contrast study may reveal the site of diverticular rupture or the presence of one or more fistulae. This examination can be done during an acute episode of diverticulitis, but must be done cautiously and without excess pressure. With precaution, complications seldom ensue.[175] Differential diagnosis include Crohn's disease, ischemic colitis, carcinoma of the colon, and the irritable bowel syndrome.

3.6.2.4. Treatment

There are no good control studies for the treatment of acute diverticulitis. Mild attacks manifested by constipation and left lower quadrant pain without fever tend to respond to a soft or liquid diet. Antibiotics are of doubtful benefit in this situation. In more severely ill patients, i.e., those with fever, abdominal pain, and leukocytosis, adequate fluid replacement is essential. A nasogastric tube is placed if nausea and vomiting are present. Antibiotic therapy is employed, but the choice of drugs is questionable. It is wise to use a combination of antibiotics that will destroy colonic flora. Many prefer gentamicin 1.0 mg/kg every 8 hr in combination with clindamycin 600 mg every 6 to 8 hr. Medical therapy is effective in two-thirds and ameliorates their need for surgery.[176] Those who fail to respond to conservative therapy usually require surgery to handle complications such as localized abscess, perforations, and fistulae formation.

3.6.2.5. Complications

Diverticulitis is the most common cause of lower gastrointestinal bleeding. Unlike other complications, it arises from an uninflamed diverticula. Spontaneous cessation of bleeding tends to occur after a slow but considerable blood loss. If conservative management and transfusion fail to control bleeding, vasopressin (0.2 unit/min) leads to temporary control in 90% of patients. About 25% will have recurrence and surgery is often necessary for those who continue to bleed. Bleeding from diverticula does not reoccur as often as from angiodysplasia, but it is more severe. Other causes of lower intestinal bleeding must be considered. In the study by Boley et al. of 99 elderly patients with lower intestinal bleeding, 43 had diverticulosis, 20 angiodysplasia, 9 colonic carcinoma, 6 radiation proctitis, and 4 ischemic proctitis.[177] In the remainder the cancer was not identified.

3.6.3. Polyposis

3.6.3.1. Incidence

Colonic polyps are a hazard for the elderly. They may cause bleeding, obstruction, and intussusception. They also constitute one of three major lesions predisposing to cancer; namely, adenomas, familial polyposis, and ulcerative colitis.[178,179]

Although the true incidence of colonic polyps is not certain, polyps become more frequent with advancing age and, in the elderly, they are more likely to be multiple. Various estimates imply that about one-half of individuals over 50 years of age have one or more polyps. Men are afflicted more frequently than women and whites have polyps more often than blacks.

3.6.3.2. Etiology

The cause of colonic polyps is unknown. Genetics and familial predisposition play roles in the familial polyposis syndromes, but not in the evaluation of solitary polyps.[180,181] Sixty percent of adenomatous polyps are found in the rectum and sigmoid colon. The remainder are scattered from the transverse colon to the cecum.[182] Pedunculated polyps are attached to the mucosa via the stalk; sessile polyps rest on the mucosa and have a broad base. Adenomas have also been classified into three histological types: (1) adenomatous polyp (tubular adenoma), (2) tubulovillous adenomas, and (3) villous adenomas (villous papilloma). The tubulovillous adenoma is a mixed type of tumor.[183] Previously adenomas were thought to rise from the crypt epithelium and villous adenomas from the surface epithelium.[184] Whitehead believes all polyps are of the same origin, i.e., a neoplastic proliferation of colonic epithelium that produces different varieties of growth patterns.[185]

Villous adenomas are papillary adenomas. Although considered benign, they have a strong tendency toward malignancy, transformation occurring in from 40 to 60%. Usually, villous adenomas are large (i.e., over 6 cm in diameter), soft and sessile. Occasionally, they may have stalks. Villous adenomas comprise 5% of all large bowel polyps. They are soft, have the same consistency as bowel tissue, and therefore are not easily palpable.

Other forms of colonic polyps include: (1) myomas arising from smooth muscles, (2) fibromas originating from supporting tissue, (3) lipomas from fatty tissue, (4) hemangiomas, and (5) lymphoid polyps.

3.6.3.3. Multiple Adenomas

The presence of one adenoma increases the chance for a second to develop later. The expected annual rate for the discovery of new adenomas is about 5% in those who have had one removed.

3.6.3.4. Relation to Cancer

Opinions have been expressed that all polyps are potentially malignant and that adenomas are usually benign although villous adenomas are usually malignant. Grinnell and Lane suggested that penetration of malignant cells beyond the muscularis mucosa is a prerequisite for metastasis.[179] Their observations are based on the finding that colonic lymphatics are only associated with the muscularis mucosa and do not extend beyond the muscularis mucosa at the time of resection offers the chance for almost a 100% cure rate.[186] Today, most agree that adenomatous polyps are premalignant lesions. What percentage develop into carcinoma, however, is unknown.

3.6.3.5. Clinical Findings

Both adenomatous polyps and villous adenomas may give rise to vague abdominal discomfort or they may be completely asymptomatic. Rectal bleeding is common to both. Large polyps with stalks may also cause intussusception or obstruction.

Villous adenomas usually occur in patients over age 50 years. Since they have large numbers of goblet cells, as they grow, they tend to secrete copious amounts of salty mucus and sometimes give rise to watery diarrhea, salt depletion, and dehydration. Fluid losses of 2 to 4 liters and salt loss of 8 to 10 g daily have been reported. Protein-losing enteropathy may also develop.

3.6.3.6. Treatment

In contrast to adenomatous polyps, villous adenomas should not be biopsied. They must be removed in one piece by local excision. If this is not possible, then part of the colon must be removed. These steps are necessary because of the tendency of this tumor to reoccur and to be malignant.

Villous adenomas must be distinguished from polypoid carcinoma of the colon and rectum, although differentiation is almost academic. Both must be removed surgically. This is not the case, however, for the benign adenoma. Three factors are related to its cancer potential, namely, a stalk, its size, and the degree of villous histologic change. A stalk suggests the lesion is benign. Adenomas less than 1 cm in diameter are usually benign. Five percent of those with a diameter of 1 to 2 cm and 10% of those over 2 cm contain invasive carcinoma.[185] Polyps over 2 cm engender a 50% chance of malignancy. Polyps greater than 1 cm, regardless of their location, should be removed. Today, colonoscopy usually permits removal of all adenomatous polyps without the need for bowel surgery. If the entire polyp cannot be removed at colonoscopy, then an open operation is necessary. Histologic examination is essential for further decision. If there is no invasion beyond the muscularis mucosa, the lesion is benign. If invasion is beyond the muscularis mucosa, a formal resection is indicated.[185]

3.6.4. Superior Mesenteric Artery Occlusion

Acute occlusion of the superior mesenteric artery (SMA) has an appallingly high mortality rate (85 to 100%). It is higher with thrombotic occlusion (97%) than with embolic occlusion (66%) or with nonocclusive ischemia (66%).[187,188]

3.6.4.1. Incidence

Acute occlusion of the SMA is relatively common among the elderly, but the true incidence is unknown.

3.6.4.2. Etiology

Occlusion of either the SMA or inferior mesenteric artery (IMA) may result from arterosclerosis, thrombosis, vasculitis, embolism, surgical ligation, and adhesions. Proximal acute occlusion of the SMA is 5 times more common than distal occlusion.[189] With main trunk occlusion, collateral linkages are usually inadequate to prevent ischemic infarction of the entire midgut loop. With distal occlusion, however, chances for survival are better because the collateral network usually guarantees the ischemic area will recover or, at worst, the infarction will be limited. With healing, these areas frequently develop strictures that may ultimately lead to bowel obstruction.

3.6.4.3. Nonocclusive Disease

Nonocclusive disease (NOD) of the SMA and the IMA has been associated with diabetes, rheumatoid arthritis, collagen vascular disease, disseminated intravascular coagulation, hypovolemia, cardiac failure, and digoxin. In this entity, there is no evidence of thrombosis or embolus at autopsy or surgery, but marked luminal narrowing of vessels occurs due to prominent intimal fibromuscular proliferation, medial hypertrophy, transmural elastosis, and focal periarteric fibrosis.[190] NOD may be precipitated by a sudden fall in cardiac output due to arrhythmias, myocardial infarction, decompensated heart failure, infection, and surgery.

3.6.4.4. Clinical Findings

These are not very helpful.[189-191] A past history of embolization or heart valve replacement or the presence of heart failure or auricular fibrillation is a potential clue. Abdominal pain is often sudden in onset and confined to the central abdominal or upper epigastrium. However, it tends to occur late in the critical period. Then, it is usually excruciating and may even exceed the pain associated with myocardial infarction. Nausea and vomiting followed by watery diarrhea result from forceful gastrointestinal emptying. Vague abdominal symptoms in elderly atherosclerotic patients and in the absence of significant abdominal signs constitute a triad considered classical for SMA. Peritoneal aspiration will yield blood-stained peritoneal fluid in over 50% of these patients.[191]

Laboratory findings are nonspecific. As intestinal ischemia increases, metabolic acidosis occurs, yielding arterial blood gas changes, electrolyte alterations, and increases in the serum amylase and alkaline phosphatase levels. Early abdominal X rays are of little help. Colonoscopy is helpful.[192] Lateral aortography provides precise information about the beginning of the SMA. If the stem is patent, the distal portions and collaterals are easily scanned. In general, emboli are located distally beyond the origin of the middle colic artery, although thrombi are found within the first few centimeters of the SMA. Viability of the involved intestine can be assessed accurately through use of the Doppler ultrasonic flowmeter. It provides useful presurgical knowledge of the involved circulation.[193,194]

3.6.4.5. Prognosis

Occlusion of the SMA has a grim prognosis. Following infarction, intestinal ileus, abdominal distention, and bloody diarrhea ensue. Serosal leakage of bacteria leads to peritonitis and eventually to vascular collapse. Unfortunately, in 40 to 80% of patients, the diagnosis is not made until vascular collapse occurs.

NOD is also found in the elderly. The average age of affected patients is 71 years.[199] Unlike acute SMA occlusion, NOD may involve any part of the gastrointestinal tract. In one series of patients with NOD, 48 had only small bowel involvement, 35 had involvement of the small intestine and colon, and 7 had involvement of the stomach and small intestine.[194]

3.6.4.6. Treatment

Surgical restoration of arterial circulation within the "critical period," i.e., the first 6-hr period after occlusion, may be curative and obviate the need for extensive bowel resection. Beyond this time, however, management becomes more difficult and mortality rises briskly. Unfortunately, 7 out of 10 patients have a delay in diagnosis beyond 12 hr and over 50% have another 12-hr delay between the time of diagnosis and laparotomy.[189,195] In part, this is due to the reticence of older patients concerning hospitalization, to dementia, or to the procrastination of the family or family physician. Surgery at the takeoff of SMA is technically complex and several approaches have been used with varying success. Embolectomy is accomplished more easily in distal areas. In 3 of 4 patients, the embolus is found at the junction of the SMA and the middle colic artery.[196] The arterial procedure of choice depends on individual findings and the surgeon's preference. The surgical management of SMA occlusion has been reviewed in detail by Ottinger and Austen.[192] Even if surgery is successful, it is often followed by massive fluid and plasma loss into the bowel lumen, a decrease in cardiac output and the appearance of vasoactive polypeptides. Metabolic acidosis and hyperkalemia ensue as the result of "acute intestinal failure." Vasopressors are contraindicated for the resulting hypotension because they cause splanchnic and portal venous vasoconstriction, further reducing the mesenteric blood supply.

3.6.5. Ischemic Colitis

Ischemic colitis is much more common than ischemic enteritis. In the elderly patient, it is also more common than inflammatory bowel disease, which is a disease of the young and middle-aged.

3.6.5.1. Etiology

Ischemic colitis results from occlusive disease involving the IMA and is usually related to arteriosclerosis. Nonocclusive colitis may be related to diabetes mellitus, collagen vascular disease, disseminated intravascular coagulation, hypovolemia, cardiac failure, arrhythmias, and digoxin. Ischemic colitis may also develop following aortoiliac surgery (2%) or after abdominal perineal resection.[199] Marston classified ischemic colitis into three types, depending upon the end result of ischemic episodes, namely, acute transitory colitis, acute nongangrenous, and gangrenous colitis.[194] The nongangrenous variety is 10 times more common than the gangrenous type.

3.6.5.2. Acute Transitory Colitis

The victims of ischemic colitis are usually the aged who have a history of heart failure and arteriosclerosis. Often their attacks follow decompensated congestive heart failure, myocardial infarction, or arrhythmia, notably auricular fibrillation. Saegesser believes that episodes of ischemic colitis which do not culminate in necrosis of the colonic wall are caused more frequently by hemodynamic disorders than by vascular occlusion.[196] Here, the crisis is often mitigated by the development of collateral circulation. This leaves the involved area vulnerable to subsequent changes in cardiac output and to subsequent stricture formation and in turn obstruction.

3.6.5.3. Acute Nongangrenous Colitis

Patients with acute ischemic nongangrenous colitis (NGC) usually have a history of left-sided lower abdominal pain that is easily confused with diverticulitis. Usually, they have no prior history of bowel diesase. Abdominal pain tends to follow passage of loose stools containing bright or dark red blood. Fever, tachycardia, left-sided abdominal tenderness, and guarding are evident. Bowel sounds are usually present and occasionally a mass is palpable. Rectal exam usually reveals dark red blood.

Differential diagnosis includes infective dysentery, diverticulitis, immunopathic proctocolitis, Crohn's disease, ulcerative colitis, volvulus, and carcinoma of the bowel.

3.6.5.4. Gangrenous Colitis

These patients tend to have a short history and to expire within the first 24 to 48 hr of illness. Abdominal pain is severe and generalized. Diarrhea is common, but rectal bleeding is seldom present. Most patients are in a state of collapse at the time of diagnosis due to generalized peritonitis and/or hypovolemia. The diagnosis is rarely made preoperatively unless the rectum and sigmoid areas are involved.

Gangrenous colitis arises from a combination of occlusive vascular damage and a fall in cardiac output. The mucosa of the large intestine is more sensitive to hypoxia and contains far more bacteria than the small intestine. The abundant bacterial flora rapidly invade any ulcerated or edematous mucosal lesion leading to localized infection and penetration of the ischemic area. In the elderly, fever, pain in the left side of the colon, bloody diarrhea, and tenesmus are more likely to be caused by ischemic colitis than by ulcerative colitis or regional enteritis. Less than 3% of patients with ischemic colitis have involvement of the rectal area per se.

3.6.5.5. Diagnosis

Leukocytosis is usually pressent. The serum alkaline phosphate, amylase, and transaminase levels become elevated in the course of an evolving metabolic acidosis.

Plain X-ray films of the abdomen often show a narrowed splenic flexure, thumb-printing, and occasionally streaks of gas in the bowel wall. The barium enema is diagnostic. It is not contraindicated in patients with acute ischemic colitis, but it must be done carefully. The most likely sites of ischemia are the splenic flexure (35 to 40%), the descending colon (30 to 35%), and the sigmoid area (10 to 20%). Involved segments are narrow and show thumb-printing. Angiography may disclose areas of vascular stenosis and occlusion. Colonoscopy reveals three stages of involvement: (1) an acute stage earmarked by petechiae, mucosal pallor, or hyperemia; (2) a subacute state characterized by ulceration and exudation; and (3) a chronic stage recognizable by stricture, haustral markings, and mucosal granularity.[203] A nonspecific prostitis is found in 5 to 10% of patients during rigid proctoscopy. Since ischemic colitis is limited to the submucosa, biopsy at the time of colonoscopy or proctoscopy is usually diagnostic.

3.6.5.6. Treatment

When gangrenous colitis is suspected, the hypovolemia must be corrected immediately and laparotomy undertaken as soon as possible in order to evaluate the extent of the disease and to ascertain the possibilities for appropriate surgical correction.

3.6.6. Constipation

Constipation has no clear-cut definition. To some, constipation means infrequent bowel movements, difficulty in passing stools, painful stools, or increasing stool hardness. To others, it is no more than the sense of abdominal discomfort. Among the aged, constipation is the most common disorder of the GI tract. One in five complain of constipation and 40 to 50% take laxatives routinely.

The problem is often compounded when the elderly become bedfast.[197] Active older people have intestinal transit times of 1 or 3 days, but bedfast, confused elderly patients may have transit times in excess of 1 or 2 weeks.[198]

3.6.6.1. Etiology

The four most common causes of primary constipation are: (1) delayed transit time, (2) incomplete bowel emptying, (3) diminished bowel awareness, and (4) neglect of call to stool. Changes in intestinal transit are usually due to alterations in colonic motility.

There are two types of colonic motility, nonpropulsive and mass propulsion. Nonpropulsive motility (rhythmic segmentation) is responsible for mixing the colonic contents. It predominates in the colon. It moves fecal material from one haustral segment to another, thereby increasing water and electrolyte absorption and preventing rapid movement of feces through the bowel. Nonpropulsive motility is enhanced by narcotics and is inhibited by epinephrine and prostaglandins.

Mass propulsive motility refers to mass movement of fecal material. This type motility may be peristaltic or antiperistaltic and it is believed to be under humoral rather than neuronal control. Experimentally, it persists in the denervated colon. The best example of mass propulsion is the "gastrocolic reflex." This reflex is associated with mass movement of feces from the cecal area to the sigmoid colon, a distance of approximately 75 cm. It occurs once or twice a day in most individuals, usually at meal time. Mass propulsive motility is decreased considerably in bedfast elderly patients. Often, they must be aided from bed to the toilet. If their call to defecation is not forthcoming, they soon lose the desire. Many develop what Brocklehurst and Kahn term, "the terminal reservoir syndrome."[199] Here, there is filling of the cecum and a gradual buildup of fecal material throughout the colon.

3.6.6.2. Secondary Constipation

Secondary constipation is due to drugs or diseases such as bowel cancer, hyperthyroidism, hypothyroism, hypercalcemia, diverticulosis, anorectal lesions, dementia, and depression. Drugs with a constipating effect include analgesics, calcium and aluminum salts, anticholernergic, and anti-parkinsonian drugs.[200]

3.6.6.3. Diagnosis

A thorough history and physical examination along with appropriate laboratory radiographic and proctoscopic examinations are essential to rule out organic bowel disease.

3.6.6.4. Treatment

Effective treatment may require alternation of bowel habits, dietary management, and breaking of the laxative habit. Mobile, healthy patients should be assured that constipation is not life-threatening and the physiology of defecation explained to them. They should be urged to defecate at the slightest urge or attempt to defecate for 5 min at the same time every day, and be encouraged to avoid laxatives. Many ingest little water, therefore, an adequate fluid intake must be ensured. Prescribe a glass or two of water on rising and one with every meal and at bedtime. Bran-containing cereals or the addition of Miller's bran (15 g) to cereal provides a high fiber diet. Hydrophilic substances such as Metamucil® or psyllium-seed preparations also increase stool bulk. If fluids aren't taken in adequate amounts, however, these preparations are ineffective. Osmotic laxatives, such as magnesium sulfate, are occasionally helpful.

For the immobile patient, stool softeners, such a dioctyl sodium sulfosuccinate (Colace®), are often effective in preventing constipation. These emollient laxatives are wetting agents that break up feces by allowing water to penetrate. Irritant purgatives such a bisacodyl (Dulcolax®) or standardized senna (Senokot®) stimulate the myenteric plexus of the colon, increase bowel motility, and inhibit mucosal transfer of fluids. Prolonged use of anthracine purgatives must be avoided for they may cause degeneration of the myenteric plexus. If stool softeners fail, these agents may be temporarily helpful.[200] Bulk producers, like bran, should not be used in the severely constipated, immobilized patient. They may compound the problem by increasing the bulk in an already distended colon. Recently, Smith and his associates found that saline infused into the stomach through a nasogastric tube over a period of several hours promptly relieves severe constipation. Furosemide is given to patients prone to congestive heart failure.[201]

3.6.6.5. Major Complications

The complications of this disease can be serious and include sudden death or cerebral vascular accidents due to straining at stool by cardiovascular patients and to fecal impaction, with its complications.

3.6.6.6. Fecal Impaction

Undiagnosed fecal impaction may lead to confusion, disorientation, and agitation in the elderly as well as tachycardia, abdominal distension, temperature elevations to 101° F, ureteral obstruction, intestinal obstruction, hepatic encephalopathy, and stercomatous perforation.[202-204] Over 90% of fecal impactions occur in the rectum or sigmoid colon. Stercomas amount for 20% of colonic perforations and may even lead to urinary tract infections. Experimentally induced impaction in animals leads to bacteruria.[205]

3.6.6.7. Treatment

This is related to the extent of the impaction, its duration, and the presence of megacolon or organic disease. Stool softeners such as dioctyl sodium sulfosuccinate, 50 mg every 8 hr, are usually sufficient for mild impactions. For more severe impactions, hypertonic phosphate or olive oil enemas in combination with syrup of dioctyl sodium sulfosuccinate are often effective. If manual removal is required, it should follow the enema. If manual removal is extremely painful, anesthesia may be necessary. If a megacolon develops, surgery with stripping of the longitudenal muscle from the distal colon may be necessary to overcome sphincter resistance and to relieve the impaction.[206]

3.6.7. Diarrhea

Diarrhea is one of man's oldest known and most distressing illnesses. Fortunately, it is usually self-limiting. In the elderly, diarrhea can quickly lead to dehydration and severe electrolyte imbalance and to increased mortality. Diarrhea lasting more than 3 weeks is either the result of a serious disorder or a functional state known as "irritable colon."

Diarrhea has been defined as a change in the frequency, fluidity, or volume of stool.[207] Clinically, it may be "functional" or "organic." Functional diarrhea is characterized by an increase in bowel movements during the day and an absence of blood, pus, or visible fat in the stools. There are no constitutional symptoms, such as weight loss or fever.

Organic diarrhea is characterized by a loss of synchronization of bowel movements with the clock. Patients may have noctural diarrhea and/or be awakened from sleep by the urge or need to defecate. Blood, pus, and fat may be found in the stool. Systemic findings, such as anemia, finger clubbing, arthritis, or weight loss, are often present.

3.6.7.1. Etiology

In the elderly, diarrhea results from infection, fecal impaction, drugs, and diseases, such as cancer, inflammatory bowel disorders, and ischemic colitis.[208,209] Utilizing new bacteriological and viral techniques, Jewkes et al. were able to identify the cause of acute diarrhea in 58% of 106 adult patients.[210] The bacterial infections most often identified were *Salmonella, Campylobacter,* and *Shigella. Clostridium difficile,* toxigenic *E. coli,* and *Vibrio parahemolyticus* were relatively rare. Rotavirus and Norwalk type viruses were recovered in 8%. *Giardia lamblia* and *Candida albicans* infections were detected in 4%. Antibiotic diarrhea characterized by sudden onset, bloody stools, colicky abdominal pain, and a rapid resolution occurred in 10%. Laxatives were responsible in 5%. Although no cultural organisms were found in 40%, Jewkes et al. suspected an infection that eluded the investigators' capabilities for culture and identification.

Sixteen of their 106 patients were found to have organic disease such as ulcerative colitis, regional enteritis, fecal impaction, pancreatic steatorrhea, irritable bowel, postvagotomy diarrhea, Stevens–Johnson syndrome, and gram-negative septicemia.

3.6.7.2. Pathogenesis of Diarrhea

There are five major types of diarrhea: (1) osmotic, (2) secretory, (3) impaired ion absorption, (4) mucosal permeability defects, and (5) motility defects.[211,212]

Osmotic diarrhea results from the ingestion of poorly soluble substances (e.g., laxatives) or maldigestion (e.g., lactase deficiency). Nonabsorbable water soluble molecules create an osmotic lumenal drag that causes a net movement of water from the plasma into the lumen.

Secretory diarrhea results from (1) increased tissue pressure, e.g., hypervolemia, (2) decreased intestinal absorption association with a high rate of normal intestinal secretion, and (3) active ion secretion by mucosal cells. Cholera is the classic example of secretory diarrhea. The cholera enterotoxin stimulates production of the enzyme adenylcyclase that converts an ATP to cyclic 3'-5'-adenosine monophosphate (AMP) that stimulates marked secretion.[213]

A mucosal permeability defect is best exemplified by celiac disease. Here, extensive mucosal surface loss leads to malabsorption. In diabetic diarrhea and in the afferent loop syndrome, decreased motility promotes stasis and leads to bacterial overgrowth. The irritable colon syndrome is the best example of altered intestinal motility.

3.6.7.3. Diagnosis

A good history and physical are essential. The history may provide clues such as antibiotic or laxative use or previous bowel surgery, or it may suggest organic bowel disease. The physical examination may indicate hyperthyroid or hyperthyroidism, diabetic diarrhea, or inflammatory bowel disease.

Often, the stool examination is the key to diagnosis. The presence of blood or pus rules out the diagnosis of "psychogenic" diarrhea immediately. Stools should be examined for pH, color, odor, leukocytes, and blood. The foul odor of fat-containing stools is well-known.

A low pH (< 5.0) suggests a fermentation diarrhea due to bacterial overgrowth or lactase or sucrase deficiency. Oil droplets are easily identified microscopically with Sudan III stains. Leukocytes, bacteria, and fungi can be seen with a Wright's stain stool preparation. The presence of polymorphic nuclear cells in the stool points to bacterial infection or inflammatory bowel disease. Stool cultures should be obtained when leukocytes are seen. Duodenal aspiration may be necessary for the diagnosis of G. lamblia. Proctoscopy is done if the diarrhea fails to subside within 4 days or immediately if there is bloody diarrhea. Preparatory enemas should be avoided. They obscure fine mucosal detail, decrease the chance of isolating parasites, and increase mucous secretion. Rectal swabs for culture are helpful in preparing slides for microscopic examination and for streaking culture plates for bacterial isolation. If a viral isolation laboratory is available, viral cultures should be taken in the absence of leukosytes. Rectal biopsy is indicated when stool leukocytes are seen. It may reveal ulcerative colitis, amebiasis, granulomatous colitis, or carcinoma. If inflammatory bowel disease or cancer is suspected, a barium enema and upper gastrointestinal series with a small bowel follow-up should be obtained. Other tests may be necessary, e.g., T3 and T4 levels, if thyroid disease is suspected, or a secretin test if pancreatic disease is considered.

3.6.7.4. Treatment

Treatment of acute diarrhea in the elderly is primarily dietary and supportive. They should stop eating solid foods or drinking milk for 24 hr and drink lots of fluids to improve hydration and replace lost electrolytes. Antibiotics may be necessary for the treatment of certian bacterial diarrheas, e.g., *Salmonella septicemia*. For shigellosis, ampicillin 100 mg/kg per day for 5 days is often effective, but resistance to this drug is increasing. The use of antibiotics in this disorder is debatable. Diphenoxylate hydrochloride (Lomotil®) is contraindicated in bacterial diarrhea because it prolongs the course of the disease. Bismuth subsalicylate (Pepto Bismol®) may be helpful in secretory diarrhea induced by *E. coli* since it impairs secretion.[214,215] Giardiasis responds readily to quinacrine hydrochloride (Atabrine®) 100 mg thrice daily for 5 days.

Lactase intolerance may be inherited. Over 90% of orientals and 20% of blacks have lactase deficiency. Cessation of lactose intake leads to cessation of this type diarrhea. Lactose intolerance may also be acquired temporarily following acute viral gastroenteritis or with giardiasis. Elimination of milk for 2 to 4 weeks is necessary for the former while treatment of giardiasis corrects the latter. Celiac sprue responds to a gluten-free diet; pancreatic steatorrhea often improves significantly with enzyme therapy, e.g., pancreatin (Viokase®), 2 g orally thrice daily. Sulfasulazine (Azulfidine®) and corticosteroids may be helpful for ulcerative colitis. Surgery may be necessary if carcinoma or regional enteritis is responsible for intractable diarrhea. Fecal evacuation is necessary when fecal incontinence due to a fecal impaction causes severe diarrhea.

3.6.8. Flatus

A common complaint of the elderly is "too much gas." The problem grows worse with age and is often a source of embarrassment. Contrary to popular belief, bloating and distension are not due to excess gas. Ordinarily, these patients have normal volume and composition of bowel gas.

3.6.8.1. Etiology

Usually the intestinal tract contains less than 200 ml of gas. Ninety percent of this consists of five gases: nitrogen, oxygen, hydrogen, carbon dioxide, and methane with nitrogen predominating. Little information is available on the odiferous gases.[216] Excessive intestinal gas is the result of air swallowing, intralumental production, or diffusion from blood into the lumen. Chronic repetitive belching is associated with air swallowing. Each belch is preceded by a swallow of air which then passes about half way down the esophagus and then is regurgitated.[217] Colonic bacteria produce hydrogen and methane. About one-third of mankind produces large amounts of methane, presumably due to differences in colonic bacteria. Hydrogen production increases when ingested carbohydrates are incompletely absorbed from the small intestine and pass through the colon. This is the basis for the hydrogen breath test for carbohydrate malabsorption.[218,219] Carbon dioxide also results from bacterial metabolism and the interaction of bicarbonate and hydrogen ions. The ingestion of large amounts of beans is known to raise carbon dioxide and hydrogen production. Under these circumstances, carbon dioxide production can increase from a normal of 1 ml/hr to 80 ml/hr.[218,219] The oligosaccharides in beans (flatulence factor) cannot be digested or absorbed from the small intestine. In the colon, the oligosaccharides are readily fermented, leading to the production of hydrogen and carbon dioxide.[220] The ingestion of wheat may also increase bacterial production of hydrogen.[221]

Intestinal gas diffuses back and forth between the lumen and the blood. The direction of infusion is related to partial pressure. The peculiar breath of certain animals and humans is due in part to gases produced in the colon and excreted by the lungs.[211]

3.6.8.2. Diagnosis

Organic disease must always be ruled out before flatulence can be considered as a functional disorder. Gas syndromes frequently induce pain sufficiently to mask angina pectoris, cholelithiasis, reflux esophagitis, and peptic ulcer disease.

3.6.8.3. Treatment

Patients should be made aware that belching is accompanied by air swallowing. Aerophagia is often due to anxiety and treatment of the latter may lead to remission.[216,218] Bloating is considered a motor disorder. Here, the volume of interstitial gas is not increased and treatment, in part, consists of restricting the quantity of carbohydrate ingested, such as lactose, legumes, and wheat, decreasing the intake of carbonated beverages, and avoidance of chewing gum. Charcoal and simethacone are sometimes helpful. Anticholergic drugs may decrease aerophagia by reducing saliva production.

3.6.9. Irritable Bowel Syndrome

Irritable bowel syndrome (IBS) is extremely common. It accounts for 40 to 70% of gastroenterologic consultation.[224]

3.6.9.1. Etiology

Although the IBS has been regarded as a psychosomatic or bowel motility disorder, its etiology is not clear. Depression is greater among patients with IBS than matched controls.[225] Psychiatric illness has been observed in 72% of office patients with IBS in contrast to 18% of controls.[226] However, 30% of presumably normal individuals also have an irritable bowellike syndrome.[227]

Thirty years ago, Almy and Tulin reported that painless diarrhea was associated with decreased colonic motility and IBS with increased sigmoid motility.[228]

Subsequently, the hypomotility pattern was found in patients with ulcerative colitis and the hypermotility pattern in patients with diverticulitis and constipation.[229] Almy now believes the altered motility patterns observed in IBS "represent a qualitative or merely a quantitative departure from the psychophysiologic reactions in healthy persons (p. 402).[230] The cramping abdominal pain in IBS coincides with colonic hypermotility while "gas" pains are due to abnormal jejunal motility.[223,231]

3.6.9.2. Clinical Findings

The IBS is found 4 times more often in women as in men. Usually, women are constipated whereas men tend to have mucous diarrhea. Constipation, diarrhea, dyspeptic symptoms, abdominal pains, and varying degrees of anxiety or depression are the most common findings. Constipation may alternate with diarrhea. Since the diarrhea is functional, it occurs during the day. Abdominal pain is poorly localized and may last from minutes to hours. Sometimes it is relieved by passage of flatus, bowel movements, or enema. The splenic flexure syndrome is believed to be a variant of the IBS.

3.6.9.3. Diagnosis

This is a diagnosis of exclusion. Sigmoidoscopy, colonoscopy, barium enema, fecal examination for ova and parasites, bacterial cultures, and lactose tolerance tests are recommended to rule out organic disease.

3.6.9.4. Treatment

This is empiric. If constipation is the primary complaint, regular dietary habits, adequate sleep, and exercise must be encouraged. A high-fiber diet and/or Metamucil® may be useful. An adequate fluid intake is essential. Laxatives are to be avoided. For diarrhea, it may be necessary to try diphenoxylate hydrochloride or codeine along with a high-fiber diet. Anxiety and depression should be treated appropriately.[232]

3.7. Lower Gastrointestinal Bleeding

3.7.1. Etiology

After age 60, vascular ectasias, diverticulosis, malignancy, and polyps, in that order, are the primary causes of major lower gastrointestinal bleeding (LGIB).[177,233] Diverticulosis, polyps, cancer, and hemorrhoids, in that order, are the primary causes of minor LGIB. Introduction of selected angiography led to recognition of angiodysplasia (vascular ectasia) as an important and common cause of LGIB.[233] In one recent study, 43 of 72 patients with LGIB had angio-dysplagia compared to 29 with diverticular bleeding.[234]

3.7.1.1. Vascular Ectasias (Angiodysplasias)

These are small ($<$ 5 mm) degenerative arteriovenous malformations that occur with aging. They are not to be confused with congenital telangiectasia[235] for they are acquired and usually restricted to the cecum and proximal descending bowel. They are not found in the upper GI tract. Vascular ectasias are usually multiple and are rarely diagnosed without angiography.

LGIB due to ectasias is recurrent and usually mild, but 15% may have massive hemorrhage. The nature and variation in the type of bleeding is due to characteristics of the ectasias. They are the result of repeated, partial, intermittent, low-grade obstruction of submucosal veins by colonic muscular contractions.[233] Eventually, the dilated submucosal veins lead to retrograde congestion of the hexagonal capillary rings surrounding the mucosal crypts. When the competency of the precapillary sphincters is lost, the result is a small arteriovenous communication. Eventually a maze of distorted dilated vascular channels may almost replace the mucosa. Bleeding varies with the stage of evolution. Since bleeding is from veins or capillaries, it is less severe than the arterial bleeding encountered in diverticulosis.[177,233] Boley et al. have reviewed the etiology, evolution, and progress of vascular ectasias in detail. About 40% of older patients who have never experienced LGIB also have vascular ectasias.[236]

3.7.1.2. Diverticulosis

Diverticular bleeding is usually experienced after age 50. This is the second most common cause of LGIB. Over one-half of patients have their bleeding lesions in the right colon. Bleeding from diverticulosis is more severe than from vascular ectasia and does not recur as often. In most instances (75%), the bleeding stops spontaneously.

3.7.1.3. Cancer

Cancer of the colon is the most common cause of malignancy in old age and the third cause of major LGIB. Its prevalence rate is 3% after age 70.[233] Synchronous cancer of the colon is present in about 3.5% of patients with newly discovered colonic cancer.[237–239]

3.7.1.4. Diagnosis

Colonoscopy is extremely valuable for localizing sites of LGIB. The flexible sigmoidoscopy with a 5.0-mm section suction port permits aspiration of 500 ml of fluid per minute, hence active bleeding can be evaluated. Vascular ectasias are easily seen when they are actively bleeding. Otherwise, they are seldom seen at colonoscopy. If endoscopy is unsuccessful in localizing a bleeding site, a technetium-99m scan may be successful and allow localization.[239] If both colonoscopy and scintigraphic studies are negative and bleeding continues, emergency angiography is the next step. If the rate of bleeding is greater than 1.5 mg/min, site localization is possible in 60% of patients with LGIB.[233] Unfortunately, angiography is not as accurate for vascular extasias as it is for other causes of LGIB.

3.7.1.5. Treatment

This is directed at locating the site of bleeding and stopping it. Vasopressin effusions through an angiographic catheter or intravenously are effective in stopping hemorrhage in 70 to 80%.[233] If vasopressin therapy is unsuccessful, transcatheter embolization may prove efficacious. Occasionally, this procedure leads to colonic infarction or stricture formation. If surgery becomes necessary, standard procedures are available for removal of malignancies, polyps, and other lesions. Segmental resection for a bleeding diverticulosis is highly successful. Angiographically, identified ectasias too can be removed successfully in 80% of patients.[177,233]

3.8. Cancer

The incidence of cancer rises with age. Cancer of the gastrointestinal tract accounts for one-third of the annual mortality due to cancer. In 1976, 169,000 of the 675,000 newly reported cancers and 102,000 of the 370,000 cancer deaths were due to malignancies of the GI tract.[240] Cancers of the colon and rectum are the most common enteric cancers followed in order by cancer of the pancreas, stomach, hepatobiliary system, and esophagus. With the exception of the esophagus and anus, most GI tract cancers are adenocarcinomas. Their spread is usually by progressive local invasion with subsequent embolization of either the lymphatics or blood vessels.

3.8.1. Cancer of the Esophagus

This is a cancer of the aged and it is more common in men than women. Almost one-half of patients are over 60 years and approximately 25% are over age 70 years.[241] Esophageal cancers are more common among the less affluent. A striking rise in the incidence has been observed among nonwhites in this country over the past several decades.[242] Morbidity is high. Among the 7500 new cases reported annually, there are 6600 fatalities.

3.8.1.1. Etiology

The etiology of this disease is unknown, but smoking, alcoholism, malnutrition, poor oral hygiene, esophageal diverticuli, Barrett's esophagus, and lye strictures are associated with an increased incidence. Patients with sideropenia tend to develop cancer of the middle esophagus.[243] Esophageal carcinoma is 7 times greater in patients with achalasia than in the general population. The rich capillary beds of the mucosa and submucosa and lack of a serosal layer allows easy dissemination of the mediastinum.

3.8.1.2. Clinical Findings

The clinical findings are vague in general, the most common being dysphagia. Initially, this is usually painless; later it is associated with difficulty in swallowing solid foods.

3.8.1.3. Diagnosis

Barium radiography reveals 90% of esophageal carcinomas. Esophagoscopy is necessary to establish a tissue diagnosis and to evaluate the extent of the disease. If the gastroesophageal junction is involved, bronchoscopy is indicated to determine if the tracheal bronchial tree is involved.

3.8.1.4. Treatment

Surgery is the principle form of therapy. Esophagogastrectomy with or without interposition of a segment of colon is the usual procedure. Unfortunately, surgery is difficult and prognosis is poor. The 5-year survival rate is less than 20%.

Radiation therapy is also disappointing. The survival rate for this form of treatment is generally less than 5%.[244]

Chemotherapy offers little therapeutic hope. In most instances, the therapeutic responses are brief and last less than 2 to 3 months.

Palliation and improved swallowing is often possible with placement of an esophageal prosthesis made from polyvinyl tubing. The prosthesis can be placed perorally within a stenosing esophageal carcinoma and may remain patent until death.[245] It reduces the incidence of aspiration pneumonia.

3.8.2. Cancer of the Stomach

This form of cancer is decreasing in the United States. It is rare before the age of 40, the highest incidence occurring in the sixth or seventh decades. Although gastric cancer may develop in any part of the stomach, it is more likely to occur in the pyloric and antral regions.[246]

3.8.2.1. Etiology

The etiology of this disease is unknown. The incidence is increased in individuals with relatives who have gastric cancer, with blood type A, achlorhydria, atrophic gastritis with pernicious anemia, and in older males.

3.8.2.2. Clinical Findings

The primary manifestations are often vague and may include epigastric pain and uneasiness following meals, anorexia, early satiety, weight loss, weakness, and blood loss. By the time the diagnosis is made, most patients have some pain. Often it is comparable to that of peptic ulcer disease and may be relieved by fluid or antacids.

3.8.2.3. Diagnosis

The mainstays of diagnosis are radiography, endoscopy, and cytology. Contrast roentgenography is extremely useful because it allows assessment of gastric mobility, distension, and wall flexibility. The diagnostic accuracy of endoscopy with biopsy is high, ranging from 85 to 99%.[247]

Ming classified gastric carcinoma into two types[247a]: (1) the expanding type wherein the carcinoma cells grow en masse and (2) the infiltrative type wherein the cancer cells invade the stomach wall individually or in small clusters. Patients with the expanding type are usually older and have less lymph node involvement than those with the infiltrative type.[248]

3.8.2.4. Treatment

Surgery is the preferred approach. The type of oeration is related to tumor location, and the surgeon's expertise. Results are related to the state of tumor. Five-year survival rate at the New York Memorial Hospital study was 57% when the neoplasm was confined to the stomach. It was only 5% when regional nodes were involved.[249] The 5-year survival rate following surgery is also better in patients with expanding type tumors (45%) than in those with infiltrating tumors (27%).[248] Gastric surgery can lead to successful results in the elderly and long-term survival is possible. Some patients live to be 80 or 90 years of age without evidence of recurrence.[250]

Radiation therapy alone is not effective therapeutically. In conjunction with chemotherapy, objective responses may be obtained.

Combination chemotherapy is superior to single drug therapy for gastric carcinoma. Among drugs known to be chemotherapeutically active, 5-fluorouracil yields a response rate of about 25%. Doxorubicin reportedly yields a 40% overall response and nitrosourea 1-3 bis(2 chloroethyl)-1-nitrosourea (BCNU), an 18%

response.[251] There is no combination of chemotherapeutic agents that leads to remarkable success.

3.8.3. Colorectal Cancer

The incidence of colorectal cancer rises significantly after age 45. Each decade thereafter, it increases by a factor of 2 until it peaks at age 75. Unfortunately, more than one-half of all patients who develop large bowel cancer die from it. In 1976, there were over 100,000 new cases of colorectal cancer reported in this country. Colon cancer was responsible for 38,900 deaths and 10,300 resulted from rectal cancer.[246]

3.8.3.1. Etiology

Although the etiology of this disease is unknown, certain environmental factors have been associated with the disease. A high-fiber diet is thought to reduce the incidence of colorectal cancer by inducing rapid transit and reducing mucosal contact time with potential carcinogens. The validity of this concept has not been substantiated, but a correlation has been observed between a high animal fat intake and large bowel carcinoma.[242] Colorectal cancer is also increased in patients with polyposis and ulcerative colitis.

3.8.3.2. Diagnosis

None of the screening tests devised for early detection of colorectal carcinoma have been shown to reduce mortality effectively by control studies. These tests include fecal occult blood tests, protosigmoidoscopy, double contrast barium enemas, and colonoscopy. The latter is the most effective means of diagnosing colorectal cancer. Further, it permits biopsy and even removal of some lesions. Carcinoma embryonic antigen is not specific. It may be elevated in inflammatory bowel disease, pancreatitis, and alcoholic liver disease. Sensitivity from the simple, easy, and cheap hemoccult test vary from 37 to 97%; but specificity ranges from 89 to 99%. False-positive reactions may occur with a red meat diet, vitamin C, and delay in developing slides.[252]

3.8.3.3. Treatment

Surgery, again, is the primary mode of therapy. The survival rate after appropriate elective surgery depends upon the extent of the cancer at the time of operation. Advanced age is not a major detriment to surgery. Five-year survival rate approaches 80% when only the mucosa is involved (Dukes Stage A); it is 60% with involvement of the muscularis mucosa (Dukes Stage B) and about 40% where there is extension through the serosa or involvement of the nodes (Dukes Stage

C).[253] The 10-year survival rate is better for patients with tumors originating in the right and transverse colon than for those whose tumors originate in the left colon.[254] Since surgery for biopsy-proven adenocarcinoma of the rectum carries a mortality rate of 2 to 10% that tends to be higher in the elderly, Gingold believes local treatment may be a more realistic therapeutic approach for the aged. He considers electrocoagulation therapy for this type of cancer superior to the results of radical surgery.[255]

Combination chemotherapy is more effective than single drug therapy. The best combination at present consists of 5-fluorouracil and methyl-CCNU (Semustine®). It is superior to regimens combining three or four chemotherapeutic agents. Even so, the response rate is low (12%) and its duration is limited to months.[256]

3.8.4. Cancer of the Pancreas

Twenty-two thousand new cases are reported annually in the United States and the incidence is increasing. Average age at onset is 56 years. Etiologically, the cause is unknown, but factors associated with the increased incidence of pancreatic carcinoma include pancreatitis, diabetes mellitus, alcoholism, and cigarette smoking.

3.8.4.1. Clinical Findings

In 75% of patients, the tumor involves the head of the pancreas. Thirty to 40% of these individuals will have an audible bruit. Classical findings include pain, particularly epigastric pain radiating through to the back and relieved by bending forward, weight loss, and progressive jaundice. Twenty to 40% of the patients have associated diabetes mellitus.

3.8.4.2. Diagnosis

There are no specific tests for carcinoma of the pancreas. Endoscopic retrograde cholangiopancreatography has improved diagnostic accuracy tremendously through direct visualization, biopsy, and aspiration for cytological material.[257] Diagnostic sensitivity is about 92% and specificity is 90%. Ultrasound is helpful if there is sufficient obstruction of the common duct to cause dilitation. It is more useful for following progressive changes than for early diagnosis. Computerized transaxial tomography is the most effective noninvasive test.[258] Percutaneous needle aspiration is difficult to perform and has been associated with clinical pancreatitis following biopsy. According to the National Cancer Institute study of 184 patients with cancer of the pancreas, computerized axial tomography, celiac angiography, the serum alkaline phosphatase levels, pancreatic scan, and ultrasonography in that order gave the greatest percentage of direct diagnosis.[259]

3.8.4.3. Treatment

A variety of surgical procedures are available including radical pancreaticod-uodenectomy (Whipple's procedure). Even in the best hands, however, mortality is high and the 5-year survival rate is low, ranging from 7 to 15%. Radiation and chemotherapy have not proven very successful.[242]

3.8.5. Hepatoma

Hepatic neoplasms arise either from the hepatic parenchymal cells or from biliary ductules.

3.8.5.1. Etiology

Primary hepatoma, a tumor of parenchymal cells, is extremely common in the Orient where the liver fluke, *Clonorchis sinensis,* is an etiologic factor. In the United States, about 4% of patients with cirrhosis develop hepatomas. The rela-tionship between alcoholism and hepatoma is not clear. Exposure to aflatoxin, a substance derived from peanuts infected with *Aspergillus flavus* and infections with hepatitis B virus have also been suggested as etiologic possibilities.[260] Hep-atitis B antigen is present in the liver cells of 74% of patients with cirrhosis and hepatoma.[261]

3.8.5.2. Clinical Findings

Onset is usually insidious and symptoms often attributed to cirrhosis. Cachexia, weakness, and weight loss are common. Malnutrition and hepatomeg-aly occur as the tumor expands. Sudden onset of hypotension or abdominal pain may occur secondary to massive hemorrhage into the tumor or the peritoneal cav-ity. Hypercalcemia, hyperglycemia, polycythemia, carcinoid syndrome, and por-phyria are some of the paraneoplastic syndromes associated with hepatoma.[262]

3.8.5.3. Diagnosis

Hepatoscans, angiography, needle biopsy, and peritoneoscopy are helpful diagnostic aids. The test for alpha I fetoprotein is positive in 30 to 50% of patients.

3.8.5.4. Treatment

In some instances, surgical resection of the involved lobe leads to relatively prolonged survival. In most instances, however, surgical resection is impossible because of advanced cirrhosis or diffuse tumor involvement.

Systemic chemotherapy is not highly successful. In those who respond to treatment, survival ranges from 7 to 9 months. Regional chemotherapy, using the Seldinger approach, or by placement into the tumor at laporotomy, also fails to yield significant survival.

3.8.6. Cancer of Gallbladder

Cancer of the gallbladder usually occurs in older women; the female-to-male ratio is 5:1. Usually, the tumor is an adenocarcinoma. Metastases occur via submucosal lymphatics or by direct extension to surrounding nodes and organs. Median survival time is 3 months.

3.8.6.1. Clinical Findings

Symptoms are similar to those found with cholecystitis or cholelithiasis and consist of right upper quadrant pain, nausea, vomiting, and weight loss. Common duct obstruction leads to jaundice. Calcification of the wall of the gallbladder may serve as an indicator of tumor.[242]

3.8.6.2. Treatment

Surgery offers the only chance for cure. The obvious link between cholelithiasis and gallbladder carcinoma has led some to suggest that elective cholecystectomy be advised to prevent further cancer. The large number of patients with gallstones in this country and the relative paucity of gallbladder carcinoma (6000 patients annually) has led others to question the need for prophylactic therapy.[242]

3.8.7. Summary

Cancer of the gastrointestinal tract is still undefeated. Surgery and radiation have not improved prognosis in the last 20 years. None of the single chemotherapeutic agents used to treat malignant tumors of the gastrointestinal tract gives an overall response greater than 30%. Moreover, none of the multidrug regimens has consistently produced response in more than 50% of the patients.[263]

References

1. Atkinson, M. A., 1976, Disorders of oesophageal motility, *Clin. Gastroenterol.* 5:49–102.
2. Palmer, E., 1976, Disorders of the cricopharyngeus muscle: A review, *Gastroenterol.* 71:510–519.
3. Paiget, F. and Fouillet, J., 1959, Le pharynx et l'oesphage senileu étude clinque, radiologique et radiocinématographique, *J. Med. Lyon* 40:951–967.

4. Orringer, M. B., 1980, Extended cervical esophagomyotomy for cricopharyngeal dysfunction, *J. Thorac. Cardiovasc. Surg.* 80:669–678.

5. Duranceau, C. A., Letendre, J., Clermont, R. J., L'Evesque, H. P., and Barbeau, A., 1978, Oropharyngeal dysphagia in patients with ovelopharyngeal muscular dystrophy, *Can. J. Surg.* 21:326–329.

6. Loizou, L. A., Small, M., and Dalton, G. A., 1980, Cricopharyngeal myotomy in motor neuron disease, *J. Neurol. Neurosurg. Psychiatry* 43:42–45.

7. Henderson, R. D. and Marryatt, G., 1977, Cricopharyngeal myotomy as a method of treating cricopharyngeal dysphagia secondary to gastroesophageal reflux, *J. Thorac. Cardiovasc. Surg.* 74:721–725.

8. Zuckerbraun, L. and Bahana, M. S., 1979, Cricopharyngeus myotomy as the only treatment for Zenker diverticulum, *Ann. Otol. Rhinol. Laryngol.* 88:798–803.

9. Rattan, S., 1981, Neural regulation of gastrointestinal motility, *Med. Clin. North Am.* 65:1129–1147.

10. Earlam, R., 1976, Pathophysiology and clinical presentation of achalasia, *Clin. Gastroenterol.* 5:73–88.

11. Selmonosky, C. A., Byrd, R., Blood, C., and Blanc, J. S., 1981, Useful triad for diagnosing the cause of chest pain, *South. Med. J.* 74:947–949.

12. Henderson, R. D., 1980, *The Esophagus: Reflux and Primary Motor Disorders,* Williams and Wilkins, Baltimore, pp. 165–166.

13. Ellis, F. H., Jr., 1976, Management of oesophageal achlasia, *Clin. Gastroenterol.* 5:89–102.

14. Lipshutz, W. H., 1979, Understanding and managing achlasia of the esophagus, *Prac. Gastroenterol.* 3:21–25.

15. Mellow, M., 1977, Symptomatic diffuse esophageal spasm. Manometric follow-up and response to cholinergic stimulation and cholinesterase inhibition, *Gastroenterology* 73:237–240.

16. Soergel, K. H., Zboralske, F. F., and Amberg, J. R., 1964, Presbyesophagus esophageal motility in nonagenarians, *J. Clin. Investig.* 43:1742–1749.

17. Hollis, J. B. and Castell, D. O., 1974, Esophaegeal function in elderly man, *Ann. Intern. Med.* 80:371–374.

18. Dimarino, A. J., Jr., 1979, Esophageal spasm: Diagnosis and management, *Prac. Gastroenterol.* 3:26–31.

19. Swamy, N., 1977, Esophageal spasm: Clinical and manometric response to nitro-glycerine and long acting nitrites, *Gastroenterology* 72:23–27.

20. Henderson, R. D. and Pearson, F. G., 1976, Reflux control following extended myotomy in primary disordered motor activity (diffuse spasm) of the esophagus, *Ann. Thorac. Surg.* 22:278–283.

21. Ellis, F. H., 1964, Surgical treatment of esophageal hypermotility disturbances, *JAMA* 188:862–866.

22. Spencer, E. S. and Andersen, H. K., 1970, Clinically evident non-terminal infections with herpes viruses and the wart virus in immunosuppressed renal allograft recipients *Br. Med. J.* 1:251–254.

23. Eras, P., Goldstein, M. J., and Sherlock, P., 1972, Candida infections of gastrointestinal tract, *Medicine,* 51:367–379.

24. Cohen, S., 1975, Recent advances in management of gastroesophageal reflux, *Postgrad. Med.* 57:97–101.

25. Behar, J., 1976, Reflux esophagitis: Pathogenesis, diagnosis and management, *Arch. Intern. Med.* 136:560–566.
26. Fisher, R. S., and Cohen, S., 1978, Gastroesophageal reflux, *Med. Clin. North Am.* 62:3–20.
27. Dodds, W. J., Hogan, W. J., Helm, J. F., and Dent, J., 1981, Pathogenesis of reflux esophagitis, *Gastroenterology*, 81:376–394.
28. Goyal, R. K., and Rattan, S., 1978, Neurohumoral, hormonal and drug receptors for the lower esophageal sphincter, *Gastroenterology* 74:598–619.
29. Castell, D. O., 1975, Lower esophageal sphincter: Physiological and clinical aspects, *Ann. Intern. Med.* 83:390–401.
30. Behor, J. and Sheahan, D. C., 1975, Histologic abnormalities in reflux esophagitis, *Arch. Pathol.* 98:387–391.
31. Dent, J., Dodds, W. J., and Friedman, R. H., 1980, Mechanism of gastroesophageal reflux in recumbent asymptomatic human subjects, *J. Clin. Invest.* 65:256–267.
32. Welch, R. W. and Drake, S. T., 1980, Normal lower esophageal spincter pressure: A comparison of rapid vs. slow pull through techniques, *Gastroenterology* 78:1446–1451.
33. Goldberg, H. I., Dodds, W. J., and Gee, S., 1969, Role of acid and pepsin in acute experimental esophagitis, *Gastroenterology* 56:223–230.
34. Henderson, R. D., Mugashe, R. L., Jeejeebhoy, K. N., Szczpanski, M. M., Cullen, J., Marryatt, G., and Boxzko, A., Synergism of acid and bile salts in the production of experimental esophagitis, *Can. J. Surg.* 16:12–17.
35. Kivilaakso, E., Fromm, D., and Silen, W., 1980, Effect of bile salts and related compounds on isolated esophageal mucosa, *Surgery* 87:280–285.
36. Fisher, R. S., Malmuel, L. S., Roberts, G. S., and Lobis, I. F., 1977, The lower esophageal spincter as a barrier to gastroesophageal reflux, *Gastroenterology* 72:19–22.
37. Bachir, G. S., Leigh-Collis, J., Wilson, P., and Pollak, E. W., 1981, Diagnosis of incipient reflux esophagitis: A new test, *South. Med. J.* 74:1072–1074.
38. Eastwood, G. L., 1977, Does early endoscopy benefit the patient with active upper gastrointestinal bleeding?, *Gastroenterology* 72(5, Pt. 1):737–739.
39. Graham, D. Y., 1980, Limited value of early endoscopy in the management of acute upper gastrointestinal bleeding, *Am. J. Surg.* 140(2):284–290.
40. Keller, R. T. and Logan, G. M., Jr., 1976, Comparison of emergent endoscopy and upper gastrointestinal series radiography in acute upper gastrointestinal hemorrhage, *Gut* 17(3):180–184.
41. Silverstein, F. E., Gilbert, D. A. Tedesco, F. J., Buenger, N. K., and Persing, J., 1981, The National ASGE survey on upper gastrointestinal bleeding. I: Study design and baseline data, *Gastrointest. Endosc.* 27(2):73–79.
42. Chang, F. C., Drake, J. E., and Farha, G. J., 1977, Massive upper gastrointestinal hemorrhage in the elderly, *Am. J. Surg.* 134(6):721–723.
43. Silverstein, F. E., Gilbert, D. A., Tedesco, F. J., Buenger, N. K., and Persing, J., 1981, The National ASGE survey on upper gastrointestinal bleeding. III: Endoscopy in upper gastrointestinal bleeding, *Gastrointest. Endosc.* 27(2):94–102.
44. Peterson, W. L., Barnett, C. C., Smith, H. J., Allen, M. H., and Corbett, D. B., 1981, Routine early endoscopy in upper-gastrointestinal tract bleeding. A randomized, controlled trial, *N. Engl. J. Med.* 304(16):925–929.

45. Inglesias, M. C., Dourdourekas, D., Adomavicius, J., Villa, F., Shobassy, N., and Steigmann, F., 1979, Prompt endoscopic diagnosis of upper gastrointestinal hemorrhage: Its value for specific diagnosis and management, *Ann. Surg.* 189(1):90–95.
46. Editorial, 1981, Why treat cirrhosis?, *Br. Med. J.* 283(6287):338.
47. Storey, D. W., Brown, S. G., Swain, C. P., Salmon, P. R., Kirkhan, J. S., and Northfield, T. C., 1981, Endoscopic prediction of recurrent bleeding in peptic ulcers, *N. Engl. J. Med.* 305(16):915–916.
48. Silverstein, F. E., Gilbert, D. A., Tedesco, F. J. Buenger, N. K., and Persing, J., 1981, The National ASGE survey on upper gastrointestinal bleeding. II: Clinical prognostic factors, *Gastrointest. Endosc.* 27(2):80–93.
49. Foster, D. N., Miloszewski, K. J. A., and Losowsky, M. S., 1978, Stigmata of recent hemorrhage in diagnosis and prognosis of upper gastrointestinal bleeding, *Br. Med. J.* 1:1173–1177.
50. Griffiths, W. J., Neumann, D. A., and Welsh, J. D., 1979, The visible vessel as an indicator of uncontrolled or recurrent gastrointestinal hemorrhage, *N. Engl. J. Med.* 300(25):1411–1413.
51. Hunt, P. S., Hansky, J., and Korman, M. G., 1979, Mortality in patients with haematemesis and melaena: A prospective study, *Br. Med. J.* 1(6173):1238–1240.
52. Lebrec, D., Nouel, O., Corbić, M., and Benhamou, J. P., 1980, Propranolol—A medical treatment for portal hypertension?, *Lancet* ii(8187):180–182.
53. Permutt, R. P., and Cello, J. P., 1982, Duodenal ulcer disease in the hospitalized elderly patient, *Dig. Dis. Sci.* 27(1):1–6.
54. Grossman, M. I., Guth, P. H., Isenberg, J. I., Passaro, E. P., Roth, B. E., Sturdevant, R. A. L., and Walsh, J. H., 1976, A new look at peptic ulcer, *Ann. Intern. Med.* 8(1):57–67.
55. Grossman, M. I., (ed.), 1981, *Peptic Ulcer: Guide for the Practicing Physician,* 1st ed., Yearbook Publishers, Inc., Chicago, pp. 10–11.
56. Elashoff, J. D., and Grossman, M. I., 1980, Trends in hospital admissions and death rates for peptic ulcer in the United States from 1970–1978, *Gastroenterology* 78(2):280–285.
57. Walsh, J. H., 1976, A new look at peptic ulcer, *Ann. Intern. Med.* 84(1):57–67.
58. Rotter, J. I., Sones, J. Q., Samloff, I. M., Gursky, J. M., Richardson, C. T., Walsh, J. H., and Rimoin, D. L., 1979, Duodenal-ulcer associated with elevated serum pepsinogen I: An inherited autosomal dominant disorder, *N. Engl. J. Med.* 300(2):63–66.
59. Cowan, W. K., 1973, Genetics of duodenal and gastric ulcer, *Clin. Gastroenterol.* 2:539–546.
60. Rotter, J. I. and Rimoin, D. L., 1977, Peptic ulcer disease—A heterogeneous group of disorders?, *Gastroenterology* 73(3):604–607.
61. Grossman, M. I. (ed.), 1981, *Peptic Ulcer: A Guide for the Practicing Physician,* 1st ed., Yearbook Medical Publishers, Chicago, pp. 21–23.
62. Steurp, K. and Mosbeck, J., 1973, Trends in mortality from peptic ulcer in Denmark, *Scand. J. Gastroenterol.* 8:49–53.
63. Pulvertaft, C. N., 1968, Comments on the incidence and natural history of gastric and duodenal ulcer, *Postgrad. Med. J.* 44:597–602.

64. Pulvertaft, C. N., 1972, Experiences with peptic ulcer in elderly men in New York, *Age Ageing* 1:24–29.
65. Romeke, O. and Loken, E., 1955, Prognosis of peptic ulcer in young patients, *Acta. Med. Scand.* 155:373–375.
66. Narayanan, M. and Steinheber, F. U., 1976, The changing face of peptic ulcers in the elderly, *Med. Clin. North Am.* 60(6):1159–1172.
67. Binder, H. J., Cocco, A., Crossley, R. J., Finkelstein, W., Font, R., Friedman, G., Groarke, J., Hughes, W., Johnson, A. F., McGuigan, J. E., Summers, R., Vlahcevic, R., Wilson, E. C., and Winship, D. H., 1978, Cimetidine in the treatment of duodenal ulcer: A multicenter double blind study, *Gastroenterology* 74:380–388.
68. Akdamar, K., Dyck, W., and Englert, A., 1981, Cimetidine versus placebo in the treatment of benign gastric ulcer: A multicenter double blind study, *Gastroenterology* 80(5, Pt. 2):1098.
69. McGuigan, J. E., 1981, A consideration of the adverse effects of cimetidine, *Gastroenterology* 80(1):181–192.
70. Ippoliti, A. F., Sturdevant, R. A. L., Elashoff, J., Cooney, C., and Isenberg, J. I., 1978, Duodenal ulcer relapse after cimetidine withdrawal, *Gastroenterology* 74:1047 (abstract).
71. Cullen, M. J., Stubrin, S. E., Hanan, M. R., Maher, J. A., and Rent, M., 1980, Cimetidine versus placebo: Complete gastric ulcer pain relief. Six week double blind control study with any antacid, *Acta Gastroenterol. Latindam.* 10:291–295.
72. Martin, F., Farley, A., Gagnon, M., and Bensewana, D., 1982, Comparison of the healing capacities of sucralfate and cimetidine in the short-term treatment of duodenal ulcer: A double blind randomized trial, *Gastroenterology* 82(3):401–405.
73. Sonnenberg, A., Muller-Lissner, S. A., Vogel, E., Schmid, P., Gonvers, J. J., Peter, P., Strohmeyer, G., and Blum, A. L., 1981, Predictors of duodenal ulcer healing and relapse, *Gastroenterology* 81(6):1061–1067.
74. Patwardhan, R. V., Johnson, R. F., Sinclair, A. P., Schenker, S., and Speeg, K. V., 1981, Lack of tolerance and rapid recovery of cimetidine-inhibited chlordiazepoxide (Librium) elimination, *Gastroenterology* 81(3):547–551.
75. Klotz, U., and Reimann, I., 1980, Delayed clearance of diazepam due to cimetidine, *N. Engl. J. Med.* 302(18):1012–1014.
76. Patwardhan, R. V., Yarborough, G. W., and Desmond, P. V., 1980, Cimetidine spares the glucuronidation of Lorazepam and Oxazepam, *Gastroenterology* 79(5 Pt. 1):912–916.
77. Roberts, R. K., Grice, J., Wood, L., Petroff, V., and McGuffie, C., 1981, Cimetidine impairs elimination of theophylline and antipyrine, *Gastroenterology* 81(1):19–21.
78. Silver, B. A., and Bell, W. R., 1979, Cimetidine potentiation of the hypoprothrombinemic effect of warfin, *Ann. Intern. Med.* 90(3):348–349.
79. Peterson, W. L., Sturdevant, R. A. L., and Frankl, H. D., 1977, Healing of duodenal ulcer with an antacid regimen, *N. Engl. J. Med.* 297(7):341–345.
80. Ippoliti, A. F. and Peterson, W., 1979, The pharmacology of peptic ulcer disease, *Clin. Gastroenterol.* 8(1):53–67.
81. Editorial, 1980, New drug for peptic ulcer disease, *Br. Med. J.* 11:95–96.

82. Brooks, J. R. and Eraklis, A. J., 1964, Factors affecting the mortality from peptic ulcer. The bleeding ulcer and ulcer in the aged, *N. Engl. J. Med.* 271:803–809.

83. Allan, R. and Dykes, P. A., 1976, A study of factors influencing mortality rates from gastrointestinal hemorrhage, *Q. J. Med.* 45(180):533–550.

84. Graham, D. Y., 1980, Limited value of early endoscopy in the management of acute upper gastrointestinal bleeding, *Am. J. Surg.* 140(2):284–290.

85. Peterson, W. L., Barnett, C. C., Smith, H. J., Allen, M. H., and Corbett, D. B., 1981, Routine early endoscopy in upper gastrointestinal bleeding: A randomized controlled trial, *N. Engl. J. Med.* 304(16):924–929.

86. Swain, C. P., Blown, S. G., Storey, D. W., Kirkham, J. S., Northfield, T. C., and Salmon, P. R., 1981, Controlled trial of argon laser photocoagulation in bleeding peptic ulcers, *Lancet* ii:1313–1316.

87. Luk, G. D., Bynum, T. E., and Hendrix, T. R., 1979, Gastric aspiration of localization of gastrointestinal hemorrhage, *JAMA* 241(6):576–578.

88. Bernuau, J., Nouel, O., Belghiti, J., and Rueff, B., 1981, Severe upper gastrointestinal bleeding. Part III: Guidelines for treatment, *Clin. Gastroenterol.* 10(1):38–59.

89. Kayasseh, L., Gyr, K., Keller, U., Stalder, G. A., and Wall, M., 1980, Somatostatin and cimetidine in peptic ulcer hemorrhage: A randomized controlled trial, *Lancet* i(8173):844–846.

90. Protell, R. L., Silverstein, F. E., Gilbert, D. A., and Feld, A. D., 1981, Severe upper gastrointestinal bleeding. Part I: Causes, pathogenesis and methods of diagnosis, *Clin. Gastroenterol.* 10(1):17–26.

91. Mattingly, S. S. and Griffen, W. O., Jr., 1980, Factors influencing morbidity and mortality in perforated duodenal ulcer, *Am. Surg.* 46(2):61–66.

92. Coleman, J. A. and Denham, M. J., 1980, Perforation of peptic ulceration in the elderly, *Age Ageing* 9(4):257–261.

93. Sirinek, K. R., Levine, B. A., Schwesinger, W. J., and Aust, J. B., 1981, Simple closure of perforated peptic ulcer: Still an effective treatment for patients with delay in treatment, *Arch. Surg.* 116:591–596.

94. Kirkpatrick, J. R. and Bouwman, D. L., 1980, A logical solution to the perforated ulcer controversy, *Surg. Gynecol. Obstet.* 150(5):683–686.

95. Lumsden, K., Maclarnon, J. C., and Dawson, J., 1970, Giant duodenal ulcer, *Gut* 11:592–599.

96. Eisenberg, R. L., Margulis, A. R., and Moss, A. A., 1978, Giant duodenal ulcers, *Gastrointest. Radiol.* 2(4):347–353.

97. Klamer, T. W. and Mahr, M. M., 1978, Giant duodenal ulcer: A dangerous variant of a common illness, *Am. J. Surg.* 135(6):760–762.

98. Dronfield, M. W., Atkinson, M., and Langman, M. J. S., 1979, Effect of different operation policies on mortality from bleeding peptic ulcer, *Lancet* i(8126):1126–1128.

99. Himal, H. S., Perrault, C., and Mzabi, R., 1978, Upper gastrointestinal hemorrhage: Aggressive management decreases mortality, *Surgery* 84(4):488–454.

100. Rossi, R. L., Braasch, J. W., Cady, B., and Sedgwick, C. E., 1981, Parietal cell vagotomy for intractable and obstructing duodenal ulcer, *Am. J. Surg.* 141(4):482–486.

100a. Palmer, E. D., 1970, *Upper Gastrointestinal Hemorrhage*, Springfield, Illinois, C. C. Thomas.

100b. Thomas, J. H., and Rees, W. E., 1954, Hematemesis and melena: A survey in a British provincial hospital (Jan. 1938–July 1951), *Gastroenterology* 26:260–267.

101. Pemberton, J. H. and Van Heerden, J. A., 1980, Vagotomy and pyloroplasty in the treatment of duodenal ulceration: Long-term results, *Mayo Clin. Proc.* 55(1):14–18.

102. Chatterfer, D., 1976, Idiopathic chronic gastritis, *Surg. Gynecol. Obstet.* 143:986–1000.

103. Siurala, M., 1974, Atrophic gastritis: A possible pre-cancerous condition, *Neoplasma* 21:253.

104. Palmer, E. D., 1981, Idiopathic gastritis, *Am. Fam. Phys.* 23(6):167–171.

105. Strickland, R. G., Fisher, J. M., Lewin, K., and Taylor, K. B., 1973, The response to prednisolone in atrophic gastritis: A possible effect on non-intrinsic factor-mediated Vitamin B 12 absorption, *Gut* 14:13–19.

106. Clearfield, H., 1981, Drug therapy of ascites, *Am. Fam. Phys.* 23(1):204–205.

107. Hoyumpa, A. M., Jr., Desmond, P. V., Avant, G. R., Roberts, R. K., and Schenker, S., 1979, Hepatic encephalopathy (clinical conference), *Gastroenterology* 76(1):184–195.

108. Webber, F. L., 1981, Therapy of portal systemic encephalopathy: The practical and promising, (editorial), *Gastroenterology* 81:174–177.

109. Tygstrup, N. and Ranek, L., 1981, Fulminant hepatic failure, *Clin. Gastroenterol.* 10(1):191–208.

110. Sumner, H. W., Holtzman, J. L., and McClain, C. J., 1981, Drug-induced liver disease, *Geriatrics* 36:83–95.

111. Wattis, J. P., 1981, Alcohol problems in the elderly, *J. Am. Geriatr. Soc.* 29:131–134.

112. MacDougall, B. R. D., Mitchell, K. J., Strunin, L., and Williams, R., 1980, Prospective controlled trial of injection sclerotherapy in patients with cirrhosis and recent variceal haemorrhage, *Lancet* ii:552–554.

113. Gonzales, C., Cochrane, A. M. G., Eddleston, A. L. W. F., and Williams, R., 1979, Mechanisms responsible for antibody-dependent, cell-mediated cytotoxicity to isolated hepatocytes in chronic active hepatitis, *Gut* 20(5):385–388.

114. Wands, J. R., Perrotto, J. L., and Albert, E., 1975, Cell-mediated immunity in acute and chronic hepatitis, *J. Clin. Invest.* 55(5):921–929.

115. Knodell, R. G., Conrad, M. E., Ishak, K. G., 1977, Development of chronic liver disease after acute non-A, non-B post-transfusion hepatitis, *Gastroenterology* 72(5 Pt. 1):902–909.

116. Koretz, R. L., Stone, O., and Gitnick, G. L., 1980, The long-term course of non-A, non-B post-transfusion hepatitis, *Gastroenterology* 79(5):893–898.

117. Dienstag, J. L. and Isselbacher, K. J., 1981, Therapy for acute and chronic hepatitis, *Arch. Intern. Med.* 141(11):1419–1423.

118. Knodell, R. G. and Farleigh, R. M., 1981, Chronic active hepatitis: A plea for conservative management, *Geriatrics* 36(4):111–115.

119. Lam, K. C., Lai, C. L., Trepo, C., and Wu, P. C., 1981, Deleterious effects of prednisolone in HBsAg-positive chronic active hepatitis, *N. Engl. J. Med.* 304(7):380–386.

120. Friedman, G. D., Kannel, W. B., and Dawber, T. R., 1966, The epidemiology of gallbladder disease: Observations in the Framingham Study, *J. Chronic Dis.* 19:273–292.
120a. Heaton, K. W., 1973, The epidemiology of gallstones and suggested aetiology, *Clin. Gastroenterol.* 2:67–83.
121. Glenn, F., 1981, Surgical management of acute cholecystitis in patients 65 years of age and older, *Ann. Surg.* 193:56–59.
122. Bouchier, I. A. D., 1969, Postmortem study of frequency of gallstones in patients with cirrhosis of the liver, *Gut* 10:705–710.
123. Heaton, K. W. and Read, A. G., 1969, Gallstones in patients with disorders of the terminal ileum and disturbed bile salt metabolism, *Br. Med. J.* 111:494–496.
124. Bouchier, I. A. D., 1973, The biochemistry of gallstone formation, *Clin. Gastroenterol.* 2:49–66.
125. Ahlberg, J., Angelin, B., and Einarsson, K., 1981, Hepatic 3-hydroxy-3-methyl-glutaryl coenzyme A reductase activity and biliary lipid composition in man: Relation to cholesterol gallstone disease and effects of cholic acid and chenodeoxycholic acid treatment, *J. Lipid Res.* 22:410–422.
126. Mok, H. Y. I., Von Bergmann, K., and Grundy, S. M., 1980, Kinetics of enteropathic circulation during fasting: Biliary lipid secretion and gallbladder storage, *Gastroenterology* 78:1023–1033.
127. Misra, P. S., and Bank, S., 1982, Gallbladder disease: Guide to diagnosis, *Hosp. Med.* 18:109–138.
128. Schoenfield, L. J., Lachin, J. M., Baum, R. A., Habig, R. L., Hanson, R. F., Hersh, T., Hightower, N. C., Jr., Hofmann, A. F., Lasser, E. C., Marks, J. W., Mekhjian, H., Okun, R., Schaefer, R. A., Shaw, L., Soloway, R. D., Thistle, J. L., Thomas, F. B., and Tyor, M. P., 1981, Chenodil (chenodeoxycholic acid) for dissolution of gallstones, The National Cooperative Gallstone Study: A controlled trial of efficacy and safety, *Ann. Intern. Med.* 95:257–282.
129. Bateson, M. C., 1982, Dissolving gallstones, *Br. Med. J.* 284:1–3.
130. Thistle, J. L., Carlson, G. L., and Hofmann, A. F., 1980, Monooctanoin, a dissolution agent for retained cholesterol bile stones: Physical properties and clinical application, *Gastroenterology* 78:1016–1022.
131. Mitzel, L., Wiederholt, J., and Wolbergs, E., 1981, Dissolution of retained duct stones by perfusion with monooctanoin via a teflon catheter introduced endoscopically, *Gastrointest. Endosc.* 27:63–65.
132. Shimada, K., Inamatsu, T., and Yamashiro, M., 1977, Anaerobic bacteria in biliary disease in elderly patients, *J. Infect. Dis.* 135:850–854.
133. Munster, A. M., Goodwin, M. N., and Pruitt, B. A., 1971, Acalculous cholecystitis in burned patients, *Am. J. Surg.* 122:591–593.
134. Morrow, D. J., Thomason, J., and Wilson, S. E., 1978, Acute cholecystitis in the elderly: A surgical emergency, *Arch. Surg.* 113:1149–1152.
135. Prian, G. W., Norton, L. W., and Eule, J., Jr., 1977, Clinical indications and accuracy of gray scale ultrasonography in the patient with suspected biliary tract disease, *Am. J. Surg.* 134:705–711.
136. Thornell, E., Jansson, R., and Svanik, J., 1982, Indomethacin intravenously: A new way for effective relief of biliary pain: A double blind study in man, *Surgery* 90:468–472.

137. Salleh, H. B. M. and Balasegaram, M., 1974, Treatment of acute cholecystitis by routine urgent operation, *Br. J. Surg.* 61:705–708.

138. MacDonald, J. A., 1974, Early cholecystectomy for acute cholecystitis, *Can. Med. Assoc. J.* 111:796–799.

139. Gagic, N., Frey, C. F., and Gaines, R., 1975, Acute cholecystitis, *Surg. Gynecol. Obstet.* 140:868–874.

140. Coppa, G. F., Lefleur, R., and Ranson, J. H., 1981, The role of chiba-needle cholangiography in the diagnosis of possible acute pancreatitis due to cholelithisis, *Ann. Surg.* 193:393–398.

141. Geokas, M. C., Von Lancker, J. L., and Kadell, B. M., 1972, Acute pancreatitis, *Ann. Intern. Med.* 76:105–117.

142. Sarles, H., 1970, Pancreatitis, in: *Symposium of Marseille* (H. Sarles ed.), Basel, Karger.

143. Renner, I. G., Rinderkneght, H., and Douglas, A. P., 1978, Profiles of pure pancreatic secretion in patients with acute pancreatitis: The possible role of proteolytic enzymes in pathogenesis, *Gastorenterology* 75:1090–1098.

144. Durbel, J. P. and Sarles, H., 1978, Multi-center survey on the etiology of pancreatic disease: Relationship between the relative risk of developing chronic pancreatitis and alcohol, protein and lipid consumption, *Digestion* 18:337–350.

145. Sarles, H. and Laugier, R., 1981, Alcoholic pancreatitis, *Clin Gastroenterol.* 10:401–415.

146. Acosta, J. M. and Ledesma, C. L., 1974, Gallstone migration as a cause of acute pancreatitis, *N. Engl. J. Med.* 290:484–487.

147. Acosta, J. M., Ross, R., and Galli, O. M. R., 1978, Early surgery for acute gallstone pancreatitis: Evaluation of a septemic approach, *Surgery* 83:367–370.

148. Fita, R. H., 1889, Acute pancreatitis, *Boston Med. Surg. J.* 120:181, 205, 229.

149. Durr, G. H. K., 1979, Acute pancreatitis, in: *The Exocrine Pancreas* (H. T. Howat and H. Sarles, eds.), W. B. Saunders & Co., Ltd., Philadelphia, pp. 352–401.

150. Multigner, L., Zigarella, C., Sahel, J., and Sarles, H., 1980, Lactoferrin and albumin in human pancreatic juice: A valuable test for diagnosis of pancreatic disease, *Dig. Dis. Sci.* 25:173–178.

151. Gauthier, A., Escoffer, J. M., Camatte, R., and Sarles, H., 1981, Severe acute pancreatitis, *Clin. Gastroenterol.* 10:209–224.

152. Ranson, J. H. C., Rifkind, K. M., Roses, D. F., Fink, S. D., Ene, K., and Spencer, F. C., 1974, Prognostic signs and the role of operative management in acute pancreatitis, *Surg. Gynecol. Obstet.* 139:69–81.

153. Ranson, J. H. C., 1981, Acute Pancreatitis—Where are we?, *Surg. Clin. North Am.* 61:55–70.

154. Warshaw, A. L., Imbembo, A. L., and Civetta, J. M., 1974, Surgical intervention in acute necrotizing pancreatitis, *Am. J. Surg.* 127:484–491.

155. Frey, C. F., 1981, Gallstone pancreatitis, *Surg. Clin. North Am.* 61:923–938.

156. Ranson, J. H. C., 1979, The timing of biliary surgery in acute pancreatitis, *Ann. Surg.* 189:654–663.

157. Frey, C. F., Lindinauer, S. M., and Miller, T. A., 1979, Pancreatic abscess, *Surg. Gynecol. Obstet.* 149:722–726.

158. Frey, C. F., 1978, Pancreatic pseudocysts: Operative strategy, *Ann. Surg.* 188:652–662.

159. Robertson, G. M., Jr., Moore, E. W., and Switz, D. M., 1976, Inadequate parathyroid response in acute pancreatitis, *N. Engl. J. Med.* 294:512–516.

160. Ranson, J. H. C., Rifkind, J. M., Turner, J. W., 1976, Prognostic signs and nonoperative peritoneal lavage in acute pancreatitis, *Surg. Gynecol. Obstet.* 143:209–219.

161. McWilliams, H. and Gross, R., 1974, Pancreatitis and the lungs, *Ann. Surg.* 40:448–452.

162. Rosenberg, I. K., Kahn, J. A., and Walt, A. J., 1969, Surgical experience with pancreatic pseudocysts, *Am. J. Surg.* 117:11–17.

163. Cameron, J. L., 1978, Chronic pancreatic ascites and pancreatic pleural effusions, *Gastroenterology* 74:134–140.

164. Sankaran, S., and Walt, A. J., 1976, Pancreatic ascites: Recognition and management, *Arch. Surg.* 111:430–434.

165. Mayo, W. J., 1930, Diverticula of the sigmoid, *Ann. Surg.* 92:739–743.

166. Connell, A. M., 1977, Pathogenesis of diverticular disease of the colon, *Adv. Intern. Med.* 22:377–395.

166a. Rankin, F. W. and Brown, P. W., Diverticulitis of the colon, *Surg. Gynecol. Obstet.* 50:836–847.

166b. Oschner, H. C. and Bargen, J. A., 1935, Diverticulosis of the large intestine: An evaluation of historical and personal observations, *Ann. Intern. Med.* 9:282–296.

166c. Willard, J. H. and Bockus, H., 1936, Clinical and therapeutic states of cases of colonic diverticulosis seen in office practice, *Am. J. Dig. Dis. Nutr.* 3:580–585.

166d. Allen, A. W., 1953. Surgery of diverticulosis of the colon, *Am. J. Surg.* 86:545–548.

166e. Smith, C. C., and Christensen, W. R., 1959, The incidence of caloric diverticulitis, *Am. J. Roentgenol.* 82:996–999.

167. Painter, N. S., 1968, Diverticular disease of the colon, *Br. Med. J.* 3(5616)475–479.

168. Painter, N. S. and Burkitt, D. P., 1975, Diverticular disease of the colon, *Clin. Gastroenterol.* 4:3–21.

169. Ornstein, M. H., Littlewood, E. R., and Baird, I. M., 1981, Are fiber supplements really necessary in diverticular disease of the colon? A controlled clinical trial, *Br. Med. J.* 282:1353–1356.

170. Barling, S., 1926, The peridiverticular state and diverticulosis, *Br. Med. J.* I:322–323.

171. Weinreich, J. and Andersen, D., 1976, Intraluminal pressure in the sigmoid colon. I: Methods and results in normal subjects, *Scand. J. Gastroenterol.* 11:557–580.

172. Eastwood, M. A., Smith, A. N., Brydon, W. G., and Pritchard, J., 1978, Colonic function in patients with diverticular disease, *Lancet* i:1181–1182.

173. Almy, T. P. and Howell, D. A., 1980, Diverticular disease of the colon, *N. Engl. J. Med.* 302:324–331.

174. Parks, T. G., 1975, Natural history of diverticular disease of the colon, *Clin. Gastroenterol.* 4:53–69.

175. Fleischner, F. G., 1966, The question of barium enema as a cause of perforation in diverticulitis, *Gastroenterology* 51:290-292.
176. Burakoff, R., 1981, An updated look at diverticular disease, *Geriatrics* 36:83-91.
177. Boley, S. J., DiBiase, A., Brandt, L. J., and Sammartano, R. J., 1979, Lower intestinal bleeding in the elderly, *Am. J. Surg.* 137:57-64.
178. Morson, B. C., 1976, Genesis or colorectal cancer, *Clin. Gastroenterol.* 5:505-525.
179. Grinnell, R. S. and Lane, N., 1958, Benign and malignant adenomatous polyps and papillary adenomas of the colon and rectum: An analysis of 1856 tumours in 1335 patients, *Surg. Gynecol. Obstet.* 106:519-538.
180. Schutte, A. G., 1973, Familial diffuse polyposis of the colon and rectum: Supplementary report on three pedigrees, *Dis. Colon Rectum* 16:517-523.
181. Smith, W. G. and Kern, B. B., 1973, The nature of the mutation space in familial multiple polyposis: Papillary carcinoma of the thyroid, brain tumors, and familial multiple polyposis, *Dis. Colon Rectum* 16:264-271.
182. Wolff, W. I. and Shinya, H., 1973, Polypectomy via the fiberoptic colonoscope: Removal of neoplasms beyond reach of the sigmoidoscope, *N. Engl. J. Med.* 288:329-332.
183. Muto, T., Bussey, H. J. R., and Morson, B. C., 1975, The evolution of cancer of the colon and rectum, *Cancer* 36:2251-2270.
184. Oohara, T., Ogino, A., and Tohma, H., 1981, Histogenesis of microscopic adenoma and hyperplastic (metaplastic) gland in non polyposis coli, *Dis. Colon Rectum* 24:375-384.
185. Whitehead, R., 1975, Rectal polyps and their relationship to cancer, *Clin. Gastroenterol.* 4:545-561.
186. Fenoglio, C. M., Kaye, G. I., and Lane, N., 1973, Distribution of human colonic lymphatics in normal, hyperplastic and adenomatous tissue. Its relationship to metastasis from small carcinomas or pedunculated adenomas, with two case reports, *Gastroenterology* 64:51-66.
187. Vellar, I. D. and Doyle, J. C., 1977, Acute mesenteric ischemia, *Aust. NZ J. Surg.* 47:54-61.
188. Ottinger, L. W., 1978, The surgical management of acute occlusion of the superior mesenteric artery, *Ann. Surg.* 188:721-731.
189. Mavor, G. E., 1972, Acute occlusion of the superior mesenteric artery, *Clin. Gastroenterol.* 1:639-654.
190. McGregor, D. H., Pierce, G. E., Thomas, J. H., and Tiezer, K. L., 1980, Obstructive lesions of distal mesenteric arteries. A light and electron microscopic study, *Arch. Pathol. Lab Med.* 104:79-83.
191. Scowcroft, C. W., Sahowski, R. A., and Kozarek, R. A., 1981, Colonoscopy in ischemic colitis, *Gastrointest. Endosc.* 27:156-161.
192. Ottinger, L. W. and Austen, W. G., 1967, A study of 135 patients with mesenteric infarction, *Surg. Gynecol. Obstet.* 124:251-261.
193. O'Donnel, J. A. and Hobson, R. W., 1980, Operative confirmation of Doppler ultrasound in evaluation of intestinal ischemia, *Surgery* 87:109-112.
194. Marston, A., 1977, *Intestinal Ischemia,* Arnold, London.
195. Renton, C. J. C., 1972, Non-occlusive intestinal infarction, *Clin. Gastroenterol.* 1:655-674.

196. Saegesser, F., 1980, The acute abdomen: Part I; Differential diagnosis, *Clin. Gastroenterol.* 10:123–176.
197. Connell, A. M., Hilton C., and Irving, G., 1965, Variations of bowel habit in two population samples, *Br. Med. J.* 5470:1095–1099.
198. Milne J. S. and Williamson, J., 1972, Bowel habit in older people, *Gerontol. Clin. (Basel)*, 14:56–60.
199. Brocklehurst, J. C. and Kahn, Y., 1969, A study of fecal stasis in old age and the use of "dorbanex" in its prevention, *Gerontol. Clin. (Basel)* 11:293–300.
200. Brocklehurst, J. C., 1980, Disorders of the lower bowel and in old age, *Geriatrics* 35:47–54.
201. Smith, R. G., Currie, J. E. J., and Walls, A. D. F., 1978, Whole gut irrigation: A new treatment for constipation, *Br. Med. J.* 6134:(2)396–397.
202. Duecher, F. and Nothiger, F., 1980, Stercoraceous perforation of the colon, *Wien. Med. Wochenschr.* 130:40–41.
203. Nelson, R. P. and Brugh, R., 1980, Bilateral ureteral obstruction secondary to massive fecal impaction, *Urology* 16:403–406.
204. Lerman, B. B., Levin, M. L., and Patterson, R., 1979, Hepatic encephalopathy precipitated by fecal impaction, *Arch. Intern. Med.* 139:707–708.
205. Breda, G., Bianchi, G. P., and Bonomi, U., 1975, Fecal stasis and bacteruria: Experimental research in rats, *Urol. Res.* 2:155–157.
206. Cefalu, C. A., McKnight, G. T., and Pike, J. I., 1981, Treating impaction: A practical approach to an unpleasant problem, *Geriatrics* 36:143–146.
207. Sheehy, T. W., 1976, Diarrhea, *J. Med. Assoc. St. Ala.* 46(3):26–31.
208. Pentland, B. and Pennington, C. R., 1980, Acute diarrhea in the elderly, *Age Ageing*, 9:90–92.
209. Smith, I. M., 1977, Infections in the elderly, *Cont. Ed. Fam. Phys.* 7:18–29.
210. Jewkes, J., Larson, H. E., Price, A. D., Sanderson, P. J., and Davis, H. A., 1981, Aetiology of acute diarrhea in adults, *Gut* 22:388–392.
211. Phillips, S. F., 1972, Diarrhea: A current view of the pathophysiology, *Gastroenterology* 63:495–518.
212. Phillips, S. F., 1975, Diarrhea—Pathogenesis and diagnostic techniques, *Postgrad Med* 57:65–71.
213. Gorbach, S. L., 1972, The toxigenic diarrheas. *Hosp. Prac.* 8:103–110.
214. Donta, S. T., 1975, Changing concepts of infectious diarrhea, *Geriatrics* 30:123–126.
215. Maasdam, C. F. and Anuras, S., 1981, Are you overlooking GI infections in your elderly patients?, *Geriatrics* 36:127–134.
216. Levitt, M. D., 1980, Intestinal gas production: Recent advances in flatology, *N. Engl. Med.* 302:1474–1475.
217. Roth, J. L. A., 1976, Gastrointestinal gas, in: *Gastroenterology*, 3rd ed., Vol. 4 (H. L. Bockus, ed.), W. B. Saunders Company, Philadelphia, pp. 652–655.
218. Bond, J. H. and Levitt, M. D., 1977, A rational approach to intestinal gas problems, *Viewpoints on Digestive Disease* 9:2 (Moon).
219. Newcomer, A. D., McGill, D. F., and Thomas, P. J., 1975, Prospective comparison of indirect methods for detecting lactase deficiency, *N. Engl. J. Med.* 293:1232–1236.

220. Steggerda, F. R., 1968, Gastrointestinal gas following food consumption, *Ann. N.Y. Acad. Sci.* 150:57–66.
221. Anderson, I. H., Levine, A. S., and Levitt, M. D., 1980, Use of breath H_2 excretion to study absorption of wheat flour, *Gastroenterology* 78:1131 (abstract).
222. Chen, S., Mahadevan, V., and Zieve, L., 1970, Volatile fatty acids in the breath of patients with cirrhosis of the liver, *J. Lab. Clin. Med.* 75:622–627.
223. Lasser, R. B., Bond, J. H., and Levitt, M. D., 1975, The role of intestinal gas in functional abdominal pain, *N. Engl. J. Med.* 293:524–526.
224. Drossman, D. A., Powell, D. W., and Sessions, J. T., Jr., 1977, The irritable bowel syndrome, *Gastroenterology* 73:811–822.
225. Hislop, I. G., 1971, Psychological significance of the irritable colon syndrome, *Gut* 12:452–457.
226. Young, S. J., Alpers, D. H., Northland, C. C., and Woodruf, R. A., Jr., 1976, Psychiatric illness and the irritable bowel syndrome: Practical implications for the primary physician, *Gastroenterology* 70:162–166.
227. Thompson, W. S. and Heaton, K. W., 1980, Functional bowel disorders in apparently healthy people, *Gastroenterology* 79:283–288.
228. Almy, T. P. and Tulin, M., 1947, Alterations in man under stress: Experimental production of changes simulating the "irritable colon," *Gastroenterology* 8:616–626.
229. Haddad, H. and Devroede-bertrand, G., 1981, Large bowel motility disorders, *Med. Clin. North Am.* 65:1377–1396.
230. Almy, T. P., 1980, The irritable bowel syndrome: Back to square 1?, *Dig. Dis. Sci.* 25:401–403.
231. Horowitz, L. and Farrar, J. T., 1962, Intraluminal small intestinal pressure in normal patients and in patients with functional gastrointestinal disorders, *Gastroenterology* 42:455–464.
232. Whitehead, W. E., 1980, Irritable bowel syndrome: Physiological and psychological differences between diarrhea-predominant and constipation-predominant patients *Dig. Dis. Sci.* 25:404–413.
233. Boley, S. J., Brandt, L. J., and Frank, M. S., 1981, Severe lower intestinal bleeding: Diagnosis and treatment, *Clin. Gastroenterol.* 10:65–91.
234. Welch, C. E., Athanasoulis, C. A., and Galdabini, J. J., 1978, Hemorrhage from the large bowel with special reference to angiodysplasia and diverticular disease, *World J. Surg.* 2:73–83.
235. Athanasoulis, C. A., Galdabini, J. J., Waltman, A. C., Novelline, R. A., Greenfield, A. J., and Ezpeleta, M. I., 1977–1978, Angiodysplasia of the colon: A cause of rectal bleeding, *Cardiovasc. Radio.* 1:3–13.
236. Nausbaum, M. and Baum, S., 1963, Radiographic demonstration of unknown sites of gastrointestinal bleeding, *Surg. Forum* 14:374–375.
237. Steinheber, F. W., 1976, Interpretation of gastrointestinal symptoms in the elderly, *Med. Clin. North Am.* 60:1141–1157.
238. Boley, S. J., Sammartano, R. J., Adams, A., DiBiase, A., Kelinhaus, S., and Sprayregen, S., 1977, On the nature and etiology of vascular ectasias of the colon. Degenerative lesions of aging, *Gastroenterology* 72:650–660.
239. Alavi, A., Dann, R. W., Baum, S., and Biery, D. N., 1977, Scintigraphic detection of acute gastrointestinal bleeding, *Radiology* 124:753–756.

240. American Cancer Society, 1980, *Cancer Facts and Figures, 1980,* American Cancer Society, New York, p. 9.
241. Miller, C., 1962, Carcinoma of the thoracic oesophagus and cardia: A review of 405 cases, *Br. J. Surg.* 49:507–522.
242. Haskell, C. M., 1980, *Cancer Treatment,* W. B. Saunders Co., Philadelphia, pp. 233–246.
243. Brocklehurst, J. C., 1978, *Textbook of Geriatric Medicine and Gerontology,* 2nd ed., Churchill-Livingston Publishing Co., New York, pp. 349–350.
244. Lowe, W. C., 1972, Survival with carcinoma of the esophagus, *Ann. Inter. Med.* 77:915–918.
245. Boyce, H. W. and Palmer, E. D., 1975, *Techniques of Clinical Gastroenterology,* C. C. Thomas, Springfield Ill., pp. 230–231.
246. Horton, J. and Hill, G. J., 1977, *Clinical Oncology,* W. B. Saunders Co., Philadelphia, pp. 247–250, 286–287.
247. Kobayashi, S., Yoshii, Y., Kzsugai, T., 1977, Biopsy and cytology in the diagnosis of early gastric cancer: 10-year experience with direct vision techniques at a Japanese institution, *Endoscopy* 8:53–58.
247a. Ming, S. C., 1977, Gastric carcinoma: A pathological classification, *Cancer* 2475–2485.
248. Riberio, M. M., Sarmento, J. A., Simoes, M. A. S., and Bostos, J. 1981, Prognostic significance of Lauren and Ming classifications and other pathological parameters in gastric carcinoma, *Cancer* 47:780–784.
249. Goldsmith, H. S. and Gnosh, B. L., 1970, Carcinoma of the stomach, *Am. J. Surg.* 120:317–319.
250. Hoerr, S. O., 1981, Long term results in patients who survive five or more years after gastric resection for primary carcimoma, *Surg. Gynecol. Obstet.* 153:820–822.
251. Moertel, C., 1974, Cancer of the gastrointestinal tract: Chemotherapy, *JAMA* 228:1290–1291.
252. Diehl, A. K., 1981, Screening for colorectal cancer, *J. Fam. Pract.* 12:625–632.
253. Silverberg, E. and Holleb, A. L., 1975, Major trends in cancer: 25 years survey, *Cancer* 25:2–8.
254. Eisenberg, B., Decosse, J. J., Harford, F. and Michel, E. K. J., 1982, Carcinoma of the colon and rectum: The natural history reviewed in 1204 patients, *Cancer* 49:1131–1134.
235. Gingold, B. S., 1981, Local treatment (electrocoagulation) for carcinoma of the rectum in the elderly, *J. Am. Geriat. Soc.* 29:10–13.
256. Engstrom, P. F., MacIntyre, J. M., Douglass, J. O., Jr., Muggia, F., and Mittleman, A., 1982, Combination chemotherapy of advanced colorectal cancer utilizing 5-flurouracil, semustine, vincristine and hydroxyurea, *Cancer* 49:1555–1560.
257. Hall, T. J., Blackstone, M. O., Cooper, M. J., Hughes, R. G., and Moossa, A. R., 1978, Prosepective evaluation of endoscopic retrograde cholangiopancreatography in the diagnosis of periampullary cancers, *Ann. Surg.* 187:313–317.
258. Haaga, J. R., Alfidi, R. J., Havrilla, T. R., Tubbs, R., Gonzalez, L., Meaney, T. F., and Corsi, M. A., 1977, Definitive role of CT scanning of the pancreas: The second year's experience, *Radiology* 124:723–730.

259. Fitzgeralt, P. J., Fortner, J. G., Watson, R. C., Schwartz, M. K., Sherlock, P., Benua, R. S., Cubilla, A. L., Schottenfeld, D., Miller, D., Sinawer, S. J., Lightdale, C. J., Leidner, S. D., Nisselbaum, J. S., Menendez-Botet, C. J., and Poleski, M. H., 1978, The value of diagnostic aids in detecting pancreas cancer, *Cancer* 41:868–879.
260. McBride, C. M., 1976, Primary carcinoma of the liver, *Surgery* 80:322–327.
261. Tan, A. Y., Law, C. H., and Lee Y. S., 1977, Hepatitus B antigen in the liver cells in cirrhosis and hepatocellular carcinoma. *Pathology* 9:57–64.
262. Knowles, D. M., II, Casarella, W. J., Johnson, P. M., and Wolff, M., 1978, Clinical, radiologic and pathologic characterization of benign hepatic neoplasms, *Medicine* 57:223–237.
263. Bedikian, A. Y., Valdivieso, M., and Bodney, G. P., 1980, Systemic chemotherapy for advanced gastrointestinal cancer, *South. Med. J.* 73:1046–1052.

Rheumatology in Geriatrics

Marc L. Miller, Fred G. Kantrowitz, and Edward W. Campion

4.1. Age-Related Changes in the Immune System

Age-related alterations in the immune system have been described in the normal population. Decrease in immune response to foreign antigens resulting in an acquired immunodeficiency state and an increase in autoantibody production occur simultaneously with aging. Much conflicting experimental evidence exists concerning the precise abnormalities responsible for these changes in immune responsiveness, but several points are clear.[1,2] Decrease in thymic function appears to be central to age-related immune changes. Involution of the thymus gland occurs in normal individuals after sexual maturation. It appears likely that the loss of thymic tissue, in which T-lymphocyte maturation and differentiation occur, and the loss of thymic hormones that exert a systemic influence on the immune system both contribute to changes in immunoregulation in aging.

Normal immune responsiveness to foreign antigens involves recognition of the antigen, processing of the antigen, presentation to immunoreactive lymphocytes, and finally effector cell response in the form of either cell-mediated or humoral immune response. This complex process involves the interaction of macrophages; T-lymphocyte subpopulations including helper, suppressor, and effector

MARC L. MILLER and FRED G. KANTROWITZ • Beth Israel Hospital; and Harvard Medical School, Boston, Massachusetts 02115.   EDWARD W. CAMPION • Geriatrics Unit, Massachusetts General Hospital; and Division on Aging, Harvard Medical School, Boston, Massachusetts 02115.

T cells; humoral substances released from T cells (lymphokines) and antibody-producing B lymphocytes. With aging the absolute numbers of T and B lymphocytes appears to remain constant or to decrease only slightly. Cell-mediated immunity (CMI) appears to be generally diminished. Some workers have found decreases in delayed hypersensitivity responses to common antigens such as PPD or candida, although others have noted no such decrease in response to antigens to which the individual had been previously exposed. There is more general agreement that aged individuals have a decreased cell-mediated response to new antigens such as dinitrochlorobenzine. Total energy is unusual, even in very aged individuals, unless there is acute illness. It is, therefore, important to test for multiple antigens before concluding that an individual has impaired CMI.

There appears to be a general decrease in naturally occurring circulating antibodies with aging. The ability to mount antibody response to a familiar antigen appears to be preserved although antibody response to a new antigen is decreased. This is mainly due to abnormal T-cell regulation of B-cell antibody production. Macrophage function appears to remain intact in aging.

The consequences of impaired immunity in aging include an increased susceptibility to infection and an increased prevalence of autoimmune phenomena such as autoantibodies. Autoantibody production in the aged is frequently without overt manifestations of autoimmune diseases such as rheumatoid arthritis (RA) or systemic lupus erythematosus (SLE). This may reflect a loss of self-tolerance that emerges with aging and have different pathologic consequences than in the young. Some have hypothesized that certain disorders of the elderly without known cause, such as atherosclerosis or neoplasia, may have an age-related autoimmune basis.[1] That immunodeficiency and increased autoimmunity both occur with aging appears to be paradoxical. The alterations in immunoregulation responsible for these phenomena remain to be more completely determined.

4.2. Laboratory Evaluation in the Rheumatic Diseases

Several laboratory tests require special interpretation in the elderly patient.

4.2.1. Erythrocyte Sedimentation Rate

The erythrocyte sedimentation rate (ESR) is an indirect measurement of the presence of acute phase reactants in plasma which accompany various inflammatory and neoplastic processes. The test measures the settling of red blood cells suspended in anticoagulated blood in a vertically positioned tube of specific dimensions for 60 min. The most accurate and, therefore, preferred method, the Westergren technique, utilizes a standard 200-mm tube.[3] Rouleaux formation, or the aggregation of red blood cells, increases the rate of settling. Large, asymmetric plasma proteins facilitate rouleaux formation. Fibrinogen is the protein responsible for this and, being an acute phase reactant, accounts for the increased ESR accompanying acute and chronic inflammatory processes. Large amounts of immunoglobulin can also increase rouleaux formation. This explains the elevated ESR in multiple-myeloma and Waldenstrom's macroglobulinemia.[3]

The normal values for ESR by the Westergren technique are generally considered to be less than 15 mm/hr for men and less than 20 mm/hr for women. In normal individuals, there is a linear increase in ESR with increasing age. In individuals over the age of 60 or 70 years, an ESR of 40 to 50 mm/hr may not carry pathologic significance.[4,5]

Markedly elevated ESRs (greater than 100 mm/hr) most commonly are associated with malignancies, both hematologic and solid tumors, acute and chronic infections, and systemic rheumatic diseases such as RA, giant-cell arteritis (GCA), and SLE.[6] Serial measurements of the ESR are valuable in monitoring the course of and managing patients with these rheumatic diseases.

4.2.2. Rheumatoid Factor

Rheumatoid factor (RF) is an antibody, usually IgM and rarely IgG or IgA, that reacts with the Fc fragment of an IgG molecule. The incidence of RF positivity and specificity for RA vary with the technique used for detection of RF and the titer considered to represent a positive test. This will vary from laboratory to laboratory.

Both the incidence and mean titer of RF increase in the normal population with increasing age. In one study, RF measured by the latex fixation method was detected in 1 to 3% of individuals less than 65 years old and 16% of individuals between ages 65 and 103 years.[7] Others have found RF in 11.4 to 25% of individuals over the age of 70.[8,9] Generally, the positive tests found in normal elderly persons are in low titers, i.e. less than 1:160.

RFs are found in 70 to 80% of patients with RA. The higher titers are more specific for RA and correlate with poorer prognosis. Other pathologic states in which RF is found include systemic rheumatic diseases such as SLE and Sjogren's syndrome; chronic infections such as syphilis, subacute bacterial endocarditis, tuberculosis, and leprosy; chronic inflammatory diseases of unknown etiology such as sarcoidosis and interstitial pulmonary fibrosis; and hematologic malignancies such as multiple myeloma and macroglobulinemia.[10]

4.2.3. Antinuclear Antibody

Antinuclear antibodies (ANA) are immunoglobulins predominantly of the IgG class that react with various constituents of the nucleus, including DNA, RNA, and nucleoprotein.[11] The most commonly used screening method for ANA involves reacting the patient's serum with mouse liver nuclei and then adding fluorescein-tagged anti-IgG antibodies. Positive fluorescence identifies the presence of

ANA. The serum can be titered by serial dilutions and a qualitative assessment of the pattern of fluorescence can be determined.[12] In addition, precipitation with particular nuclear components can further identify the specific nature of the ANA.[13]

As with RF, ANA can be found in a small percentage of normal individuals, and this incidence increases with age. In one study, 16% of individuals aged 60 to 91 years had evidence of ANA.[14] Typically, ANAs in normal individuals are low in titers. A variety of drugs, particularly those assoicated with a lupuslike syndrome, can also induce the formation of ANA.[15]

The specific staining pattern and the precipitin present show some specificity for disease, although no one pattern is most commonly present in the normal elderly individual and in drug-induced situations. The rim or peripheral pattern is associated with SLE although the speckled pattern is suggestive of SLE, scleroderma, or Sjogren's syndrome.[16] Antibodies to double-stranded DNA, detected in an assay using DNA from the protozoa *Crithidia luciliae,* is the single most specific test for SLE.[17] Changes in its titer also correlate most clearly with SLE activity.[18]

The value of testing ANA as a screen for SLE is qualified by its predictive value in a given setting. In those situations where the clinical suspicion of SLE is either very low or very high, the incidence of falsely positive or falsely negative results respectively reduce the usefulness of the test. The test is most useful when there is a moderate clinical suspicion of the diagnosis of SLE.[19]

4.3. Rheumatoid Arthritis

RA is a systemic disease characterized by synovitis and a variety of extraarticular manifestations such as pulmonary and pleuropericardial disease, subcutaneous nodules, vasculitis, Sjogren's syndrome, and Felty's syndrome. Although a variety of immunologic markers and abnormalities have been found in association with RA, its etiology and pathogenesis remain unknown.[20]

4.3.1. Epidemiology

Probable, definite, or classical RA as defined by the American Rheumatism Association criteria[21] has been estimated to occur in approximately 1 to 3% of the population greater than 15 years old[8,22–24] with an annual incidence rate of 67 new cases/100,000 population. Although RA has often been considered an affliction of young and middle-aged adults,[24,25] a comprehensive study of the general population of Olmstead County, Minnesota, showed that both the peak incidence and prevalence rates of RA occurred in the population greater than 70 years. The annual incidence was 157.6 cases/100,000 population in the over-70 group compared to 40.8 and 74.2/100,000 in the 30 to 39 and 40 to 49 groups, respectively.[24]

Prevalence rates increased with age in the Tecumseh, Michigan,[8] and National Health Survey[22] studies as well. It is not surprising that the prevalence rate increased with age in a disease such as RA in which there are many long-term survivors. However, the high annual incidence of new cases in the elderly is of note. Overall, 39% of the RA patients in the Minnesota study had the onset of their disease after the age of 60.[24] Other studies have found from 5.7% to 30% of all RA patients with onset at this age.[26]

The sex ratio of RA patients varies with age of onset. The female predominance observed in those with younger onset decreased[27] or, in fact, disappeared[28] in those with onset after age 60. However, others have found no change in the extent of female predominance between the two age groups.[24]

4.3.2. Clinical Manifestations

In general, the clinical manifestations of RA in the elderly are not different from cases presenting at an earlier age.[27] The joint involvement is typically a symmetric polyarthritis involving the metacarpophalangeal and proximal phalangeal joints of the hands and fingers, carpus, elbows, shoulders, hips, knees, and ankles; the metatarsophalangeal joints of the feet; and the cervical spine. Distinct from osteoarthritis, the distal interphalangeal joints and lumbosacral spine are spared.

Two studies have found a higher incidence of shoulder involvement in older RA patients than in those under 60 years with an otherwise similar distribution of joint involvement.[27,28] The higher incidence of shoulder problems may relate to higher occurrence of periarticular processes such as rotator cuff tears, tendonitis, and acromioclavicular joint disease in the elderly rather than rheumatoid synovitis of the true shoulder joint.[27]

The majority of elderly-onset RA patients will follow a clinical course similar to younger RA patients. The natural history of RA is highly variable with improvement over time seen in 50% of cases, no change in 25%, and worsening in 25%.[29] Poor prognostic factors include female sex, RF positivity, extraarticular manifestations, persistently elevated ESR, anemia or hypoalbuminemia, prolonged duration of illness, and insidious onset.[30]

This last characteristic is of particular interest because several authors have commented on a subgroup of elderly RA patients with an abrupt onset with a benign outcome.[31,32] Approximately 20 to 30% of elderly RA patients will have an abrupt onset, i.e., patients present within a few days of the onset of symptoms.[27,32,33] In one series of 29 RA patients older than 60 years with abrupt onset, all were in remission by 18 months from the onset of their disease. All of these patients presented with severe constitutional illness in addition to arthritis with fever, night sweats, anorexia, malaise, markedly elevated ESR, anemia, and hypoalbuminemia. The diagnosis of polymyalgia rheumatica (PMR) was considered in six patients because of presentation with myalgias and involvement of the neck and shoulders before the more typical findings of RA appeared. The acute phase of the illness was managed with hospitalization, joint splinting, and antiin-flammatory drugs. Ten patients received systemic corticosteroids and two chry-sotherapy.[32] This course may also be seen with younger RA patients, but appears to be more common in the elderly. Two other series, however, could find no difference in outcome related to mode of onset.[33,34]

The differential diagnosis of rheumatoid arthritis in the elderly patient can be extensive. Osteoarthritis, PMR, primary amyloidosis, SLE, subacute bacterial endocarditis, hypothyroidism, and Parkinson's disease can all present as a polyar-thropathy that must be distinguished from RA on the basis of history, distribution of joint involvement, and specific diagnostic tests.

4.3.3. Management

The management of RA in the elderly, as in younger RA patients, centers around the basic principle of preserving and improving functional capacity while attempting to put the disease into remission. Essential is the multidisciplinary approach involving rheumatologist, general internist, orthopedic surgeon, physical and occupational therapist, podiatrist, visiting nurse, and social worker together with the patient and family.[35] The mainstays of therapy are antiinflammatory medications[36] and intraarticular corticosteroid injections to relieve symptoms and allow increased mobility; disease-remitting agents including gold salts, plaquenil, penicillamine, and azathioprine;[37] joint reconstruction and replacement as neces-sary; and a physical therapy program of joint splinting, exercises, and aids to the activities of daily living. The management program for each individual patient needs to be individualized allowing for the specific distribution and activity of the disease as well as the expectations for the patient's outcome. For example, the goals of therapy and therefore the specifics of the program will be different for an active, fully employed 65-year-old with new onset disease than for a bedridden 65-year-old with a 20-year history of RA, in whom pain relief, rather than pre-vention or correction of deformities, will be most important.

Because of the frequency of coexistent illnesses such as congestive heart fail-ure, osteoporosis, and renal insufficiency, the elderly RA patient may be particu-larly sensitive to the toxicities of the various therapeutic agents such as corticoste-roids and nonsteroidal antiinflammatory drugs (NSAIDs). Furthermore, the elderly RA patient is at increased risk for the complications of prolonged bedrest. Therefore measures should be taken to prevent or shorten such an occurrence and restore the patient to a more independent level of function. Low-dose corticoste-roids, 10 mg/day or less, despite their potential toxicity in this group, may be efficacious for those with an abrupt onset, in whom a more self-limited course might be predicted, and for those patients severely disabled by symptoms related to active inflammation, in whom remission-inducing agents are being started or in whom they have failed. Extreme caution must be taken that systemic corticoste-roids be given only to those patients with active inflammatory disease rather than with symptoms due to secondary osteoarthritis, and then only for the shortest duration possible.

4.4. Systemic Lupus Erythematosus

SLE is a multisystem disorder of unknown etiology with clinical manifestations that include constitutional signs and symptoms such as fever, weight loss, and fatigue,[38–41] cutaneous,[42] pulmonary,[43] pleuropericardial, musculoskeletal,[44] hematologic,[45] renal,[46] and neurologic[47] involvement. A working hypothesis of the pathogenesis of SLE holds that a complex interaction of genetic and environmental factors results in abnormal immune response that mediates tissue destruction.[48] Abnormalities in lymphocyte numbers and function,[48] reticuloendothelial system dysfunction,[49] circulating immune complexes[18] and autoantibodies,[11] and associations with certain alleles of the HLA system[50] have been documented.

SLE is a clinical diagnosis. Because of its protean manifestations with different expression in different patients, there is a wide range of presentations and courses. The diagnosis depends on the presence of a constellation of clinical and laboratory abnormalities. The ARA criteria serve as a rough guide. These were established to define comparable populations for clinical investigation.[51] Of course, other etiologies and explanations for the observed abnormalities must always be excluded. The role of ANA testing has been overemphasized in recent years in making the diagnosis. The ANA is not a specific test for SLE, and it must be interpreted in the clinical context of the individual patient.[19]

4.4.1. Epidemiology

While SLE is generally considered a disease of adolescence and young adulthood with peak incidence in the second and third decades, in 7 to 18% of the cases in reported series, the disease has had its onset after the age of 50 or 55.[52–56] Racial and sex differences have been found between groups of older- and younger-onset SLE patients. Several series have shown a higher incidence in whites than blacks in the older groups, which differs from the predominance of blacks in younger patients.[54,56,57] Another study, however, could find no racial difference between the two groups.[52] Although women predominate at all ages, men constitute a larger percentage of the elderly group than of the younger group.[53,56] This reflects the peak incidence in women at an early age, although the incidence in men appears to change little throughout all age groups.[58]

4.4.2. Clinical Manifestations

Differences in clinical presentation and manifestations between older- and younger-onset patients have been studied. Several series[52,54,59] suggest that, in some elderly patients, the onset of SLE may be insidious with longer intervals from onset of initial manifestations to diagnosis. Constitutional symptoms or musculo-skeletal complaints might be ignored more readily by the elderly patient or be misinterpreted by the physician, leading to delay or error in diagnosis. Early SLE in the elderly may be confused with RA, PMR, osteoarthritis (OA), or malignancy.

Older-onset patients may have a higher frequency of serositis and pneumo-nitis.[56,59] One recent study could find no significant difference in renal, central nervous system, cutaneous, or hematologic manifestations between the two groups.[56] In general, although there may be differences when comparing groups of patients, the clinical manifestations of SLE in any given elderly patient may be identical to those of a younger patient.

SLE with onset in the elderly may, in general, follow a more benign course. The absolute 5-year survival rate does not appear to differ from younger SLE patients, but when both groups are compared to age-matched controls, there is a relatively longer survival in the elderly.[56]

4.4.3. Management

In view of the morbidity of corticosteroid therapy in the elderly and the more benign nature of the disease, a more conservative approach to therapy in this age group has been suggested.[54] Treatment in SLE should be determined by the clin-ical course of the individual patient. In evaluating a SLE patient with a new symptom or sign, it is imperative to exclude other diagnoses such as intercurrent infection or drug-induced disorders. Many flares in disease activity may be self-limited and respond to rest and antiinflammatory therapy in the form of salicylates or NSAIDs.[40] Corticosteroids should be reserved for life-threatening or severe complications. Although corticosteroids are widely used and are felt to improve the outcome of nephritis and central nervous system involvement, this has not been fully proven by controlled trials. It appears that influenza and pneumococcal vac-cines can be safely and effectively administered to SLE patients.[60,61]

4.4.4. Drug-Induced Systemic Lupus Erythematosus

Drug-induced SLE occurs most frequently in the elderly population and reflects the pattern of drug use in the population.[62] Procainamide and hydralazine are the most commonly involved agents, but the list of reported drugs is exten-sive.[63,64] Use of isoniazid does not seem to result in age-related increase in the frequency of induction of ANA.[65] ANA induction has been reported in 50 to 70% of patients treated with procainamide for at least 12 months.[64] The clinical lupus syndrome may occur in 5 to 29% of patients developing ANA.[64,66] Because of the low incidence of clinically apparent disease, the drug may be continued in the absence of symptoms despite the appearance of ANA. Likewise, it is not necessary to monitor routinely all patients on procainamide or hydralazine for the development of ANA. A lupuslike syndrome has been reported to occur in 2 to 21% of patients treated with hydralazine.[64] The development of the syndrome may be related to the cumulative dose of hydralazine, with most cases occurring after a total dosage of 100 g[67] and rarely occurring in patients on less than 200 mg/day.[68]

Induction of ANA and development of the lupus syndrome with isoniazid, hydralizine, and procainamide are associated with the slow acetylator phenotype.[69–71] N-acetylprocainamide induces ANA formation at a slower rate than does procainamide and might be useful in the treatment of patients with significant arrhythmias who have developed the syndrome on procainamide.[72,73] These drugs should probably be used with caution in patients with idiopathic SLE. One study has demonstrated the use of hydralazine in idiopathic SLE patients on corticosteroids without exacerbation of SLE activity.[74]

4.4.4.1. Clinical Manifestations

The diagnosis of drug-induced SLE is based on the same criteria as idiopathic SLE. The presence of a positive ANA is the hallmark of the disorder. Joint complaints, fever, and pleuropulmonary involvement are most important in the drug-induced syndrome; renal, neurologic, and hematologic manifestations occur with decreased frequency.[64,75] Hypocomplementemia and antibodies against double-standard DNA have been reported, but generally do not occur in the drug-induced syndrome. The diagnosis of drug-induced SLE should always be considered in a patient on a medication known to be associated with the disorders who develops unexplained fever, arthritis, pneumonia, or pleuropericarditis. Other features of SLE should be sought and the serum tested for the presence of ANA.

4.4.4.2. Management

The signs and symptoms of the syndrome resolve within days to weeks after discontinuation of the offending drug although the ANA may remain positive for much longer. Generally, the syndrome can be managed by discontinuing the drug and instituting a NSAID.

Occasionally, a short course of corticosteroids may be necessary to control severe symptoms. In cases where the offending drug cannot be easily or safely discontinued, the use of antiinflammatory medications may control the syndrome despite continued exposure to the drug.

4.5. Sjogren's Syndrome

Dry eyes secondary to decreased lacrimal gland secretion is designated keratoconjuctivitis sicca (KCS). KCS together with xerostomia are designated as the sicca complex. When the sicca complex is the result of lacrimal and salivary gland dysfunction to lymphocytic infiltration of the glands, Sjogren's syndrome (SS) is said to be present.

4.5.1. Epidemiology

The sicca complex may also be seen as a manifestation of aging in which atrophy of the lacrimal and salivary glands is the mechanism rather than an immunologic mechanism as in SS. Tear production and salivary secretion fall progressively with aging.[76] KCS was found in 16.7% of men and women and xerostomia in 18.2% of women and 2.8% of men by clinical history in an elderly population.[77] In a recent study, 19 of 34 patients with documented KCS attending an ophthalmologic clinic had no evidence of SS. Their median age of onset was 44 years compared to a group with sicca complex and evidence of SS with a median age of 36 years.[78]

4.5.2. Diagnosis

Objective measures of diminished lacrimal and salivary secretion allow better documentation of the presence of the sicca complex than the patient's history alone. The Schirmer test (measurement of wetting a strip of filter paper placed on the inside of the lower eyelid for 5 min) is a rough screening test with many falsely positive tests, particularly in older patients. However, a result of less than 5 mm of wetting at any age is probably significant. Direct visualization of devitalized corneal epithelium with rose bengal or fluorescein dyes examined via the slit lamp provides more definitive information. Objective signs of xerostomia are a dry, poorly papillated tongue with absent or diminished saliva pool beneath the tongue. Various techniques including scialography, nuclear scans, and salivary flow studies are available to assess parotid gland function but are seldom used in clinical practice.[79] Biopsy of the minor salivary glands of the lip, the preferred objective measure of xerostomia, is easily performed and provides histopathologic confirmation of the diagnosis.[80,81] Diuretics, anticholinergic or antihistaminic drugs, and infiltrative disorders such as amyloidosis or sarcoidosis may also produce or exacerbate sicca symptoms and signs, but will be distinguished from SS by history and labial biopsy.[82]

Because of the multiple causes of the sicca complex, the diagnosis of SS depends on the presence of two of the following three criteria: (1) sicca complex, (2) associated rheumatic or lymphoproliferative disorder, and (3) labial biopsy showing lymphocytic infiltration.[82]

4.5.3. Clinical Associations

SS is often present in patients with RA or SLE and less commonly in patients with polymyositis and progressive systemic sclerosis. It is also associated with graft-versus-host disease and autoimmune diseases including Grave's disease, chronic active hepatitis, primary biliary cirrhosis, dermatitis herpetiformis, and celiac disease. SS is predominantly a disease of middle-aged and elderly females with a very wide range of onset including patients in the seventh and eighth decades. The age of onset in primary SS (no associated disease) is higher than in secondary SS, reflecting the younger age of onset of the associated rheumatic illness.[81,83]

4.5.4. Clinical Manifestations

The clinical manifestations of SS in the elderly resemble the general SS population. Symptoms of KCS include a burning sensation of the eyes, a sensation of grittiness or of a foreign body in the eye, photosensitivity, eye fatigue, dryness of the eyes and inability to make tears, or paradoxically, increased tear production early in the course of the disease in reaction to increased ocular irritation. Ocular signs include dilation of the conjunctival vessels, pericorneal injection, corneal exudate, ptosis, and dullness of the conjunctiva or cornea. Corneal ulcers, corneal perforation, or bacterial conjunctivitis may result from long-standing KCS.[83]

Diminished salivary flow results in dryness of the mouth and lips with development of fissures and ulcers of the lips and tongue. The patient may complain of difficulty eating dry foods such as crackers or will complain of requiring frequent ingestion of liquids in order to remain comfortable. Loss of taste and smell, acceleration of the development of caries, and dysphagia due to pharyngeal dryness and irritation may occur. Swelling of the salivary glands, particularly the parotids, occur in 30 to 50% of patients and is the result of lymphocytic infiltration.[82]

Generalized lymphocytic infiltration in SS may be manifest as dry skin due to dysfunction of sweat glands, nonthrombocytopenic hyperglobulinemic purpura, nasal dryness, chronic nonproductive cough, pleurisy and pleural effusions, pulmonary fibrosis, dysparenuria in women, hyposthenuria and renal tubular acidosis, pancreatitis, myositis, hepatitis, and vasculitis with skin ulcers and neuropathy.[76]

4.5.4.1. Natural History

The lymphocytic infiltration in SS may be viewed as a spectrum ranging from benign infiltration of various exocrine glands, to extraglandular organ infiltration with a benign appearance termed pseudolymphoma, to a frank malignant lymphoproliferative process.[84] Paralleling this progression is a transformation of the lymphocyte population from polyclonal to monoclonal B lymphocytes, and in some cases a precipitous drop in IgM rheumatoid factor or in a previously elevated immunoglobulin class is seen.[85] The risk of lymphoma in SS is clearly elevated with 43.8 times the expected incidence described in a series from the National Institutes of Health.[86]

4.5.4.2. Immunologic Correlates

A number of immunologic abnormalities have been observed in SS. RF is found in 75 to 90% of cases, with ANA in 50 to 80%.[82] Precipitating antibodies to SS-A (Ro) and SS-B (La, Ha) antigens have been associated with SS and may be preferentially associated with primary rather than secondary SS.[88,89] A defect in the clearance of IgG-coated red blood cells by the Fc receptor of reticuloendothelial cells has been identified in one series of SS patients and was associated with the presence of extraglandular manifestations.[89] Immunogenetic studies have demonstrated an association between HLA–DR3 and primary SS. As with the total RA population, patients with RA and SS have a higher frequency of HLA–DR4 when compared to normal controls.[88]

4.5.4.3. Management

The management of SS is directed at symptomatic relief of KCS and xerostomia. Frequent applications of methylcellulose artificial tears, sugarless sour candies or slippery elm lozenges, and artificial saliva preparations may ameliorate symptoms and prevent complications such as corneal ulcers. Corticosteroids and immunosuppressive therapy are reserved for patients with severe organ dysfunction.

4.6. Amyloidosis

Amyloidosis is a syndrome characterized by the deposition of β-pleated sheet protein fibrils and an associated pentagonal glycoprotein termed P-component in diffuse organ sites. The β-pleated sheet structure of amyloid deposits is unique in vertebrate tissues.[90] A variety of biochemically distinct proteins, disease associations, and clinical presentations exist.

4.6.1. Biochemistry of Amyloid

Primary generalized amyloidosis (without associated disease) and amyloidosis-complicating plasma cell dyscrasias share clinical and biochemical characteristics. In both, the amyloid fibrils have been shown to consist of intact immunoglobulin light chains or fragments of the variable region of immunoglobulin light chains and are designated AL protein.[90] An antigenically related serum immunoglobulin may be detected in these patients, suggesting an amyloid precursor protein is produced by a benign or malignant plasma cell proliferation that deposits in tissues as amyloid fibrils.[91] The amyloid fibrils of secondary amyloidosis (associated with chronic infections, inflammatory diseases, and neoplasms other than multiple myeloma) and the amyloidosis complicating Familial Mediterranean Fever contain AA protein that is biochemically distinct from AL protein. AA protein is antigenically related to a much larger serum protein, SAA. A portion of the SAA polypeptide is identical to the AA sequence. The cell of origin of SAA is unknown, but it appears to be produced in response to an immunologic stimulus such as chronic infections or inflammatory disorders, undergoes proteolytic cleavage, and is then deposited as AA fibrils in tissue.[90]

SAA occurs in low levels in normal individuals and increases abruptly in the population over 60 to 70 years.[92,93] Elevated SAA levels are also seen in chronic infections such as tuberculosis or osteomyelitis, chronic inflammatory diseases such as RA, and in neoplastic disease. In addition, SAA rises in acute infections, during pregnancy, and in postoperative patients and returns to the normal range with resolution of the acute process.[92] A close correlation between SAA level and ESR, C-reactive protein, and serum complement in acute and chronic inflammatory processes has been found.[92,93]

Amyloid fibrils consisting of protein immunologically identical to prealbumin are found in familial Portuguese neuropathy. Localized amyloid deposits have been found in endocrine tumors. In one of these, medullary carcinoma of the thyroid, the protein is a fragment of procalcitonin.[90] Localized amyloid deposits are also found in a variety of tissues in the elderly. The protein composition of these deposits is not fully determined, but is distinct from AL or AA and appears to differ from one tissue site to another.[94,95]

4.6.2. Clinical Amyloid Syndromes

4.6.2.1. Primary Generalized Amyloidosis

Primary generalized amyloidosis (PGA), multiple myeloma-associated amyloidosis, and localized senile amyloidosis are the syndromes of particular relevance to the elderly population. PGA is a disease of middle-aged and elderly individuals with a mean age at diagnosis of 55, 61, and 62 in three large series.[96,98] Men predominate. Amyloidosis complicates 6 to 15% of the cases of patients with multiple myeloma and up to 20 to 24% in cases of light-chain oyeloma.[90]

Major presenting symptoms are fatigue, weight loss, edema, dyspnea, paresthesias, and syncope.[97] The clinical manifestations of amyloid depend on the location of the amyloid deposits, and are protean. The major clinical syndromes include[90,97,99]: (1) peripheral and autonomic neuropathy; (2) restrictive cardiomyopathy with congestive heart failure, low EKG voltage, and conduction defects; (3) cutaneous involvement with pinch purpura, skin induration, and postproctoscopic periorbital purpura; (4) macroglossia; (5) hepatosplenomegaly; (6) nephrotic syndrome; (7) carpal tunnel syndrome; (8) acquired Factor-X deficiency with bleeding tendencies; and (9) a polyarthropathy that may resemble RA.

Amyloid arthropathy may present as a symmetic polyarthropathy involving large and small joints. Typically, there are few signs of inflammation despite joint swelling. A unique feature is massive amyloid deposition in the glenohumeral joint producing the characteristic "shoulder pad" sign. Synovial fluid tends to be viscous and may be xanthochromic. Both electrophoretic M components and amyloid fibrils have been detected in the synovial fluid and fluid sediment. Synovial fluid leukocyte counts range from a few hundred to 10,000/mm³ with a predominance of mononuclear cells. Synovial biopsy reveals amyloid deposits. Radiographs may show osteopenia and lytic lesions due to either amyloid infiltration or myeloma, but the typical marginal erosions of RA are absent. Most cases of amyloid arthropathy have been seen in association with a malignant plasma cell dyscrasia, and, in most cases, a serum or urine paraprotein and Bence Jones proteinuria can be detected.[100]

4.6.2.2. Amyloidosis of Aging

Localized amyloid depositions, sometimes called "senile amyloid," have been detected at autopsy in the cerebrum, heart, pancreas, and great vessels of elderly patients, and the incidence increases with increasing age.[90,99,101] Usually these deposits are of no clinical significance. It has been proposed that amyloid deposition in neuritic plaques and cerebral vessels may be related to the development of Alzheimer's disease.[102,103] Extensive cardiac deposition may occasionally occur and result in congestive heart failure and conduction defects.[104]

4.6.3. Diagnosis

Amyloid fibrils, regardless of fibril protein type, characteristically show green birefringence under polarizing microscopy when stained with Congo red. The diagnosis of amyloidosis can be established by demonstrating typical fibrils from any tissue site in a clinical situation consistent with amyloidosis in which no alternative diagnosis exists. Site of biopsy may be directed by location of clinical involvement. Rectal biopsy, positive in about 80% of patients with generalized amyloidosis,[97] is the preferred approach when a more directed biopsy is not possible. Aspiration of the abdominal wall subcutaneous fat pad may prove to be a less invasive alternative.[105,106]

4.6.4. Management

All patients with generalized amyloidosis should be investigated for an associated malignant plasma cell dyscrasia with serum and urine immunoelectrophoresis and bone marrow aspiration. The treatment of primary amyloidosis with cytotoxic agents is controversial.[99] Myeloma-associated amyloidosis may respond to the treatment of the underlying plasma cell dyscrasia, but this is not invariable. The prognosis of primary amyloidosis is poor with average survival time of about 14 months. The average survival of myeloma patients is shortened when amyloidosis is present.[90]

4.7. Crystal-Induced Arthropathies

4.7.1. Hyperuricemia and Gout

4.7.1.1. Epidemiology

Serum uric acid level remains at a stable low level until puberty at which time it rises to a stable level that is maintained in men from approximately age 20 onward. There is an increase in level in women at the time of menopause. At all ages after puberty, the mean level is higher in men than women.[107] The prevalence of hyperuricemia in the hospitalized population is higher because of the higher frequency of complicating factors such as medications and renal insufficiency.[110]

The prevalence of gouty arthritis has been estimated at 1% with the peak incidence in the fourth to sixth decades.[108,109] The development of gouty arthritis depends on deposition of monosodium urate crystals in tissue over time. There is a correlation between high levels of serum uric acid and presentation of gout at an earlier age.[111] The frequency of gout is considerably lower in women than men and is extremely unusual in premenopausal women reflecting the lower uric acid levels.[110]

Large population studies have demonstrated associations between obesity, hyperuricemia, and gout. Diabetes mellitus, hypertriglyceridemia, and hypertension are also more common in hyperuricemic or gout patients, but these disorders appear to be related to obesity or underlying renal disease rather than being independently associated factors.[110]

Drugs used frequently in the elderly, particularly diruetics, and renal insufficiency are two common causes of secondary hyperuricemia. Most hyperuricemic patients, however, have no identifiable cause. In the majority of these cases, there is decreased urinary excretion of uric acid. Less than 10% of patients with primary gout are overproducers of uric acid as defined by renal excretion of greater than 699 mg/24 hr of uric acid while on a purine-restricted diet.[111] The new onset of, or extremely high levels of, serum uric acid should raise the suspicion of an underlying lymphoproliferative or myeloproliferative disorder.

4.7.1.2. Clinical Manifestations

Clinical attacks of gout in the elderly do not differ from attacks in younger individuals. A common setting for acute gouty arthritis is in the immediate postoperative period or in association with other medically stressful situations such as myocardial infarction, stroke, or infection. Acute gout often occurs with fluctuations in the serum uric acid level, particularly with decreasing levels,[112] hence the association with onset of uric acid-lowering therapy or with stress in which renal handling of uric acid is altered.[113] In one study of patients with polyarticular gout, the mean age at the time of the attack was 60 years suggesting that it is a manifestation seen more commonly in older patients.[114] Fever and leukocytosis were commonly seen. In 40% of the patients, the polyarticular attack was the first manifestation of gout. In almost 38%, the serum acid level was normal at the time of the attack. Polyarticular gout should be considered in the differential diagnosis of patients with polyarthritis, and even in the absence of a history of gout or an elevated serum uric acid level, the synovial fluid should be examined for crystals.

4.7.1.3. Management

The indications for treatment of hyperuricemia include recurrent uric acid nephrolithiasis, tophaceous deposits, frequent recurrent attacks of gouty arthritis, and initiation of chemotherapy in patients with lympho- or myeloproliferative disorders. Asymptomatic hyperuricemia itself is not an indication for therapy[115] and does not appear to be associated with significant decreases in renal function over time.[116,117] Some would recommend treating extreme elevations of hyperuricemia such as greater than 13 mg% in an otherwise asymptomatic individual.

Acute gouty attacks can be managed with NSAIDs other than salicylates, intravenous colchicine, or local corticosteroids. Patients should be maintained on oral colchicine or a NSAID for 4 to 6 weeks after an acute attack resolves before uric acid lowering agent is begun in those patients in whom it has been decided to treat the hyperuricemia. The colchicine or NSAID should then be continued for 6 months after the serum uric level has normalized to prevent an acute flare. In those patients in whom no specific hyperuricemic therapy is planned, the therapy of the acute attack can be tapered shortly after the attack has resolved.[118] Chronic maintenance colchicine, 0.6 mg twice a day, is an alternative to uric acid lowering therapy in patients with recurrent attacks of gout without evidence of tophi or joint erosions, thus avoiding the greater toxicity of allopurinol or a uricosuric gout.[119]

4.7.2. Calcium Pyrophosphate Dihydrate Crystal Deposition Disease

4.7.2.1. Epidemiology

Calcium pyrophosphate dihydrate (CPPD) crystals may be deposited in articular cartilage and be accompanied by radiographic evidence of calcium deposition (chondrocalcinosis) and arthritis. Autopsy studies have revealed the presence of CPPD deposits in the knee cartilage of 5% of adults at the time of death.[120] Chondrocalcinosis increased in prevalence with advancing age,[121] and in one study 27.6% of 58 unselected patients ranging in age from 70 to 90 years radiographic evidence of chondrocalcinosis.[122]

4.7.2.2. Clinical Manifestations

CPPD crystal deposition has been shown to have six distinct clinical presentations.[120] Type A, termed pseudogout, is marked by acute monarticular or polyarticular attacks of arthritis and is seen in about 25% of the CPPD deposition cases. The attacks are self-limited, predominantly affecting the knees, wrists, elbows, and ankles. Clinically, the attacks resemble acute gout and are frequently provoked by surgery or major medical illness.[123] The diagnosis is established by the indentification of weakly positive birefringent rhomboid-shaped CPPD crystals in synovial fluid. The acute synovitis results from the phagocytosis of CPPD crystals by synovial polymorphonuclear leukocytes, the elaboration of a crystal-induced chemotactic factor, and subsequent inflammatory response.[122]

Type B, or pseudorheumatoid arthritis, occurs in approximately 5% of patients with CPPD deposition disease. These patients have subacute polyarticular attacks lasting weeks to months. The presence of morning stiffness, synovial thickening, and limited joint range of motion due to inflammation or flexion contractures resemble the manifestations of RA.

Approximately 50% of cases resemble osteoarthritis with progressive degeneration of multiple joints, commonly in a symmetric distribution. The knee is the most commonly involved joint, but other affected joints include the wrists, metacarpophalangeal joints, hips, shoulder, elbows, and ankles. The involvement of wrists, shoulders, elbows, and ankles is distinct from the pattern of joint involvement in primary generalized OA. Osteoarthritic involvement in this distribution should raise the suspicion of underlying CPPD crystal deposition. If there are superimposed attacks of pseudogout, the pattern is classified Type D; without acute attacks, Type C.

Type E refers to patients with radiographic evidence of chondrocalcinosis who are entirely asymptomatic. This group comprises about 20% of the total. The Type F, or pseudo-Charcot joint, pattern is a severe, destructive arthropathy usually of the knees occurring either with or without a neurologic deficit.

4.7.2.3. Etiology and Pathogenesis

CPPD deposition disease is seen in sporadic cases, as in inherited disease in families or in association with a metabolic disorder.[124] The sporadic form constitutes the vast majority of cases.[125] Several informative families have been studied. The pattern of inheritance for these families conformed to an autosomal dominant pattern. There was a spectrum of clinical severity in these families ranging from asymptomatic chondrocalcinosis to a mild oligoarthritis to severe polyarthritis with repeated pseudogout attacks and joint destruction usually occurring in younger patients.[126–128] A generalized increase in intracellular pyrophosphate concentration has been found in one family and may represent the underlying inherited metabolic defect in these families.[129]

4.7.2.4. Associated Disorders

The metabolic disorders reported in association with CPPD deposition include hyperparathyroidism, hemochromatosis, Wilson's disease, hypophosphatasia, hypomagnesemia, ochronosis, and hypothyroidism.[130] The mechanism of the associations are not completely understood, but it has been postulated that disease-related factors such as elevated cations seen in Wilson's disease, hemochromatosis, and hyperparathyroidism, elevation of parathyroid hormone and decreased alkaline phosphatase in hypophosphatasia may all result in altered pyrophosphate metabolism in cartilage, causing chondrocyte damage or altering proteoglycans, thus promoting CPPD crystal formation and deposition.[125] When evaluating patients with chondrocalcinosis, appropriate screening tests should be obtained for these metabolic disorders.

There appears to be a close association between CPPD deposition and OA, but the exact nature of the relationship is unclear. It has not been shown that the prevalence of OA is higher in patients with chondrocalcinosis than in age-matched controls.[130] Abnormal pyrophosphate metabolism in OA cartilage might account for increased CPPD deposition secondary to OA.[131,132] In addition, alteration of normal cartilage response to stress, because of chondrocalcinosis or cartilage damage following repeated attacks of pseudogout, could lead to OA secondary to CPPD deposition. This concept is supported by the observations that chondrocalcinosis can appear in joints prior to any evidence of OA[133] and that joints not usually involved in primary OA are affected in CPPD deposition.[134]

4.7.2.5. Management

Episodes of pseudogout can be managed with NSAIDs or intravenous colchicine. Severe attacks respond well to joint aspiration and intraarticular corticosteroids. Treatment is continued until the attack resolves. Acute episodes must be distinguished from septic arthritis by examination and culture of synovial fluid. The presence of typical crystals does not entirely exclude the diagnosis of sepsis, as the two can coincide in the same joint, making Gram stain and culture of the fluid critical. The subacute and chronic presentations of CPPD deposition disease are managed in a way similar to OA.[10]

4.7.3. Hydroxyapatite Deposition Disease

Hydroxyapatite (HA), the calcium phosphate component of normal bone, may be deposited in periarticular structures such as tendon insertions and joint capsules or in articular cartilage. Acute calcific periarthritis is characterized by painful, tender swelling and radiographic evidence of amorphous calcification of extraarticular structures.[135] The shoulder and wrist are common sites, but any joint may be involved.

More recently, HA crystals have been identified in the synovium and synovial fluid of patients with acute and chronic arthritis, often associated with OA.[136-138] Clumps of HA crystals may be identified by light microscopy, but individual crystals are below the resolution of the light microscope and definitive identification requires electronmicroscopy or X-ray diffraction.[137] HA arthritis is indistinguishable clinically from gout or pseudogout. HA crystals may be the cause of some of the sudden exacerbations seen occasionally in patients with OA. The pathogenesis of inflammation is felt to be the same as for the other crystal-induced arthropathies. The management is the same as for pseudogout.

4.8. Osteoarthritis

OA is a condition marked pathologically by deterioration of articular cartilage, changes in subchondral bone, and evidence of new bone formation. Radiographically, there is loss of normal joint space, subchondral sclerosis, cysts, and osteophyte formation. Clinically, there is pain and progressive joint deformity.[139-141] It is the end result of numerous complex interacting mechanical, biochemical, cellular, genetic, and metabolic factors, which are not fully understood.

4.8.1. Epidemiology

Population studies in both England and the United States showed a high prevalence of OA in the general population.[142-143] Prevalence increases with age. Radiographic evidence of OA has been seen in 10% of a study population between ages 55 and 64 years.[142,143] Overall, the prevalence is equal between men and women with men predominating below the age of 45 years and women above the age of 45 years. Localized trauma probably explains the increased rate in young men.[142] With age, both the radiographic severity and number of joints involved increase.[143] Prevalence figures are considerably lower if the diagnosis is based upon clinical symptoms rather than radiographic abnormalities.[139,145]

4.8.2. Biology of Normal Cartilage

Normal cartilage consists of chondrocytes, cells derived from mesenchymal tissue, embedded in an organic matrix composed of type II collagen and proteoglycans (PG).[146] PGs are macromolecules with keratin sulfate and chondroitin sulfate gycosaminoglycan polymers attached to a central protein core.[147,148] PGs are highly hydrophilic and normal cartilage function depends on its high water content which accounts for 70 to 80% of the total cartilage weight.[149] A small amount of hyaluronic acid is also present which is essential for PG aggregation.[150] Normal cartilage function also depends on the physiologic interaction of collagen and PGs, the former providing tensile strength and the latter compressibility. Normal cartilage is highly resilient. Together with subchondral bone, periarticular structures, and muscles, it forms the mechanism for absorbing and dissipating large mechanical forces applied to joints in normal use.[151,152]

Cartilage is the site of active metabolism and matrix turnover. Collagen and PG units are synthesized and deposited by chondrocytes. Likewise, the chondrocyte releases degradative enzymes active against both collagen and PGs.[151] Normal cartilage is avascular and therefore depends upon diffusion of nutrients chiefly from the synovial fluid. It is felt that the normal repetitive compression and decompression of articular cartilage with normal use facilitates this diffusion process.

4.8.3. Pathology of OA and Age-Related Changes in Cartilage

Early pathologic findings in OA occur in the articular cartilage matrix and include both quantitative and qualitative changes. At first, there is an increase in water content, perhaps reflecting a decrease in the supporting capacity of collagen, but, at later stages, the water content falls.[153,154] There is an overall decrease in the content of PGs[155] while the synthetic rate of PGs as well as the rate of chondrocyte replication actually increases as measured by isotope labeling studies.[156] This would suggest an even greater increase in the rate of PG degradation. In OA cartilage, the percentage composition of chondroitin sulfate falls while keratin sulfate increases.[157] The length of glycosaminoglycan polymers is reduced and there is a decrease in the capacity of PGs to form aggregates.[158] By contrast, changes in articular cartilage collagen do not seem to be a prominent part of the pathologic process.

The OA joint shows softening and fibrillation of the articular cartilage in its early stages. Vertical clefts appear and can penetrate through to the subchondral bone. There are changes in the staining characteristics of the cartilage consistent with the biochemical changes present and an increase in the mitotic activity of chondrocytes.[139] The cartilage loses its normal resilience and hence its ability to dissipate mechanical forces optimally. In the subchondral bone, microfractures, cysts, and subsequent collapse result. Progressive loss of cartilage occurs. In repose a reparative reaction begins, resulting in vascularization of cartilage and new bone or osteophyte formation. Ultimately chondrocyte death occurs and there is complete loss of cartilage with gross joint deformity of supporting structures, resulting in joint instability.[140]

Although there are well-documented changes in nonarticular cartilage with aging that resemble those seen in OA (i.e., decrease in water content and relative increase in keratin sulfate to chondroitin sulfate), there is less certainty about age-related changes in articular cartilage. Some have found age-related decreases in the chondroitin sulfate to keratin sulfate ratio[159,160] but others have found no age-related change in water, collagen, protein or PG content. Cellularity and chondrocyte function likewise appear unchanged with normal aging.[151] One study has shown an abnormality in PG aggregation in morphologically normal cartilage from hips of patients aged 69 to 81 years.[161] The significance of this finding in the development of OA is unknown. This paucity of age-related findings in the articular cartilage of humans suggests that OA might not be an inevitable consequence of aging in all persons, but rather that OA is related to aging in certain predisposed individuals. Alternatively, cartilage changes might be an inevitable consequence of senescence given sufficient time, but with the length of time varying among individuals.

4.8.4. Pathogenesis

Explanations of the pathogenesis of OA are complex and must account for the numerous etiologic factors that appear to exist and for the various clinical correlates of OA. One operational model is that the basic lesion in OA is damaged or the chondrocyte function is altered, resulting in release of various lysosomal enzymes that degrade the cartilage matrix.[162] Mechanical stresses applied to joints as the result of unusually forceful activity or as the result of uneven distribution of force across a joint due to an anatomic derangement could exceed a tolerable level of force applied to the chondrocyte.[152] The biochemical changes thus produced would decrease the ability of the articular cartilage to dissipate force and establish a cycle of increased cartilage stress leading to further degradation of the normal matrix. Genetic factors, sex-related factors, subtle age-related factors, systemic metabolic disorders such as associated with chondrocalcinosis, previous cartilage damage secondary to a septic or inflammatory process and other unrecognized factors could alter the normal articular cartilage in such a way as to render it more susceptible to mechanical stress.[151,163]

4.8.5. Clinical Manifestations

The clinical and radiographic manifestations of OA are well described and are not different in the aged than the general population.[139,140,164] OA is characterized clinically by pain, deformity, and limitation of joint motion. Generally, there is a gradual onset with slow progression of symptoms and signs. Characteristically, pain is exacerbated by use and weight-bearing and relieved by rest. During the later stages of the disease, however, symptoms can become persistent and occur at rest. Morning stiffness may occur, but is not as prominent as in RA. Pain is due to inflammation, trabecular microfractures, pressure on nerves, muscle spasm, and capsular distention. Sudden exacerbations with marked signs of inflammation, joint effusions, warmth, tenderness, and erythema occasionally occur, probably in relation to the release of mediators of inflammation from damaged cartilage[165] or to shedding of HA or CPPD crystals into the synovium with subsequent crystal-induced synovitis.[136,137] Progressive loss of joint range of motion develops related to muscle spasm, deformity, loss of normal articulating surface and chronic effusions.

OA can be divided clinically into primary and secondary forms based on whether or not precipitating factors can be identified. Primary generalized OA, described in the early 1950s, has a predisposition for women, may be genetically determined (autosomal dominant in women and autosomal recessive in men). It has a distinct joint distribution involving the distal interphalangeal joints (Heberden's nodes), the proximal interphalangeal joints (Bouchard's nodes), the first carpometacarpal joint, the knees, and the spine.[166–168] That primary generalized OA occurs in elderly patients suggests that repetitive joint use over time contributes to the expression of disease in susceptible individuals. Similarly, it has been shown that repetitive activities involving the small joints of the hands in female factory workers probably contributes to OA changes in the hands that would ordinarily be considered to be primary or idiopathic.[169]

Secondary OA may involve any joint. OA localized to one joint or to a few joints or to a joint not usually involved in primary OA should raise the suspicion of an underlying process. Underlying factors include anatomic abnormalities such as angulation deformities, congenital and developmental hip disorders, or posttraumatic derangements; prior cartilage and joint damage secondary to septic or inflammatory synovitis; metabolic disorders such as hemachromatosis,[170] Wilson's disease,[171] ochronosis,[172] chondrocalcinosis,[173] and hypothyroidism[174] changes in the underlying bone as in Paget's disease[175] and osteonecrosis.[176] Occupational exposure to excessive joint stresses is associated with OA changes in the ankles of ballet dancers, the shoulders and elbows of penumatic drill operators, and the knees of coal miners. Subtle subclinical anatomic abnormalities are thought to underlie over 80% of osteoarthritic hips[177,178] suggesting that the hips are not generally part of primary generalized OA. Obesity is a secondary factor that is related to increased OA of the knees.[142,143,179] Curiously, the ankle, despite being a weight-bearing joint, is generally spared of OA. This has been attributed to a more effective dissipation of joint stress across the ankle's articular surface.[180]

4.8.6. Management

The general goal of improved functional capacity in OA is approached by efforts to increase joint motion and reduce pain.[164,181] For the elderly patient, this might make possible the ability to live or ambulate independently or to enjoy a relatively sedentary existence without pain. For others, the ability to perform one's job or household chores might be the goal. Weight loss in obese patients, correction of anatomic abnormalities, avoidance of traumatic occupational and recreational activities, appropriate joint rest with splinting and assistive devices, and good muscular conditioning all help relieve the patient of excessive joint stress, thereby preventing or slowing progression of the disease and alleviating symptoms. Exercises that involve active motion without excessive joint loading such as swimming or bicycling may strengthen muscles without further injuring articular surfaces. Heat therapy may relieve pain and muscle spasm.

Analgesic and antiinflammatory medications play a major role in relief of symptoms. As OA is a chronic disorder, narcotic analgesics are best avoided. In some patients, adequate relief may be obtained from acetominophen. Others may require a salicylate or other NSAID. Joint aspiration and intraarticular cortico-steroids are effective, particularly in patients with large effusions or signs of acute inflammation. Because of the potential for a deleterious effect on articular carti-lage with frequent repeated use, corticosteroid injections should be used only infre-quently. Sepsis must always be ruled out beforehand.

Coincidental nonarticular sources of pain such as anserine bursitis of the knee, carpal tunnel syndrome, or tendonitis should be looked for and treated spe-cifically as they may be the major source of symptoms even in a patient with obvious signs of OA.

Surgical management of OA is reserved for those patients with severe and persistent symptoms despite medical management, particularly those with rest and nocturnal symptoms. Joint stabilization with fusion, osteotomy to transfer weight-bearing forces to a different part of the articular surface, and joint replacement are the major alternatives available. Considerations such as the location of joint involvement, health status, and operative suitability of the patient and the appro-priateness of the goals for the individual patient are necessary in patient selection for surgery. Advanced age itself is not a contraindication.

4.9. Seronegative Spondyloarthropathies

Ankylosing spondylitis (AS), Reiter's syndrome, psoriatric arthritis, reactive arthritis related to bacterial dysentery, and the arthropathy associated with inflammatory bowel disease are known collectively as the seronegative spondy-loarthropathies. These disorders share the clinical manifestations of sacroilitis and spondylitis, often in association with the HLA–B27 antigen. Although these dis-orders generally have their onset in young and middle-aged individuals, several aspects are of relevance to the elderly. AS typically presents in the second or third decades. Onset of symptoms of AS (and other spondyloarthropathies when they involve the back) are morning stiffness and pain in the back that is worse at rest and improves with activity. The onset is usually insidious. Asymmetric involve-ment of peripheral joints, particularly of the hips and knees, may be present.[182]

The approach to *new* onset back pain in an elderly patient first involves determining if the process is inflammatory (stiffness, pain at rest, improvement with exercise, insidious onset, diffuse radiation) or mechanical (pain relieved by rest, worsening with activity, acute onset, radicular radiation). Inflammatory back pain in this age group suggests an underlying process other than primary AS such as psoriasis or inflammatory bowel disease.[113]

Although AS presents in younger patients, the diagnosis may be delayed many years in mild cases. Some of the sequelae of AS occur after many years of disease activity and will be present in elderly AS patients. The development of upper lobe fibrobullous pulmonary lesions has been reported in 1 to 2% of AS patients at the Mayo Clinic. All were men with an average age of 60 years at the time of detection of the lung lesion. There was an average interval of 21 years from the onset of spondylitis to onset of pulmonary manifestations. In all but one of the 28 cases, the patient no longer was symptomatic with pain from the AS. Unless complicated by infection, the fibrobullous lesion was asymptomatic. Aspergilloma developed in preexisting bullae in five cases.[184]

Another late complication of AS is spinal fracture. Minor trauma insufficient to produce a fracture in a normal spine often precedes a fracture of an ankylosed, osteoporotic spine in AS. In a recent review of reported cases, the average age of fracture was 54.6 years (range 33 to 85 years) and the mean duration of AS was 24 years prior to the fracture.[185] The diagnosis is often missed or delayed because changes in symptoms may be regarded as increased disease activity rather than a new process, and radiographic evidence of fracture may be obscured by spinal deformity and osteoporosis. In patients with ankylosed spines, sudden increases in pain, new neurologic complaints, and sudden increase in spinal range of motion should prompt a search for a spinal fracture. Spinal tomograms and bone scans may be helpful when plain radiographs are unrevealing. At times, it may be necessary to manage the patient as if a fracture has occurred even when it cannot be demonstrated if the clinical setting strongly suggests that diagnosis. Conservative therapy with traction and immobilization is usually effective with spine stability occurring by 3 months of conservative therapy in 47 of 49 patients. Surgical fusion is indicated if progressive neurologic defects occur or if immobilization cannot be obtained. The mortality associated with spine fracture in AS is substantial.[185]

Cardiac complications have been seen in 10% of AS patients with 15 to 30 years of disease duration. The most common lesions are aortic insufficiency due to dilation of aortic valve ring and conduction abnormalities. Cardiac complications are more common in patients with severe spondylitis, prominent systemic manifestations, and marked peripheral joint disease.[182] Cauda equina syndrome may result from advanced lumbar spondylitis. Surgical decompression may be necessary.[186,187]

Management of AS aims primarily to maintain functional posture and relieve pain. There is no disease-remitting therapy. Range-of-motion exercises, attention to good posture, avoidance of certain activities such as bicycling which promotes spinal flexion, and avoidance of a pillow while sleeping may help to maintain upright posture and function. Antiinflammatory agents may relieve pain and permit more effective exercise therapy.

The spondyloarthropathies accompanying Reiter's syndrome, psoriasis, and inflammatory bowel disease occur rarely in the elderly and the clinical presentations do not differ from younger patients.

4.10. Polymyalgia Rheumatica and Giant-Cell Arteritis

PMR and GCA are disorders of the elderly. They affect the same population and often the same patient. As such, they have been considered to be manifestations of the same disease although others view them as two coincidental disorders or as two disorders linked by a common etiology.[188-193] An incidence of 11.7 cases/ 100,000 population age 50 years or older and prevalence of 133 cases/100,000 population older than 50 years has been found for GCA.[192] Accurate figures are not available for PMR, but, in one center, the diagnosis of PMR was made 3 times more frequently than GCA.[194]

4.10.1. Clinical Manifestations

PMR is a clinically defined syndrome marked by proximal myalgias and stiffness. The syndrome occurs almost exclusively after the age of 50 years and affects females twice as often as males.[189] The myalgias are experienced in the posterior neck, intrascapular region, and shoulder or hip girdle. Symptoms are often worse in the morning and there is frequently morning stiffness. The onset may be either abrupt or insidious and symptoms should generally be present for more than four weeks before the diagnosis is accepted in order to exclude self-limited viral syndromes. Although joint motion is usually preserved and symptoms are localized to muscles rather than joints, sensitive nuclear scans have shown increased synovial uptake, suggesting synovitis with referred pain to proximal muscles are the source of the myalgias.[194] Likewise, muscle strength, muscle enzymes, electromyograms, and biopsies of involved muscles are all normal or show only minor abnormalities, in distinct contrast to polymyositis.[195] Occasionally, frank peripheral arthritis, most often of the knees, is seen in cases where PMR is distinguished from RA only by the clinical course or development of other features of RA such as nodules, RF, and persistent, deforming, erosive arthritis.[196]

GCA is a vasculitis of unknown etiology involving any artery of the body but most commonly involving the cranial branches of arteries arising from the aortic arch.[197] In addition to PMR symptoms, patients with GCA have signs and symptoms related to the underlying arteritis. Headache, scalp tenderness, jaw claudication, and visual symptoms are commonly seen. The headache and scalp tenderness may be unilateral and localized to a tender, indurated, swollen temporal artery. More commonly, both are nonspecific and diffuse, and the arteries are normal to palpation. Visual symptoms include blurring, diplopia, ptosis, and loss of acuity ranging to blindness. Although sudden blindness may occasionally be the presenting ocular symptom, most commonly there are preceding transient visual disturbances. Visual disturbance is due to involvement of the posterior ciliary artery and less often to vasculitis of the central retinal artery.[189,181,197] GCA involvement of the vertebrobasilar system can present brainstem infarctions. Involvement of the rest of the intracranial circulation is uncommon presumably because of the loss of the elastic lamina of the walls of vessels after they have penetrated the dura mater.[198] Involvement of the aorta or its major branches may present as extremity claudication, Raynaud's phenomenon, ruptured aortic aneurysm, chest pain due to coronary arteritis, or hematuria due to renal artery involvement. Diminished pulses and bruits over involved arteries may be present.

Large artery manifestations may be the presenting manifestations or may occur later in the course of GCA.[199]

Fever, weight loss, anorexia, fatigue and depression commonly accompany both GCA and PMR.[188,190,197] The constitutional symptoms may be present without the features of PMR or GCA. They may dominate the clinical picture with fever of unknown origin or findings suggestive of an occult malignancy.[200] Temporal artery biopsy should be strongly considered in patients over the age of 50 years presenting with fever of unknown origin in whom no other etiology is found after basic clinical and laboratory evaluations have been performed.[201]

Both PMR and GCA are almost invariably associated with an elevated ESR, often greater than 100 mm/hr (Westergren). Normochromic, normocytic anemia, hypoalbuminemia, and elevated alkaline phosphatase with normal transaminases and bilirubin are commonly seen.[195] Even in patients with elevated alkaline phosphatase liver biopsy is normal or nonspecific. Granulomatous hepatitis has been described. The alkaline phosphatase returns to normal with treatment.[202,203] The routine use of liver biopsy in PMR/GCA patients with only alkaline phosphatase elevations is not recommended.

4.10.2. Diagnosis

Temporal artery biopsy is positive in up to 40 to 50% of patients presenting with PMR, with or without arteritic symptoms. If those with any arteritic symptoms are eliminated, the frequency falls.[189] The histology of the involved artery is a necrotizing vasculitis with destruction of the internal elastic membrane accompanied by a mononuclear cell infiltrate. Giant cells are not invariably present.[195] Involvement of the artery may be segmental and, therefore, long specimens should be obtained and serially sectioned to reduce the frequency of false-negative biopsies.[204] The use of temporal artery angiography to localize abnormal segments is not recommended.[205]

4.10.3. Management

The goals of management in PMR and GCA are to relieve symptoms and prevent complications of the vasculitis. Patients with PMR should be questioned and examined for the presence of arteritic symptoms and signs. If present, a temporal artery biopsy should be performed. In the absence of GCA, PMR patients can be managed with low doses of corticosteroids. There is often a rapid and dramatic response to 10 to 15 mg of prednisone per day. Within 1 to 2 weeks, the symptoms resolve and the ESR returns to baseline. If this should fail to occur, one should perform temporal artery biopsy to look for GCA or reconsider the diagnosis.

If GCA is proven by biopsy or if there is sufficiently high clinical suspicion of the diagnosis even in the absence of a positive biopsy, corticosteroids should be administered in high dose, generally 40 to 60 mg/day. In patients presenting with signs or symptoms of arteritis, therapy should be initiated immediately. Biopsy results will not be altered provided the biopsy is performed within several days. This is particularly important in patients with visual symptom or who have lost the vision in one eye already. Progressive visual loss can be stopped. Vision may improve in eyes with partial deficits and involvement of the contralateral eye can be avoided with therapy.[206]

Both PMR and GCA are chronic disorders and may require therapy for many years. Corticosteroids are tapered when symptoms resolve and the ESR has returned to baseline. Tapering is gradual, with reductions of approximately 10% of the dose/week. Recurrences of PMR and GCA or the new development of GCA in a treated PMR patient may occur at any time in the course of therapy[207] so patients should have regular follow-up, be carefully monitored during steroid tapering, and be educated to report promptly any new or changing symptom or sign.

4.11. Malignancies and Rheumatic Diseases

Because of the increased prevalence of neoplastic disease in the elderly, a discussion of the rheumatic disease association with malignancies is warranted.

4.11.1. Hypertrophic Osteoarthropathy

Hypertrophic osteoarthropathy (HO) is characterized by clubbing, periostitis with pain, tenderness, and warmth particularly over the long bones of the extremities, symmetrical polyarthralgias or polyarthritis involving the metacarpophalangeal joints, wrists, elbows, knees, and ankles. Radiographs show periosteal new bone formation along the shafts of long and short bones. Bone scans may show uptake in involved areas before radiographic changes are apparent.[208] Synovial fluid analysis shows a noninflammatory fluid with leukocyte counts less than 500 cells/mm^3, but with a tendency to form a spontaneous clot suggestive of a fibrinogen leak into the synovial fluid.[209] The patient may also develop acromegalic features with coarse, thickened, deeply furrowed skin and facial features, hyperkeratosis of the palmar skin, and gynecomastia.[210,211]

HO may be either primary, with no associated disease, or secondary to associated diseases including both malignant and benign neoplasms, chronic cardiopulmonary disorders, and numerous others.[208] Those cases associated with malignancies are said to have a more abrupt onset of clubbing and arthritis with markedly painful fingertips, more painful joints, and more prominent skin changes than those associated with benign lesions.[210] The rheumatic manifestations of HO may precede those of the associated neoplasm and therefore should prompt an investigation for an underlying malignancy. Intrathoracic malignancies are most common, but almost all neoplasms have been implicated.[208]

The HO symptoms generally respond dramatically to removal or effective treatment of the associated malignancy. HO also responds to NSAIDs such as aspirin or indomethacin and to corticosteroids.[208,209,212] The syndrome may relapse with recurrence of the tumor. Several pathophysiologic mechanisms have been proposed for HO. A reflex neurovascular mechanism has been supported by response of the syndrome to vagotomy or chronic atropine therapy.[213] Other mechanisms proposed include a response to circulating immune complexes related to the tumor,[209,214] a remote effect of increased estrogen in view of the associated gynecomastia and increased vascularity of the nailbeds, and a response to elevated growth hormone.[215]

4.11.2. Malignancy-Related Polyarthritis

A polyarthritis resembling RA has been described in association with malignancy. There is evidence to support this as more than just a coincidence of two disorders. The polyarthritis associated with malignancy in two uncontrolled series demonstrated several atypical features including explosive onset, and asymmetric joint involvement with sparing of the hands and wrists. Typically, there is a close temporal relationship to the discovery of the malignancy. Rheumatoid nodules and RF factor are absent, and the synovial biopsy shows mild nonspecific inflammation and perivascular infiltrates without typical rheumatoid proliferation.[216,217] The true frequency of polyarthritis occuring as a manifestation of a malignancy is not known, but it is a relatively infrequent event. Nevertheless, a polyarthritis presenting in an elderly patient with features atypical of RA should increase one's suspicion of an underlying neoplasm.[218] In one report, breast cancer constituted 80% of the underlying malignancies in women while no predominant type was noted in men.[217] As with HO, the pathophysiologic mechanism or mechanisms is unknown for this paraneoplastic syndrome.

Typical RA does not appear to be associated with a significant increase in malignancies.[219,220] However, it will be important to monitor this rate as more RA patients are treated with immunosuppressive agents.[221,222]

4.11.3. Polymyositis and Dermatomyositis

Inflammatory muscle disease may be associated with malignancy. Polymyositis, characterized by proximal muscle weakness, elevated muscle enzymes, abnormal electromyograms, and muscle biopsy showing necrosis and inflammation may occur alone or together with features of another systemic rheumatic disease such as RA, SLE or scleroderma (termed an "overlap syndrome") or with a characteristic skin rash, termed dermatomyositis.[223]

A malignancy has been estimated to occur in 8 to 14% of all patients with polymyositis or dermatomyositis.[223-225] This is approximately 5 to 7 times greater than in the general population.[226] Those patients at highest risk for an associated malignancy are: (1) older-onset patients,[223-225] (2) those patients with dermatomyositis,[226,227] and possibly, (3) men.[224] Both dermatomyositis and polymyositis have been associated with occult malignancies. The average age of onset of myositis with malignancy is in the sixth and seventh decades while age of onset in all myositis cases peaks in the fifth decade.[223,225]

Lung and breast carcinomas are the most commonly found tumors. There may be an excess of ovarian, uterine, and gastric tumors and a decreased number of colon carcinomas compared to the general cancer population.[226] One study found an overwhelming predominance of adenocarcinomas.[225]

Investigation for an underlying malignancy in a patient with myositis can generally be limited to a detailed history and physical examination; screening blood, urine, and stool for occult blood studies; and subsequent follow-up of any abnormal findings. An extensive invasive search of all patients with myositis is not warranted.[225,227]

The onset of the myopathy may precede, coincide with, or follow the presentation of the underlying malignancy although, in most cases, the two appear within 1 year of each other.[226] In some cases, the myositis improves coincidentally with effective treatment of the underlying malignancy, but this is variable and unpredictable. Response to corticosteroids is said to be less marked and more short-lived than in cases not complicated by malignancy.[223,226] The underlying malignancy is more often the cause of death than progressive weakness from the myositis.[223]

4.11.4. Metastatic Disease

Metastatic disease may present as an arthritis, most commonly as a monoarthritis but occasionally involving multiple joints and simulating RA. The joint effusion may be hemorrhagic or serosanguinous and is usually noninflammatory. Any hemorrhagic, noninflammatory monoarthritis that is persistent should arouse the suspicion of malignancy involving the joint. The suspicion may be confirmed by careful cytologic examination of synovial fluid or by synovial biopsy.[228]

4.11.5. Leukemia

Leukemic infiltration of the synovium in both acute and chronic forms of leukemia may present as arthritis that is typically polyarticular with predilection for the knees, shoulders, and ankles. There is a close correlation between the arthritis and activity of the leukemia. Radiographs may be normal or may show nonspecific abnormalties. Synovial biopsy shows leukemic infiltration.[229]

4.11.6. Carcinoma of the Pancreas

Carcinoma of the pancreas may be complicated by a syndrome of arthritis, usually polyarticular and asymmetric and subcutaneous nodules. Both the nodules and arthritis appear to be secondary to local fat necrosis due to pancreatic lipases released into the circulation. The arthritis is resistent to therapy.[230,231]

4.12. Medications for the Treatment of Rheumatic Diseases

This section describes the therapeutic effects, metabolism, and drug interactions of agents used in the management of rheumatic diseases. Aspirin and other NSAIDs, corticosteroids, gold compounds, and allupurinol will be reviewed.

4.12.1. General Principles of Drug Therapy

Several aspects of drug therapy must be considered in the elderly patient. The elderly may be more sensitive to the physiologic effects of pharmaceutical preparations than younger individuals. Therefore, treatment should be started at low doses, which should be increased only gradually. Elderly individuals may suffer from a variety of medical problems and take multiple medications, thus increasing the risk of drug complications and interactions. Finally, elderly individuals may have difficulty understanding and complying with instructions; thus, single drug schedules are preferable whenever possible.[232]

4.12.2. Nonsteroidal Antiinflammatory Drugs

These include salicylates in their various forms (acetylated and nonacetylated), propionic acid derivatives (ibuprofen, narpoxen, fenoprofen calcium), idoleacetic acid derivatives (indomethacin and sulindac), tolmetin sodium (structurally related to indomethacin), anthranilic acid derivatives (fenamates such as meclofenamate sodium), and the enolic acids, which are divided into the pyrazolines (oxypenbutazone and phenylbutazone) and the oxicams (piroxicam).

4.12.2.1. Mechanisms of Action

These agents reduce inflammation by interacting with a number of processes: phagocytosis, chemotactic stimuli, lysosomal enzyme release, and activation of various pathways including clotting, fibrinolytic, kinin, and complement.[233] Aspirin and other NSAIDs inhibit the enzyme cyclooxygenase (prostaglandins synthetase), which converts arachidonic acid to prostaglandins, thromboxane A2, and prostacyclin. Prostaglandins are potent inflammatory agents that appear to sensitize blood vessels to bradykinin and histamine, increase permeability of the vessel wall, and augment pain perception. Superoxide and hydroxyl free radicals are also produced during the synthesis of prostaglandins. These are capable of causing tissue damage. NSAIDs inhibit phosphodiesterase, which increases the intracellular levels of cyclic AMP,[234] thus stabilizing lysosomal membranes, and which decreases superoxide generation.[235]

4.12.2.2. Metabolism

Salicylates and other NSAIDs are absorbed in the stomach and proximal small intestine and metabolized by the hepatic microsomal system or kidney to various degrees. The drugs are excreted in the urine or bile as free drug conjugates or metabolites.[236] Underlying hepatic or renal disease can therefore result in toxic blood levels if the dose is not reduced. Salicylates are metabolized to salicyluric acid, salicylic phenolic, and acyl glucuronide. Since the enzymes responsible for conversion to salicylurate become saturated at high doses, the blood salicylate level is not a simple linear function. When the enzyme system becomes saturated, small increments in dose result in abrupt elevations of salicylate blood levels.[36]

4.12.2.3. Side Effects and Hypersensitivity Reactions

Therapeutic serum salicylate levels range from 15 to 30 mg/100 ml. In young and middle-aged individuals, tinnitus and high-frequency hearing loss are often relied upon as signs of salicylate toxicity. However, elderly individuals with baseline hearing problems, even if clinically inapparent, may not note these changes.[36] The elderly are also more sensitive to central nervous system effects such as delirium, psychosis, stupor, and coma than are younger individuals.[237]

Salicylates and other NSAIDs can result in mucous membrane irritation.[238] Resulting side effects include epigastric discomfort, nausea, and vomiting, which may be minimized by concomitant use of an antacid. Superficial erosions result in occult gastrointestinal blood loss and iron-deficiency anemia, especially in an individual on an iron-poor diet. Serious erosions can result in major bleeding in hypotension which can precipitate myocardial infarction, stroke, or acute renal tubular necrosis. NSAIDs cause erosions by disrupting the gastric mucosal barrier, allowing back diffusion of hydrogen ions[239] and possibly by reducing blood flow to the gastric mucosa.[240] NSAIDs also interfere with hemostasis through inhibition of platelet aggregation, altering the physiochemical properties of platelet membranes, decreasing platelet release of adenosine diphosphonate, and inhibiting platelet synthesis of thromboxane A2 which facilitates platelet aggregation.[232] Since aspirin inactivates platelet cyclooxygenase by an irreversible acetylation process, the dysfunction lasts as long as the life of the platelet, 7 to 10 days after the drug is stopped.[241] Since other NSAIDs reversibly inhibit cyclooxygenase, the resulting platelet dysfunction lasts only as long as the offending agent is present.[242]

The use of NSAIDs can result in sodium and fluid retention. Prostaglandins facilitate cortical renal blood flow. A decrease in postaglandin biosynthesis, therefore, may result in a decreased glomerular filtration rate with resulting sodium retention. The use of NSAIDs may result in congestive heart failure and pulmonary edema, particularly in individuals with impaired cardiac function. Although phenylbutazone is probably the worst offender, significant sodium retention can be seen as a side effect of all of the NSAIDs.[232] Inhibition of renal prostaglandin synthesis may also result in renal dysfunction, particularly in someone with underlying renal disease.[243]

Central nervous system effects of NSAIDs such as headache, dizziness, confusion, light-headedness, agitation, delirium, somnolence, lethargy, stupor, and coma are more common in the elderly than in younger individuals.[236] The relatively high prevalence of such side effects secondary to indomethacin serves as a relative contraindication to the use of this drug in the elderly.[232] One variable that may contribute to toxic drug manifestations is the serum albumin level. Since toxicity is a function of free drug levels, patients with low serum albumin concentrations may experience toxicity at a lower serum concentration than those with normal serum albumin levels.[36] Bone marrow suppression secondary to phenylbutazone occurs more frequently in individuals over 70 years old.[244] Because of this and the occurrence of other serious adverse reactions, such as fluid retention, phenylbutazone should be avoided in the elderly.[245] NSAIDs may precipitate asthma in individuals with the syndrome of bronchial asthma, vasomotor rhinitis, and nasal polyposis. It may also cause urticaria or angioedema. Both reactions are caused by prostaglandin inhibition.[246] Since nonacetylated salicylates are very weak inhibitors of prostaglandin synthesis, they do not produce these hypersensitivity reactions.[247]

4.12.2.4. Drug Interactions

Since NSAIDs are strongly protein bound, they interfere with drugs also bound to plasma proteins such as oral hypoglycemics, and warfarin.[248] Because piroxicam is effective in relatively low doses, the associated low plasma concentration minimizes displacement of drugs bound to plasma proteins,[250] thus minimizing drug interactions. Aspirin blocks the diuretic action of spironolactone by binding to the same renal tubule receptor.[249]

4.12.2.5. Drug Administration

Although the NSAIDs have similar mechanisms of action and toxicities, the response of any given patient is quite variable. A patient may achieve little relief and experience bothersome side effects with one NSAID and react quite differently with another.[232] Since a correlation has been demonstrated between patient compliance and the number of times a drug must be taken,[251] drugs such as naproxen and sulindac, which are taken twice daily, and piroxicam, which is only taken once daily, may prove advantageous, especially in the elderly individual. Piroxicam has the added advantage of remaining at therapeutic levels if a dose is missed.[250]

4.12.3. Corticosteroids

Steroids aggravate a variety of problems that are particularly prevalent in the elderly. These include sodium and fluid retention, hypertension, confusional states, hyperglycemia, and osteoporosis.[244,252] When used with gastric irritants they can retard the healing of gastric mucosal erosions.[253] Steroids cause osteoporosis by inhibiting bone formation and stimulating resorption by interfering with intestinal calcium absorption,[254] which stimulates parathyroid hormone secretion.[255] Treatment with supplemental vitamin D may enhance calcium absorption and suppress parathyroid hormone secretion and bone resorption.[254] It should also be noted that steroids may aggravate the potassium wasting of diuretics such as thiazides and furosemide. Their antiinflammatory effects may also mask the signs of an infection in the elderly, who have a blunted fever response to septic processes even without steroids.[232]

4.12.4. Gold Therapy

Intramuscular gold sodium thiomalae (Myochrysine®) occasionally causes vasomotor reactions, termed *nitritoid reactions*. These are characterized by facial flushing, dizziness, fainting, weakness, malaise, sweating, headache, nausea, and vomiting,[232] and have been implicated in causing myocardial ischemia and infarction.[256] Since aurothioglucose (Solganal®) rarely causes such reactions,[257] it is the gold preparation of choice in the elderly patient.

4.12.5. Allopurinol

Since allopurinol inhibits the catabolism of 6-mercaptopurine and azathioprine, the dose of these drugs should be reduced to 25% of the original dose when used with allopurinol to prevent severe bone marrow depression.[258] Allopurinol also increases the half-life of bishydroxycoumarin by inhibiting hepatic microsomal enzymes responsible for its catabolism. The prothrombin time must be monitored carefully when these drugs are used concurrently.[253] Allopurinol is excreted primarily by the kidney. Severe reactions (rashes, liver function abnormalities, toxic epidermal necrolysis, and vasculitis) have occurred in some patients with underlying renal disease or on thiazide diuretics.[232,259]

References

1. Weksler, M. E., 1981, The senescence of the immune system, *Hosp. Prac.* 16:53–64.
2. Trentham, D. E., 1982, The immune system and how it changes with age, in: *Rheumatic and Metabolic Bone Disease in the Elderly* (D. F. Giansiracusa and F. G. Kantrowitz, eds.), The Collamore Press, Lexington, Massachusetts, pp. 3–9.
3. Kusher, I., 1981, The acute phase reactants and the erythrocyte sedimentation rate, in: *Textbook of Rheumatology* (W. N. Kelly, E. D. Harris, Jr., S. Ruddy, and C. B. Sledge, eds.), W. B. Saunders Company, Philadelphia, pp. 669–676.

4. Bottiger, L. E. and Svedberg, C. A., 1967, The normal erythrocyte sedimentation rate and age, *Br. Med. J.* 2:85–87.
5. Hayes, G. S. and Stinson, I. N., 1976, Erythrocyte sedimentation rate and age, *Arch. Ophthalmol.* 94:939–940.
6. Zacharski, L. R. and Kyle, R. A., 1967, Significance of extreme elevations of erythrocyte sedimentation rates, *JAMA* 202:264–266.
7. Cammarata, P. G., Rodnan, G. P., and Fennell, R. H., 1967, Serum anti-gammaglobulin and anti-nuclear factors in the aged, *JAMA* 199:455–458.
8. Mikkelson, W. M., Dodge, H. J., Duff, I. V., and Kato, H., 1967, Estimates of the prevalence of rheumatic disease in the population of Tecumseh, Michigan 1950–50, *J. Chronic Dis.* 20:351–369.
9. Litwen, S. D. and Singer, J. M., 1965, Studies of the incidence and significance of anti-gammaglobulin factors in aging, *Arthritis Rheum.* 8:538–550.
10. Giansiracusa, D. F. and Kantrowitz, F. G., 1982, Pseudogout: Calcium pyrophosphate dihydrate deposition disease, *Rheumatic and Metabolic Bone Diseases in the Elderly,* The Collamore Press, Lexington, Massachusetts, pp. 45–54.
11. Fernandez-Madrid, F. and Mattioli, M., 1976, Anti-nuclear antibodies (ANA): Immunologic and clinical significance, *Sem. Arth. Rheum.* 6:83–124.
12. Friou, G. J. and Quismorio, F. P., 1975, The LE cell factor and antinuclear antibodies, in: *Laboratory Diagnostic Procedures in the Rheumatic Diseases,* 2nd ed. (A. S. Cohen, ed.), Little, Brown and Company, Boston, pp. 159–206.
13. Notman, D. D., Kurata, N., and Tan, E. M., 1975, Profiles of antinuclear antibodies in systemic rheumatic disease, *Ann. Intern. Med.* 83:464–469.
14. Svec, K. H. and Viet, B. C., 1967, Age-related anti-nuclear factors: Immunologic characteristics and associated clinical aspects, *Arthritis Rheum.* 10:509–516.
15. Alarcon-Segovia, D. and Fishbein, E., 1975, Patterns of anti-nuclear antibodies and lupus activating drugs, *J. Rheumatol.* 2:167–171.
16. Davis, J. S., 1981, Anti-nuclear antibodies (ANA), in: *Textbook of Rheumatology,* (W. N. Kelley, E. D. Harris, Jr., S. Ruddy, and C. B. Sledge, eds.) W. B. Saunders Company, Philadelphia, pp. 694–697.
17. Chubick, A., Sontheimer, R. D., Gilliam, J. N., and Ziff, M., 1978, An appraisal of tests for native DNA antibodies in connective tissuse disease, *Ann. Intern. Med.* 89:186–192.
18. Lloyd, W. and Schur, P. H., 1981, Immune complexes, complement, and anti-DNA in exacerbations of systemic lupus erythematosus (SLE), *Medicine* 60:208–217.
19. Richardson, B. and Epstein, W. V., 1981, Utility of the flourescent anti-nuclear antibody test in a single patient, *Ann. Intern Med.* 95:333–338.
20. Harris, E. D., Jr., 1981, Pathogenesis of rheumatoid arthritis, in: *Textbook of Rheumatology* (W. N. Kelley, E. D. Harris, Jr., S. Ruddy, and C. B. Sledge, eds.), W. B. Saunders Company, Philadelphia, pp. 896–927.
21. Ropes, M. W., Bennett, G. A., Cobb, S., Jacox, R., and Jessar, R. A., 1958, 1958 revision of diagnostic criteria for rheumatoid arthritis, *Bull. Rheum. Dis.* 9:175–176.
22. Engel, A., Roberts, J., and Burch, T. A., 1966, Rheumatoid arthritis in adults in the United States 1960–1962, in: *Vital and Health Statistics,* Series 11, Data from the National Health Survey, Number 17, National Center for Health Statistics, Washington, D.C.

23. Cathcart, E. S. and O'Sullivan, J. B., 1970, Rheumatoid arthritis in a New England town: A prevalence study in Sudbury, Massachusetts, *N. Engl. J. Med.* 282:421–424.

24. Lenos, A., Worthington, J. W., O'Fallon, W. M., and Kurland, L. T., 1980, The epidemiology of rheumatoid arthritis in Rochester, Minnesota: A study of incidence, prevalence, and mortality, *Am. J. Epidemiol.* 111:87–98.

25. Christian, C. L., 1979, Rheumatoid arthritis, in: *Textbook of Medicine* (P. Beeson, W. McDermott, and J. B., Wyngaarden, eds.), W. B. Saunders Company, Philadelphia, pp. 186–187.

26. Moesmann, G., 1968, Subacute rheumatoid arthritis in old age, 1., *Acta. Rheum. Scand.* 14:14–23.

27. Erlich, G. E., Katz, W. A., and Cohen, S. H., 1970, Rheumatoid arthritis in the elderly, *Geriatrics,* 25:103–113.

28. Brown, J. W. and Sones, D. A., 1967, The onset of rheumatoid arthritis in the aged, *J. Am. Geriat. Soc.* 15:873–881.

29. Pearson, C. M., Barnett, E., Kroening, R., Mormor, L., Murray, J. F., Peter, J. B., and Salick, A., 1966, Rheumatoid arthritis and its systemic manifestations, *Ann. Intern. Med.* 65:1101–1130.

30. Short, C. L., 1968, Rheumatoid arthritis: Types of course and prognosis, *Med. Clin. N. Am.* 52:549–557.

31. Lockie, L. M. and Talbot, J. H., 1956, Arthritis in the aged, *JAMA* 162:1514–1517.

32. Corrigan, A. B., Robinson, R. G., Terenty, T. R., Dick-Smith, J. B., and Walters, D., 1974, Benign rheumatoid arthritis of the aged, *Br. Med. J.* 1:444–445.

33. Deal, C., Goldenberg, D., Meenan, R., Sack, B., Pastan, R., and Cohen, A. S., 1981, Elderly onset rheumatoid arthritis: A comparison with earlier onset, matched for disease duration, *Arthritis Rheum.* 24:599 (abstract).

34. Jacoby, R. K., Jayson, M. I. V., and Cosh, J. A., 1973, Onset, early stages and prognosis of rheumatoid arthritis: A clinical study of 100 patients with 11-year follow-up, *Br. Med. J.* 2:96–100.

35. Ruddy, S., 1981, The management of rheumatoid arthritis, *Textbook of Rheumatology* (W. N. Kelley, E. D. Harris, Jr., S. Ruddy, and C. B. Sledge, eds.),W. B. Saunders Company, Philadelphia, pp. 1000–1014.

36. Simon, L. S. and Mills, J. A., 1980, Nonsteroidal anti-inflammatory drugs, *N. Engl. J. Med.* 302:1179–1185, 1237–1243.

37. Bunch, T. W. and O'Duffy, J. D., 1980, Disease-modifying drugs for progressive rheumatoid arthritis, *Mayo Clin. Proc.* 55:161–179.

38. Dubois, E. L., 1974, *Lupus Erythematosus: A Review of the Current Status of Disease and Systemic Lupus Erythematosus,* 2nd ed. University of Southern California Press, Los Angeles.

39. Fries, J. F. and Holman, H. R., 1975, *Systemic Lupus Erythematosus,* W. B. Saunders Company, Philadelphia.

40. Ropes, M. W., 1976, *Systemic Lupus Erythematosus,* Harvard University Press, Cambridge, Massachusetts.

41. Rothfield, N., 1981, Clinical features of systemic lupus erythematosus, in: *Textbook of Rheumatology,* (W. N. Kelley, E. D. Harris, Jr., S. Ruddy, and C. B. Sledge, eds.) W. B. Saunders Company, Philadelphia, pp. 1106–1132.

42. Rothfield, N. F., 1979, Lupus erythematosus, in: *Dermatology in General Medicine,* 2nd ed. (T. Fitzpatrick, ed.), McGraw-Hill Book Company, New York, pp. 1273–1298.

43. Matthay, R. A., Schwarz, M. I., Petty, T. L., Stanford, R. E., Gupta, R. C., Sahn, S. A., and Steigerwald, T. C., 1974, Pulmonary manifestations of systemic lupus erythematosus: Review of 12 cases of acute lupus pneumonitis, *Medicine* 54:397–409.

44. Labowitz, B. and Schumacher, H. R., 1971, Articular manifestations of systemic lupus erythematosus, *Ann. Intern. Med.* 74:911–921.

45. Budman, D. R. and Steinberg, A. D., 1977, Hematologic aspects of systemic lupus erythematosus, *Ann. Intern. Med.* 86:220–229.

46. Baldwin, D. S., Gluck, M. C., Lowenstein, J. and Gallo, G. R., 1977, Lupus nephritis, *Am. J. Med.* 62:12–30.

47. Feinglass, E. J., Arnett, F. C., Dorsch, C. A., Zizic, T. M., and Stevens, M. B., 1976, Neuropsychiatric manifestations of systemic lupus erythematosus: Diagnosis, clinical spectrum and relationship to other features of the disease, *Medicine* 55:323–339.

48. Steinberg, A. D., 1979, Studies of immune regulation, in: *Systemic Lupus Erythematosus; Evolving Concepts* (J. Decker, moderator), *Ann. Intern. Med.* 91:587–592.

49. Frank, M. M., Hamburger, M. I., Lawley, T. J., Kimberly, R. P., and Plotz, P. H., 1979, Defective Fc-receptor function in lupus erythematosus, *N. Engl. J. Med.* 300:518–523.

50. Reinertsen, J. L., Klippel, J. H., Johnson, A. H., Steinberg, A. D., Decker, J. L., and Mann, D. L., 1978, B-lymphocyte alloantigens associated with systemic lupus erythematosus, *N. Engl. J. Med.* 299:515–518.

51. Cohen, A. S., Reynolds, W. E.. Franklin, E. L., Kulka, J. P., Ropes, M. L., Shulman, L. E., and Wallace, S. N., 1971, Preliminary criteria for the classification of systemic lupus erythematosus, *Bull. Rheum. Dis.* 21:643–648.

52. Foad, B. S. I., Sheon, R. P., and Kirsner, A. B., 1972, Systemic lupus erythematosus in the elderly, *Arch. Int. Med.* 130:743–746.

53. Dimant, J., Ginzler, E. M., Schlesinger, M., Diamond, H. S., and Kaplan, D., 1979, Systemic lupus erythematosus in the older age group: Computer analysis, *J. Amer. Geriat. Soc.* 27:58–61.

54. Baker, S. B., Rovera, J. R., Campion, E. W., and Mills, J. A., 1979, Late onset systemic lupus erythematosus, *Am. J. Med.* 66:727–732.

55. Wilson, H. A., Winfield, J. B., Hamilton, M. E., Spyker, D. A., Brunner, C. M., and Davis, J. S., 1979, Serologic studies in late onset systemic lupus erythematosus, *Arthritis Rheum.* 22:674 (abstract).

56. Ballou, S. P., Khan, M. A., and Kirshner, I., 1982, Clinical features of systemic lupus erythematosus: Differences related to race and age of onset, *Arthritis Rheum.* 25:55–60.

57. Siegel, M. and Lee, S. L., 1973, The epidemiology of systemic lupus erythematosus, *Sem. Arth. Rheum.* 3:1–54.

58. Maddock, R. K., 1965, Incidence of systemic lupus erythematosus by age and sex, *JAMA* 191:137–138.

59. Urowitz, M. B., Steven, M. D., and Shulman, L. E., 1967, The influence of age on

the clinical pattern of systemic lupus erythematosus, *Arthritis Rheum.* 10:319–320 (abstract).

60. Hess, E. V. and Hahn, B., 1978, Influenza immunization in lupus erythematosus: Safe, effective?, *Ann. Intern. Med.* 88:833–834.

61. Klippel, J. H., Karsh, J., Stahl, N. I., Decker, J. L., Steinberg, A. D., and Schiffman, G., 1979, A controlled study of pneumococcal polysaccharide vaccine in systemic lupus erythematosus, *Arthritis Rheum.* 22:1321–1325.

62. Alarcon-Segovia, D., 1975, Drug-induced systemic lupus erythematosus and related syndromes, *Clin. Rheum. Dis.* 1:573–582.

63. Lee, S. L. and Chase, P. H., Drug induced systemic lupus: A critical review, *Sem. Arth. Rheum.* 5:83–103.

64. Giansiracusa, D. F. and Kantrowitz, F. G., 1982, Systemic Lupus Erythematosus and drug-induced lupuslike syndromes, *Rheumatic and Metabolic Bone Diseases in the Elderly,* The Collamore Press, Lexington, Massachusetts, pp. 69–82.

65. Rothfield, N. F., Bierer, W. F., and Garfield, J. W., 1978, Isoniazid induction of antinuclear antibodies, *Ann. Intern. Med.* 88:650–652.

66. Blomgren, S. E., Condemi, J. J., and Bignall, M. C., 1969, Antinuclear antibody induced by procainamide. A prospective study, *N. Engl. J. Med.* 281:64–66.

67. Hildreth, E. A., Biro, C. E., and McCreary, T. A., 1960, Persistence of the "hydralazine syndrome": A follow-up study of eleven cases, *JAMA* 173:657–660.

68. Perry, H. M., Jr., 1972, Late toxicity to hydralazine resembling systemic lupus erythematosus or rheumatoid arthritis, *Am. J. Med.* 54:58–72.

69. Alarcon-Segovia, D., Fishbein, E., and Alcala, H., 1971, Isoniazid acetylation rate and development of antinuclear antibodies upon isoniazid therapy, *Arthritis Rheum.* 14:748–752.

70. Perry, J. M., Jr., Tan., E. M., Carmody, S., and Sakamoto, A., 1970, Relationship of acetyltransferase activity to anti-nuclear and toxic symptoms in hypertensive patients treated with hydralazine, *J. Lab. Clin. Med.* 76:114–125.

71. Woolsey, R. L., Drayer, D. E., Reidenberg, M. M., Nies, A. S., Carr, K., and Oates, J. A., 1978, Effect of acetylator phenotype on the rate at which procainamide induces anti-nuclear antibodies and the lupus syndrome, *N. Engl. J. Med.* 298:1157–1159.

72. Lahita, R., Kluger, J., and Drayer, D. E., 1979, Antibodies to nuclear antigens in patients treated with procainamide or acetylprocainamide, *N. Engl. J. Med.* 301:1387–1388.

73. Kluger, J., Drayer, D. E., Reidenberg, M. M. and Lahita, R., 1981, Acetylprocainamide therapy in patients with previous procainamide-induced lupus syndrome. *Ann. Intern. Med.* 95:18–23.

74. Reza, M. J., Dornfeld, L., and Goldberg, L. S., 1975, Hydralazine therapy in hypertensive patients with idiopathic systemic lupus erythematosus, *Arthritis Rheum.* 18:335–338.

75. Blomgren, S. E., Condemi, J. J., and Vaugh, J. H., 1972, Procainamide-induced lupus erythematosus: Clinical and laboratory observations, *Am. J. Med.* 52:338–348.

76. Giansiracusa, D. F. and Kantrowitz, F. D., 1982, Sjogren Syndrome, *Rheumatic and Metabolic Bone Diseases in the Elderly,* The Collamore Press, Lexington, Massachusetts, pp. 83–90.

77. Whaley, K., Williamson, J., Wilson, T., McGavin, M. M., Hughes, G. R. U., Hughes, H., and Schmulian, L. R., 1972, Sjogren's syndrome and autoimmunity in the geriatric population, *Age Aging,* 1:197–206.

78. Forstot, J. Z., Forstot, S. L., Greer, R., and Tan, E. M., 1982, The incidence of Sjogren's sicca complex in a population of patients with keratoconjunctivitis sicca, *Arthritis Rheum.* 25:156–160.

79. Daniels, T. E., Powell, M. R., Sylvester, R. A., and Talal, N., 1979, An evaluation of salivary scintigraphy in Sjogren's syndrome, *Arthritis Rheum.* 22:809–814.

80. Greenspan, J. S., Daniels, T. E., Talal, N., and Sylvester, R. A., 1974, The histopathology of Sjogren's syndrome in labial salivary gland biopsies, *Oral Surg.* 37:217–229.

81. Daniels, T. E., Silverman, S., Michalski, J. P., Greenspan, J. S., Sylvester, R. A., and Talal, N., 1975, The oral component of Sjogren's syndrome, *Oral Surg.* 39:875–885.

82. Strand, V. and Talal, N., 1979–80, Advances in the diagnosis and concept of Sjogren's syndrome (autioimmune exocrinopathy), *Bull. Rheum. Dis.* 30:1046–1052.

83. Whaley, K., Williamson, S., Chrisholm, D. M., Mason, D. K., and Buchanan, W. W., 1973, Sjogren's Syndrome, *Q. J. Med.* 42:279–304.

84. Anderson, L. G. and Talal, N., 1971, The spectrum of benign to malignant lymphoproliferation in Sjogren's syndrome, *Clin. Exp. Immunol.* 9:199–221.

85. Whaley, K., Webb, J., McAvoy, B. A., Hughes, G. R. V., Lee, P., MacSween, R. N. M., and Buchanon, W. N., 1973, Sjogren's syndrome II. Clinical associations and immunological phenomena, *Q. J. Med.* 42:513–548.

86. Kassan, S. S., Thomas, T. L., Moutsopoulos, H. M., Hoover, R., Kimberly, R. P., Budman, D. R., Costa, J., Decker, J. L., and Chused, T. M., 1978, Increased risk of lymphoma in sicca syndrome, *Ann. Intern. Med.* 89:888–892.

87. Alspaugh, M. A., Talal, N., and Tan, E. M., 1976, Differentiation and characterization of autoantibodies and their antigens in Sjogren's syndrome, *Arthritis Rheum.* 19:216–222.

88. Moutsopoulos, H. M., Chused, T. M., Mann, D. L., Klippel, J. H., Fauci, A. S., Frank, M. M., Lawley, J. J., and Hamburger, M. I., 1980, Sjogren's syndrome (sicca syndrome): Current issues, *Ann. Intern. Med.* 92:212–226.

89. Hamburger, M. I., Moutsopoulos, H. M., Lawley, T. J., and Frank, M. M., 1979, Sjogren's syndrome: A defect in reticuloendothelial system Fc-receptor-specific clearance, *Ann. Intern. Med.* 91:534–538.

90. Glenner, G. G., 1980, Amyloid deposits and amyloidosis: The B-fibrilloses, *N. Engl. J. Med.* 302:1283–1292,1333–1343.

91. Isersky, L., Ein, D., Page, A. L., Harada, M., and Glenner, G. G., 1972, Immunochemical cross-reactions of human amyloid proteins with immunoglobulin light polypeptide chains, *J. Immunol.* 108:486–493.

92. Rosenthal, C. J. and Franklin, E. C., 1975, Variations with age and disease of an amyloid A protein-related serum component, *J. Clin. Invest.* 55:746–753.

93. Benson, M. D. and Cohen, A. S., 1979, Serum amyloid A protein in amyloidosis, rheumatic and neoplastic diseases, *Arthritis Rheum.* 22:36–42.

94. Westermark, P., Natvig, J. B., and Johansson, B., 1977, Characterization of an amyloid fibril protein from senile cardiac amyloid, *J. Exp. Med.* 146:631–636.

95. Cornwall, G. G., Natvig, J. B., Westermark, P., and Husby, G., 1978, Senile car-

diac amyloid: Demonstration of a unique fibril protein in tissue sections, *J. Immunol.* 120:1385-1388.

96. Bandt, K., Cathcart, E. S., and Cohen, A. S., 1968, A clinical analysis of the course and prognosis of 42 patients with amyloidosis, *Am. J. Med.* 44:955-969.

97. Kyle, R. A. and Bayrd, E. D., 1975, Amyloidosis: Review of 236 cases, *Medicine,* 54:271-299.

98. Pruzanski, W. and Katz, A., 1976, Clinical and laboratory findings in primary generalized and multiple-myeloma-related amyloidosis, *Can. Med. Assoc. J.* 115:906-909.

99. Ignaczak, T. F., 1981, Amyloidosis, in: *Textbook in Rheumatology* (W. N. Kelley, E. D. Harris, Jr., S. Ruddy, and C. B. Sledge, eds.), W. B. Saunders Company, Philadelphia, pp. 1511-1530.

100. Gordon, D. A., Pruzanski, W., Ogryzlo, M. A., and Little, H. A., 1973, Amyloid arthritis simulating rheumatoid disease in five patients with multiple myeloma, *Am. J. Med.,* 55:142-154.

101. Wright, J. R., Calkins, E., Breen, W. J., Stolte, G., and Schultz, R. T., 1969, Relationship of amyloid to aging, *Medicine,* 48:39-60.

102. Mandybur, T. I., 1975, The incidence of cerebral amyloid angiopathy in Alzheimer's disease, *Neuropathy,* 25:120-126.

103. Glenner, G. G., 1979, Congophilic microangiopathy in the pathogenesis of Alzheimer's syndrome, *Med. Hypoth.* 5:1231-1236.

104. Wright, J. R. and Calkins, E., 1975, Amyloid in the aged heart: Frequency and clinical significance *J. Am. Geriat. Soc.* 23:97-103.

105. Stenkvist, B., Westermark, P., and Wibell, L., 1974, Simple method of diagnostic screening for amyloidosis, *Ann. Rheum. Dis.* 33:75-76.

106. Libbey, C. A., Canoso, J. M., Skinner, M. O. Sipe, J. D., and Cohen, A. S., 1981, Diagnosis of amyloidosis and differentiation of secondary amyloid by analysis of abdominal fat tissue aspirate, *Arthritis Rheum.* 24:125 (abstract).

107. Mikkelson, W., Dodge, H. J., Valkenburg, H., and Hines, S., 1965, The distribution of serum uric acid values in a population unselected as to gout or hyperuricemia, *Am. J. Med.* 39:242-251.

108. Hall, A. P., Barry, P. E., Dawber, T. R., and McNamara, P. M., 1967, Epidemiology of gout and hyperuricemia: A long-term population study. *Am. J. Med.* 42:27-37.

109. O'Sullivan, J. B., 1972, Gout in a New England town: A prevalence study of uric acid levels in Sudbury, Massachusetts, *Ann. Rheum. Dis.* 31:166-169.

110. Wyngaarden, J. B. and Kelley, W. N., 1976, *Gout and Hyperuricemia,* Grune and Stratton, New York.

111. Kelley, W. N., 1981, Gout and related disorders of purine matabolism, in: *Textbook of Rheumatology* (W. N. Kelley, E. D. Harris, Jr., S. Ruddy, and C. B. Sledge, eds.), W. B. Saunders Company, Philadelphia, pp. 1397-1437.

112. Rodman, G. P., 1980, The pathology of Alderman's gout: Procatarctic role of fluctuations in serum urate concentration in gouty arthritis provoked by feast and alcohol, *Arthritis Rheum.* 23:737 (abstract).

113. Snaith, M. L. and Scott, J. T., 1972, Uric acid excretion and surgery, *Ann. Rheum. Dis* 31:162-165.

114. Hadler, N. M., Franck, W. A., Bress, N. M., and Robinson, D. R., 1974, Acute polyarticular gout, *Am. J. Med.* 56:715-719.

115. Liang, M. W. and Fries, J. F., 1978, Asymptomatic hyperuricemia: The case for conservative management, *Ann. Intern. Med.* 88:666–670.

116. Berger, L. and Yu, T. F., 1975, Renal function in gout: An analysis of 524 gout subjects including long-term follow-up, *Am. J. Med.* 56:665–675.

117. Fessel, W. J., 1979, Renal outcomes in gout and hyperuricemia, *Am. J. Med.* 67:74–82.

118. Kelley, W. N., 1981, Approach to the patient with hyperuricemia, in: *Textbook of Rheumatology,* (W. N. Kelley, E. D. Harris, Jr., S. Ruddy, and C. B. Sledge, eds.) W. B. Saunders Company, Philadelphia, pp. 494–500.

119. Gutman, A. B., 1972, Medical management of gout, *Postgrad. Med.* 51:61–66.

120. McCarty, D. J., 1976, Calcium pyrophosphate dehydrate deposition disease, 1975, *Arthritis Rheum.* 19:275–285.

121. Rubinstein, H. M. and Shah, D. M., 1972–1973, Pseudogout, *Sem Arth. Rheum.* 2:259–280.

122. Ellman, M. H. and Levin, B., 1975, Chondrocalcinosis in elderly persons, *Arthritis Rheum.* 18:43–47.

123. O'Duffy, J. D., 1976, Clinical studies of acute pseudogout attacks, *Arthritis Rheum.* 19:349–352.

124. McCarty, D. J. and Kozin, F., 1975, An overview of cellular and molecular mechanisms in crystal-induced inflammation, *Arthritis Rheum.* 18:757–765.

125. Howell, D. S., 1981, Diseases due to the deposition of calcium pyrophosphate and hydroxyapatite, in: *Textbook of Rheumatology* (W. N. Kelley, E. D. Harris, Jr., S. Ruddy, and C. B. Sledge, eds.), W. B. Saunders Company, Philadelphia, pp. 1438–1456.

126. Vanderkorst, J. and Geerards, J., 1976, Articular chondrocalcinosis in a Dutch pedigree, *Arthritis Rheum.* 19:405–409.

127. Reginato, A. M., 1976, Articular chondrocalcinosis in the Chiloe islanders, *Arthritis Rheum.* 19:395–404.

128. Bjelle, A., Edvinsson, U., and Hagstun, A., 1982, Pyrophosphate anthropathy in two Swedish families, *Arthritis Rheum.* 25:66–74.

129. Lust, G., Faure, G., Nelter, P., Gaucher, A., and Seegmiller, J. E., 1981, Evidence of a generalized metabolic defect in patients with hereditary chondrocalcinosis, *Arthritis Rheum.* 24:1517–1521.

130. Hamilton, E. B. D., 1976, Diseases associated with calcium pyrophosphate dihydrate deposition disease, *Arthritis Rheum.* 19:353–357.

131. Howell, D. S., Muniz, O., Pita, J. L., and Enis, J. E., 1976, Pyrophosphate release by osteoarthritis cartilage incubates, *Arthritis Rheum.* 19:488–494.

132. Tennenbaum, J., Muniz, O., and Schumacher, H. R., 1981, Comparison of phosphohydrolase activities from articular cartilage in calcium pyrophosphate dihydrate deposition disease and primary osteoarthritis, *Arthritis Rheum.* 24:492–500.

133. Genant, H. K., 1976, Roentgenographic aspects of calcium pyrophosphate dihydrate crystal deposition disease, *Arthritis Rheum.* 19:307–328.

134. Resnick, D., Nuwayama, G., Goergen, T. G., Utsinger, P. D., Shapiro, R. F., Haselwood, D. H., and Wiesner, K. B., 1977, Clinical, radiographic, and pathologic abnormalities in calcium pyrophosphate dihydrate deposition disease (CPPD): Pseudogout, *Radiology* 122:1–16.

135. McCarty, D. J. and Gatter, R. A., 1966, Recurrent acute inflammation associated with focal apatite crystal deposition, *Arthritis Rheum.* 9:804–819.

136. Dieppe, P. A., Crocker, P., Huskisso, E. C., and Willoughby, D. A., 1976, Apatite deposition disease—A new anthropathy?, *Lancet* i:266-269.
137. Schumacher, H. R., Somlyo, A. P., Tse, R. L., and Maurer, K., 1977, Arthritis associated with apatite crystal, *Ann. Intern. Med.* 87:411-416.
138. Fam, A. G., Pritzker, K. P. H., Stein, J. L., Houpt, J. B., and Little, A. H., 1979, Apatite-associated arthropathy: A clinical study of 14 cases and of 2 patients with calcific bursitis, *J. Rheumatol.* 6:461-471.
139. Sokoloff, L., 1979, Pathology and pathogenesis of osteoarthritis in: *Arthritis* (D. J. McCarty, ed.) Lea and Febiger, Philadelphia, pp. 1135-1153.
140. Moskowitz, R. W., 1979, Clinical and laboratory findings in osteoarthritis, in: *Arthritis* (D. J. McCarty, ed.) Lea and Febiger, Philadelphia, pp. 1161-1180.
141. Bland, J. H. and Stolbert, S. D., 1981, Osteoarthritis: Pathology and clinical patterns, in: *Textbook of Rheumatology* (W. N. Kelley, E. D. Harris, Jr., S. Ruddy, and C. B. Sledge, eds.), W. B. Saunders Company, Philadelphia, pp. 1471-1490.
142. Kellgren, J. H. and Lawrence, J. S., 1958, Osteo-arthrosis and disc degeneration in an urban population, *Ann. Rheum. Dis.* 17:388-397.
143. Lawrence, J. S. Brenner, J. M., and Bier, F., 1966, Osteo-arthrosis prevalence in the population and relationship between symptoms and x-ray changes, *Ann. Rheum. Dis.* 25:1-24.
144. Gordon, T., 1968, Osteoarthrosis in United States adults, in: *Population Studies of the Rheumatic Disease* (P. H. Bennett and P. H. N. Woods, eds.), Excerpta Medica Foundation, New York, pp. 391-397.
145. Kellgren, J. H. and Lawrence, J. S., 1952, Rheumatism in miners, Part II: X-ray study, *Br. J. Ind. Med.* 9:127-207.
146. McDewitt, C. A., 1973, Biochemistry of articular cartilage: Nature of proteoglycans and collagen of articular cartilage and their role in aging and in osteoarthrosis, *Ann. Rheum. Dis.* 32:364-378.
147. Lamberg, S. I. and Stoolmiller, A. C., 1974, Glycosaminoglycans. A biochemical and clinical review, *J. Invest. Derm.* 63:433-449.
148. Lindahl, U. and Hook, M., 1978, Glycosaminoglycans and their binding to biologic macromolecules, *Ann. Rev. Biochem.* 47:385-417.
149. Hardingham, T. E. and Muir, H., 1974, Hyaluronic acid in cartilage and proteoglycan aggregation, *Biochem. J.* 139:565-581.
150. Maroudas, A., Muir, H., and Wingham, J., 1969, The correlation of fixed negative charge with glycosaminoglycan content of human articular cartilage, *Biochem. Biophys. Acta* 177:492-500.
151. Brandt, K. D., 1981, Pathogenesis of osteoarthritis (OA), in: *Textbook of Rheumatology* (W. N. Kelley, E. D. Harris, Jr., S. Ruddy, and C. B. Sledge, eds.), W. B. Saunders Company, Philadelphia, pp. 1457-1470.
152. Radin, E. L., 1976, Mechanical aspects of osteoarthritis, *Bull. Rheum. Dis.* 26:862-868.
153. Bollet, A. J. and Nance, J. L., 1966, Biochemical findings in normal and osteoarthritic articular cartilage II. Chondroitin sulfate concentration and chain length, water, and ash contents, *J. Clin. Invest.* 45:1170-1177.
154. Mankin, H. J., 1974, The reaction of articular cartilage to injury and osteoarthritis, *N. Engl. J. Med.* 291:1285-1292, 1335-1340.
155. Mankin, H. J. and Lippiello, L., 1970, Biochemical and metabolic abnormalities

in articular cartilage from osteoarthritic human hips, *J. Bone Joint Surg.* 52A:424–434.

156. Mankin, H. J., Dorfman, H., Lippiello, L., and Zarius, A., 1971, Biochemical and metabolic abnormalities in articular cartilage from osteoarthritic hips, *J. Bone Joint Surg.* 53A:523–537.

157. Mankin, H. J. and Lippiello, L., 1971, The glycosaminoglycans of normal and arthritic cartilage, *J. Clin. Invest.* 50:1712–1719.

158. Brandt, K. D. and Palmoski, M., 1976, Organization of ground substance proteoglycans in normal and osteoarthritic knee cartilage, *Arthritis Rheum.* 19:209–215.

159. Bayliss, M. T. and Ali, S. Y., 1978, Age-related changes in the composition and structure of human articular cartilage proteoglycans, *Biochem. J.* 176:683–693.

160. Roughly, P. J. and White, R. J., 1980, Age-related changes in the structure of proteoglycan subunits from human articular cartilage, *J. Biol. Chem.* 225:217–225.

161. Perricone, E., Palmoski, M. J., and Brandt, K. D., 1977, Failure of proteoglycans to form aggregates in morphologically normal aged human hip cartilage, *Arthritis Rheum.* 20:1372–1380.

163. Bollet, A. J., 1969, An essay on the biology of osteoarthritis, *Arthritis Rheum.* 12:152–163.

163. Lee, P., Rooney, P. J., Sturrock, R. D., Kennedy, A. L., and Dick, W. C., 1974, The etiology and pathogenesis of osteoarthritis: A review, *Sem. Arth. Rheum.* 3:189–218.

164. Giansiracusa, D. F. and Kantrowitz, F. G., 1982, Articular cartilage: Changes associated with aging and osteoarthritis, in: *Rheumatic and Metabolic Bone Disease in the Elderly,* The Collamore Press, Lexington, Massachusetts, pp. 27–43.

165. Goldstein, I. M., Perez, H. D., and Weksler, B. B., 1981, Oxygen-derived free radicals and inflammation: Role of arachadonic acid, *Sem. Arthritis Rheum.* 11:99–101.

166. Kellgren, J. H. and Moore, R., 1952, Generalized osteoarthritis and Heberden's nodes, *Br. Med. J.* 1:181–187.

167. Stecher, R. M., 1955, Heberden's nodes: A clinical description of osteoarthritis of the finger joints, *Ann. Rheum. Dis.* 14:1–10.

168. Kellgren, J. H., Lawrence, J. S., and Bier, F., 1963, Genetic factors in generalized osteoarthrosis, *Ann. Rheum. Dis.* 22:237–255.

169. Hadler, N. M., Gillings, D. B., Imbers, H. R., Leviton, P. M., Makur, D., Utsinger, P. D., Yount, W. J., Slusser, D., and Moscovitz, N., 1977, Hand structure and function in an industrial setting, *Arthritis Rheum.* 21:210–220.

170. Schumacher, H. R., 1964, Hemochromatosis and arthritis, *Arthritis Rheum.* 7:41–50.

171. Feller, E. R. and Schumacher, H. R., 1972, Osteoarticular changes in Wilson's disease, *Arthritis Rheum.* 15:259–266.

172. Schumacher, H. R. and Holdsworth, D. E., 1977, Ochronotic arthropathy. I. Clinicopathologic studies, *Sem. Arthr. Rheum.* 6:207–246.

173. McCarty, D. J., 1979, Calcium pyrophosphate crystal deposition disease: Pseudogout: Articular chondrocalcinosis, in: *Arthritis* (D. J. McCarty, ed.),Lea and Febiger, Philadelphia, p. 1279–1299.

174. Dorwart, B. B. and Schumacher, H. R., 1975, Joint effusion, chondrocalcinosis and other rheumatic manifestations in hypothyroidism: A clinical study, *Am. J. Med.* 59:780–790.

175. Franck, W. A., Bress, W. M., Singer, F. R., and Krane, S. M., 1974, Rheumatic manifestations of Paget's disease of bone, *Am. J. Med.* 56:592–603.
176. Kenzora, J. E. and Gilmcher, M. J., 1981, Osteonecrosis, in: *Textbook of Rheumatology* (W. N. Kelley, E. D. Harris, Jr., S. Ruddy, and C. B. Sledge, eds.),W. B. Saunders Company, Philadelphia, pp. 1755–1779.
177. Murray, R. O., 1965, The etiology of primary osteoarthritis of the hip, *Br. J. Radiol.* 38:810–824.
178. Solomon, L., 1976, Patterns of osteoarthritis in the hip, *J. Bone Joint Surg.* 58B:176–183.
179. Leach, R. E., Baumgard, S., and Broom, J., 1973, Obesity: Its relationship to osteoarthritis of the knee, *Clin. Orthop. Rel. Res.* 93:271–273.
180. Greenwald, A. S. and Matejczyk, M. B., 1978, Articular cartilage contact areas of the ankle, *Ann. Rheum. Dis.* 37:482 (abstract).
181. Moskowitz, R. W., 1981, Management of osteoarthritis, *Bull. Rehum. Dis.* 31:31–35.
182. Calin, A. 1981, Ankylosing spondylitis, in: *Textbook of Rheumatology* (W. N. Kelley, E. D. Harris, Jr., S. Ruddy, and C. B. Sledge, eds.),W. B. Saunders Company, Philadelphia, pp. 1017–1032.
183. Giansiracusa, D. F. and Kantrowitz, F. G., Articular cartilage: Changes associated with aging and osteoarthritis, *Rheumatic and Metabolic Bone Disease in the Elderly,* The Collamore Press, Lexington, Massachusetts, pp. 119–134.
184. Rosenow, E. L., Strimlan, C. V., Meehan, J. R., and Ferguson, R. H., 1977, Pleuropulmonary manifestations of ankylosing spondylitis, *Mayo Clin. Proc.* 52:641–649.
185. Hunter, T. and Dubo, H., 1978, Spinal fractures complicating ankylosing spondylitis, *Ann. Intern. Med.* 88:546–549.
186. Russell, M. L., Gordon, D. A., Ogryzlo, M. A., and McPhedran, R. S., 1973, The cauda equina syndrome of ankylosing spondylitis, *Ann. Intern. Med.* 78:551–554.
187. Gordon, A. L. and Yudell, A., 1973, Cauda equina lesion associated with rheumatoid spondylitis, *Ann. Intern. Med.* 78:555–557.
188. Sorensen, P. S. and Lorenzen, I., 1977, Temporal arteritis and polymyalgia rheumatica, *Acta Med. Scand.* 201:207–213.
189. Ettlinger, R. E., Hunder, G. G., and Ward, L. E., 1978, Polymyalgia rheumatica and giant cell arteritis, *Ann. Rev. Med.* 29:15–22.
190. Goodman, B. W., 1979, Temporal arteritis, *Am. J. Med.* 67:839–852.
191. Bengtsson, B. and Malmwall, B., 1981, The epidemiology of giant cell arteritis including temporal arteritis and polymyalgia rheumatica, *Arthritis Rheum.* 24:899–904.
192. Huston, K. A., Hunder, G. G., Lie, J. T., Kennedy, R. H., and Elveback, L. R., 1978, Temporal arteritis: A 25 year epidemiologic, clinical, and pathologic study, *Ann. Intern. Med.* 88:162–167.
193. Calamia, K. T. and Hunder, G. G. 1980, Clinical manifestations of giant cell arteritis, *Clin. Rheum. Dis.* 6:389–403.
194. O'Duffy, D. J., Wanner, H. W., and Hunder, G. G., 1976. Joint imaging in polymyalgia rheumatica, *Mayo Clin. Proc.* 51:519–524.
195. Hunder, G. G. and Hazleman, B. L., 1981, Giant cell arteritis and polymyalgia rheumatica, in: *Textbook of Rheumatology* (W. N. Kelley, E. D. Harris, Jr., S.

Ruddy, and C. B. Sledge, eds.),W. B. Saunders Company, Philadelphia, pp. 1189–1198.

196. Giansiracusa, D. F. and Kantrowitz, F. G., 1982, Polymyaglia rheumatica and giant cell arteritis, in: *Rheumatica and Metabolic Bone Disease in the Elderly*, The Collamore Press, Lexington, Massachusetts, pp. 97–105.

197. Hunder, G. G. and Allen, G. L., 1978–1979, Giant cell arteritis: A review, *Bull. Rheum. Dis.* 29:980–987.

198. Williamson, I. M. S. and Russel, R. W. R., 1972, Arteritis of the head and neck in giant cell arteritis: A pathological study to show the pattern of arterial involvement. *Arch. Neurol.* 27:378–391.

199. Klein, R. G., Hunder, G. G., Stanson, A. W., and Sheps, S. G., 1975, Larger artery involvement in giant cell (temporal) arteritis, *Ann. Intern. Med.* 83:806–812.

200. Healy, L. A. and Wilske, K. R., 1980, Presentation of occult giant cell arteritis, *Arthritis Rheum.* 23:641–643.

201. Calamia, K. T. and Hunder, G. G., 1981, Giant cell arteritis (temporal arteritis) presenting as fever of unknown origin, *Arthritis Rheum.* 24:1414–1418.

202. Long, R. and James, O., 1974, Polymyalgia rheumatica and liver disease, *Lancet* i:77–79.

203. Litwack, K. D., Bohan, A., and Silverman, L., 1977, Granulomatous hepatitis and giant cell arteritis, *J. Rheumatol.* 4:307–312.

204. Klein, R. G., Campbell, R. J., Hunder, G. G., and Carney, J. A., 1976, Skip lesions in temporal arteritis, *Mayo Clin. Proc.* 51:504–510.

205. Sewell, R. R., Allison, D. J., Tarin, D., and Hughes, G. L., 1980, Combined temporal arteriography and selective biopsy in suspected giant cell arteritis, *Ann. Rheum. Dis.* 39:124–128.

206. Schneider, H. A., Weber, A. A., and Ballen, P. A., 1971, The visual prognosis in temporal arteritis, *Ann. Ophthal.* 3:1215–1230.

207. Jones, J. G. and Hazleman, B. L., 1981, Prognosis and management of polymyalgia rheumatica, *Ann. Rheum. Dis.* 40:1–5.

208. Altman, R. D. and Tennenbaum, J., 1981, Hypertrophic osteoarthropathy, in: *Textbook of Rheumatology* (W. N. Kelley, E. D. Harris, Jr., S. Ruddy, and C. B. Sledge, eds.),W. B. Saunders Company, Philadelphia, pp. 1647–1657.

209. Schumacher, H. R., 1976, Articular manifestations of hypertrophic pulmonary osteoarthropathy in bronchogenic carcinoma, *Arthritis Rheum.* 19:629–636.

210. Calabro, J. J., 1967, Cancer and arthritis, *Arthritis Rheum.* 10:553–567.

211. Robinson, D. R. and Vickery, A. L., Jr., 1978, Case record, *N. Engl. J. Med.* 299:708–714.

212. Evans, W. K., 1980, Reversal of hypertrophic osteoarthropathy after chemotherapy for bronchogenic carcinoma, *J. Rheumatol.* 7:93–97.

213. Lopez-Enriquez, E. Morales, A. R., and Robert, F., 1980, Effect of atropine sulfate in pulmonary hypertrophic osteoarthropathy, *Arthritis Rheum.* 23:822–824.

214. Auerback, M. D. and Brooks, P. M., 1981, Role of immune complexes in hypertrophic osteoarthropathy and non-metastatic polyarthritis, *Ann. Rheum. Dis.* 40:470–472.

215. Rees, L., 1975, The biosynthesis of hormones by nonendocrine tumors, *J. Endocrinol.* 67:143–175.

216. MacKenzie, A. H. and Scherbel, A. L., 1963, Connective tissue syndromes associated with carcinoma, *Geriatrics* 18:745–753.

217. Sheon, R. P., Kirsner, A. B., Tangsintanapas, P., Samuel, F., Garg, M. L., and Finkel, R. I., 1977, Malignancy in rheumatic disease: Interrelationships, *J. Am. Geriat. Soc.* 25:20-27.

218. Bennett, R. M., Ginsberg, M. H., and Thomsea, S., 1976, Carcinomatous polyarthritis. The presenting symptoms of an ovarian tumor and association with platelet activating factor, *Arthritis Rheum.* 19:953-958.

219. Isomaki, H. A., Mutru, O., and Koota, K., 1975, Death rates and causes of death in patients with rheumatoid arthritis, *Scand. J. Rheumatol.* 4:205-208.

220. Lewis, R. B., Castor, C. W., Kinsley, R. E., and Boles, G. G., 1976, Frequency of neoplasia in systemic lupus erythematous and rheumatoid arthritis, *Arthritis Rheum.* 19:1256-1260.

221. Kinlea, L. J., Sheil, A. G. R., Peto. J., and Doll, R., 1979, Collaborative United Kingdom-Australiasian study of cancer in patients treated with immunosuppressive drugs, *Br. Med. J.* 2:1461-1466.

222. Lewis, D., Hazleman, B. L., Hanka, R., and Roberts, S., 1980, Cause of death in patients with rheumatoid arthritis with particular reference to azathioprine, *Ann. Rheum. Dis.* 39:457-461.

223. Bohan, A., Peter, J. B., Bowman, R. L., and Pearson, C. M., 1977, A computer-assisted analysis of 153 patients with polymyositis and dermatomyositis, *Medicine* 56:255-286.

224. DeVere, R. and Bradley, W. G., 1975, Polymyositis: Its presentation, morbidity and mortality, *Brain* 98:637-666.

225. Callen, J. P., Hyla, J. F.. Boles, G. G., Jr., and Kay, D. R., 1980, The relationship of dermatomyositis and polymyositis to internal malignancy, *Arch Derm.* 116:295-298.

226. Barnes, B. E., 1976, Dermatomyositis and malignancy: A review of the literature, *Ann. Intern. Med.* 84:68-76.

227. Callen, J. P., 1981, The value of malignancy evaluation in patients with dermatomyositis, *Arthritis Rheum.* 24:S103 (abstract)

228. Murray, G. C. and Persellin, R. H., 1980, Metastatic carcinoma presenting as monoarticular arthritis, *Arthritis Rheum.* 23:95-100.

229. Spilberg, I. and Meyer, G. J., 1972, The arthritis of leukemia, *Arthritis Rheum.* 15:630-635.

230. Virshup, A. M. and Sliwinski, A. J., 1973, Polyarthritis and subcutaneous nodules in a patient with carcinoma of the pancreas, *Arthritis Rheum.* 16:388-392.

231. Morgan, G. J., Jr., 1981, Panniculitis and erythema nodosum, in: *Textbook of Rheumatology* (W. N. Kelley, E. D. Harris, Jr., S. Ruddy, and C. B. Sledge, eds.), W. B. Saunders Company, Philadelphia, pp. 1203-1207.

232. Giansiracussa, D. F. and Kantrowitz, F. G., 1982, Medication used in the management of rheumatic diseases, in: *Rheumatic and Metabolic Diseases in the Elderly,* Collamore Press, Lexington, Massachusetts, pp. 145-156.

233. Ferreira, S. H. and Vane, J. R., 1974, New aspects of the mode of action of non-steroidal anti-inflammatory drugs, *Ann. Rev. Pharmacol. Toxicol.* 14:57-73.

234. Weiss, B. and Hait, W. N., 1977, Selective cyclic nucleotide phosphodieterase inhibitors as potential therapeutic agents, *Ann. Rev. Pharmacol. Toxicol.* 17:441-477.

235. Lehmeyer, J. E. and Johnston, R. B. Jr., 1978, Effect of anti-inflammatory drugs and agents that elevate intraceullar cyclic AMP in the release of toxic oxygen

metabolites by phagocytes; studies in a model of tissue bound IgG, *Clin. Immunol. Immunopathol.* 9:482–490.

236. New drugs for arthritis, 1976, *Med. Lett.* 18:77–79.

237. Woodbury, D. M., 1971, Analgesics, antipyretics, anti-inflammatory agents, and inhibitors or uric acid synthesis, in: *The Pharmacological Basis of Therapeutics* (L. S. Goodman and A. Gilman, eds.), The MacMillan Co., New York, pp. 325–366.

238. Mann, N. S. and Sachdeu, A. J., 1977, Acute erosive gastritis, induced by aspirin, ketoprofen, ibuprofen, and naproxen: Its prevention by metiamide and cimetadine, *South Med. J.* 70:562–564.

239. Baskin, W. N., Ivey, K. J., Krause, W. J., Jeffrey, G. E., and Gemmell, R. T., 1976, Aspirin-induced ultrastructural changes in human gastric mucosa, *Ann. Intern. Med.* 85:299–303.

240. Kivilaakso, E. and Silen, W., 1979, Pathogenesis of experimental gastric-mucosal injury, *N. Engl. J. Med.* 301:364–369.

241. Famaey, J. P. Brooks, P. M., and Carson. D. W., 1975, Biological effects on non-steroidal anti-inflammatory drugs, *Sem. Arthr. Rheum.* 5:63–81.

242. Zucher, M. B. and Peterson, J., 1970, Effect of acetylsalicylic acid, other nonsteroidal anti-inflammatory agents, and dipyridanole in human blood platelets. *J. Lab. Clin. Med.* 76:66–75.

243. Kimberly, R. P., Bowden, R. E., Keisner, H. R., and Plotz, P. H., 1978, Reduction of renal function by newer nonsteroidal anti-inflammatory drugs, *Am. J. Med.* 64:804–807.

244. Huskisson, E. C., 1975, Anti-inflammatory drugs, *Sem. Arthr. Rheum.* 7:1–20.

245. Fowler, P., 1975, Indomethacin and phenylbutazone, *Clin. Rheum. Dis.* 1:267–283.

246. Szczeklik, A., Gryglewski, R. M., and Czerniawksa-Mysik, G., 1977, Clinical patterns of hypersensitivity to nonsteroidal anti-inflammatory drugs and their pathogenesis, *J. Allergy Clin. Immunol.* 60:276–284.

247. Weinberger, M., 1978, Analgesic sensitivity in children with asthma, *Pediatrics* 62:910–915.

248. Salmon, J. E. and Kimberly, R. P., 1981, Formulary, in: *Manual of Rheumatology and Outpatient Orthopedic Disorders* (J. F. Beary, C. C. Christian, and T. P. Sculco, eds.), Little Brown and Co., Boston, Massachusetts.

249. Hoffman, L. M., Krupnick, M. I., and Garcia, H. A., 1972, Interactions of spironolactone and hydrochlorthiazide with aspirin in the dog and rat, *J. Pharmacol. Exp. Ther.* 180:1–5.

250. Wiseman, E. H. and Hobbs, D. C., 1982, Review of pharmacokinetic studies with Piroxicam, *Am. J. Med.* (Supplement) 2:9–17.

251. Smith, A., Mucklow, J. C., and Wandless, I., 1979, Compliance with drug treatment, *Br. Med. J.* 2:1335–1336.

252. Axelrod, L., 1976, Glucocorticoid therapy, *Medicine* 55:39–65.

253. Buckingham, R. B., 1978, Interactions involving anti-rheumatic agents, *Bull. Rheum. Dis.* 28:960–966.

254. Hahn, T. J. and Hahn, B. H., 1976, Osteopenia in patients with rheumatic disease: Principles of diagnosis and therapy, *Sem. Arthr. Rheum.* 6:165–188.

255. Fucik, R. F., Kukreja, S. C., Hargis, G. K., Bowser, E. N., Hunderson, W. J., and Williams, G. A., 1975, Effect of glucocorticoids in function of the parathyroid glands in man, *J. Clin. Endocrinol. Metab.* 40:152–155.

256. Gottlieb, W. C. and Brown, H. E., 1972, Acute myocardial infarction following gold sodium thiomalate induced vasomotor (nitritoid) reaction, *Arthritis Rheum.* 20:1026–1028.
257. Lintz, R. M., 1941, Toxic reactions with gold salts in treatment of rheumatic arthritis, *J. Lab. Clin. Med.* 26:1629–1634.
258. Greenberg, M. S. and Zambrano, S. S., 1972, Aplastic agranulocytosis after allopurinol therapy, *Arthritis Rheum.* 15:413–416.
259. Young, J. L., Boswell, R. B., and Nies, A. S., 1974, Severe allopurinol hypersensitivity; association with thiazides and prior renal compromise, *Arch. Intern. Med.* 134:553–558.

Genitourinary Problems in the Elderly

Stephen C. Jacobs and Joseph B. Murphy

5.1. Renal Function

5.1.1. Renal Changes with Aging

The kidneys reach their maximum size in early adult life and then gradually shrink approximately 20% by age 70. The number of glomeruli also decrease such that by age 70, only 50 to 70% of the 800,000 to 1,000,000 present at birth remain. In addition, the basement membrane of the glomerulus thickens with aging and tubular surface area decreases. Renal loss is scattered throughout the kidney, but a disproportionate loss occurs among the juxtamedullary nephrons, perhaps explaining some of the loss of urinary concentrating ability in elderly subjects.[1] These changes appear to occur as part of the normal aging process without the presence of other systemic diseases. Obviously, common disorders of the elderly, such as hypertension and diabetes, will superimpose significant renal disease on the normal aging kidney.

From a functional standpoint, a reduction in creatinine clearance begins in the 30s and accelerates in the 60s and 70s. Rowe et al.[2] found the creatinine clear-

STEPHEN C. JACOBS • Department of Urology, The Medical College of Wisconsin, Milwaukee, Wisconsin 53226; and Urology Section, Surgery Service, Wood Veterans Administration Medical Center, Wood, Wisconsin 53193. JOSEPH B. MURPHY • Department of Urology, The Medical College of Wisconsin, Milwaukee, Wisconsin 53226.

ance fell 30% from the fourth decade to the eighth decade. Interestingly, the serum creatinine varied little throughout life despite the fall in creatinine clearance, an indication of a parallel fall in muscle mass with aging.

Renal blood flow also decreases with age. Although slowly changing in early adult life, this decline accelerates after age 50, such that by the eighth decade, total renal blood flow is only one-half of its peak value.[1] The decrease in renal blood flow is in excess of the decrease in renal weight. This may help explain why aged kidneys are more susceptible to further ischemic insult that may occur with renal surgery, sepsis, or hypotension.

For many years, it has been known that renal concentrating ability is diminished in the aged, i.e., the maximum specific gravity that urine can reach is decreased. For this reason, the elderly may not be able to retain water as well during a period of dehydration. Similarly, the clearance of free water may be impaired leading to an increased tendency for hyponatremia during a period of water excess. The kidney of the aged person seems able to maintain acid–base equilibrium normally within a narrow range; if faced with a large acid or base load, however, return to a normal serum pH will be slower in the elderly.

5.1.2. Acute Renal Failure

Acute renal insufficiency can best be described as a rapid deterioration of glomerular filtration with resultant accumulation of nitrogenous wastes in the body. Often, but not always, there is a decreased urinary flow rate. The causes of acute renal failure can be classified as prerenal, postrenal, or renal parenchymal in origin.

5.1.2.1. Prerenal Azotemia

Prerenal azotemia results from underperfusion of the renal arterioles. The kidney responds approximately to underperfusion by retaining sodium to reexpand effective circulating blood volume. Since the kidney retains salt in an effort to reexpand blood volume, the urinary concentration of sodium will be low (0 to 20 meq/liter).

Extracellular fluid volume may be expanded (congestive heart failure) or contracted (dehydration, nephrotic syndrome, hepatorenal syndrome). There is, however, always decreased effective renal artery perfusion.

Urine osmolality is greater than serum osmolality in prerenal azotemia. Reabsorption is stimulated in patients with prerenal azotemia. Since the kidney can reabsorb urea, BUN rises relatively more than the serum creatinine. Despite this relative stability, serum creatinine does rise in association with severe renal underperfusion. The BUN:creatinine ratio is usually > 10 in prerenal azotemia.

In response to underperfusion, the kidney produces renin to vasoconstrict the arterial system and raise renal artery blood pressure. Secondary aldosteronism accompanies the contraction of effective arterial blood volume causing urinary potassium levels to be high.

Since prerenal azotemia is always secondary to some other problem, treatment should be aimed at the primary cause of renal underperfusion. Fluid losses from the GI tract, GU tract (excessive diuresis), skin, or secondary to hemorrhage must be replaced. If done prior to ischemic renal injury, renal function can be restored to the level existing prior to the insult. However, if the underperfusion is due to a decrease in effective rather than absolute blood volume (as in congestive heart failure), then administration of fluids may be contraindicated. In the latter case, renal function will be restored only when cardiac function is improved.

Although diuretics are appropriate in the treatment of isolated congestive heart failure, the use of diuretics in prerenal azotemia is in general contraindicated. The use of powerful loop diuretics (furosemide, ethacrynic acid) to produce a urine output only makes the effective blood volume and prerenal azotemia worse, especially in the elderly who may already have reduced extracellular and intracellular volume.

5.1.2.2. Acute Parenchymal Renal Failure

Acute parenchymal renal failure may result from acute tubular necrosis (ATN), toxin-induced renal failure,[3] glomerulonephritis, hypertension, renal artery occlusion, and a multitude of disorders affecting the intrarenal vasculature, glomeruli, tubules, and interstitium. ATN is often seen in the absence of identifiable histologic abnormality and might better be thought of as reversible acute tubular dysfunction. Pathophysiologically, ATN results from volume contraction secondary to hypotension, cardiovascular collapse, hemorrhage, or toxins, often combined with hemolysis or rhabdomyolysis. Prevention of ATN can best be accomplished by the prevention of volume contraction. Once the insult has occurred, the patient must be carefully supported until recovery occurs as attempts at lessening the severity of ATN with diuretics or fluid challenges usually are ineffective.

Since the tubules are diseased, there is impaired urinary concentrating ability and decreased reabsorption of sodium. The urine osmolality tends to equal that of the plasma with a sodium concentration < 40 meq/liter. Classically, the urine may contain casts or renal tubular epithelial cells. Usually, ATN can be divided into an early oliguric phase and a late diuretic phase. Some patients, however, develop acute renal failure without the initial oliguric phase. The oliguric phase lasts from days to weeks during which time the 24-hr urine volume is usually between 50 to 400 ml/day. Oliguria rarely lasts longer than 1 month. The presence of anuria is atypical and should suggest another disorder (cortical necrosis, urinary tract obstruction, or renal artery occlusion). The oliguric phase ends with a gradual increase in urine volume, resulting from a diuresis of accumulated edema fluid and not from the inability to conserve fluids and electrolytes as some might think; accumulated urea may also act as an osmotic diuretic. Occasionally, however, diuresis may be massive requiring large amounts of replacement fluid. Recovery of glomerular function may lag behind in the diuretic phase and the initial urine volume increase may not be accompanied by a fall in BUN or creatinine. After several days, however, BUN and creatinine should fall if the correct diagnosis has been made. BUN rises first and falls last, making it a more sensitive indicator of renal failure.

5.1.2.3. Postrenal (Obstructive) Uropathy

Postrenal (obstructive) uropathy must be considered in any patient who develops acute renal failure or even diminished urinary output. Permanent impairment of renal function develops if total upper tract obstruction persists more than 7 days. Early diagnosis is desirable and prevents many unnecessary medical assaults on the patient. An intravenous pyelogram should be obtained in the hydrated patient. Renal visualization may be obtained even with a serum creatinine as high as 5 to 7 mg%. There is no longer a need to dehydrate patients prior to receiving contrast material. Renal and abdominal examination must be performed as part of the initial physical examination of all patients. If there is a question of bladder distention or prostatic enlargement, a catheter should be sterily placed per urethra. If the renal pelvis and ureters have not been visualized by intravenous pyelography, then prompt bilateral retrograde pyelography should be performed.

A postobstructive diuresis may follow relief of urinary tract obstruction. This results from an osmotic diuresis due to the accumulated BUN and a water diuresis to clear accumulated edema fluid. Replacement of large amounts of fluid and electrolytes at this time will only perpetuate these two diureses. Occasionally, impaired tubular reabsorption of salt and water will also be present due to long-standing obstruction. In this situation, circulatory collapse may occur if fluid and electrolytes are not replaced promptly. One method of replacing fluids is to give 80 to 90% of the previous hour's urine output using 0.45 normal saline.

5.1.3. Management of Acute Renal Failure

From the moment potential renal failure is diagnosed, one must prepare for potential vascular access needs. Age is not in itself a criterion for altering treatment. One arm should have all lines removed and be marked "do not touch" with no blood drawing or lines of any sort permitted. Close adherence to this policy of sparing one arm for vascular access can prevent the patient, the dialysis unit, and the vascular surgeon from facing major problems in the course of the renal failure. Dialysis should be performed early in acute renal failure. Management will be more difficult if the patient is allowed to become uremic before dialysis is instituted. There is little to be gained by heroic attempts to manage renal failure without dialysis. Patients with acute renal failure, especially postoperatively or following trauma, need frequent dialysis. Hemodialysis is preferred to peritoneal dialysis in patients who have suffered extensive tissue destruction (trauma, postoperative), resulting in the release of large amounts of K^+ into the extracellular fluid and in patients who are severely catabolic.

Peritoneal dialysis uses the peritoneal membrane to separate the dialysate from the blood stream. Since a foreign body is being implanted transcutaneously, maintenance of sterility of the peritoneal dialysis is extremely important. Implantation of the silastic catheter may be performed surgically under anesthesia or at the bedside using the trocar. The bladder must be empty. Patients with skin infections or any GI disorder (ileus, intraabdominal adhesions) are best not treated with peritoneal dialysis. After catheter placement, antibiotics are added to standard dialysate which is warmed to 38°C and sterily run in and out of the peritoneal cavity in 500- to 1000-ml exchanges at two exchanges per hour. Later, in chronic peritoneal dialysis, this is increased to 2000-ml exchanges at three exchanges per hour. Standard peritoneal dialysate contains 130 meq/liter Na^+, 96.5 meq/liter Cl^-, 3.5 meq/liter Ca^{++}, 38 meq/liter acetate, 15 g/liter dextrose. This fluid will remove Na^+, Cl^-, K^+, phosphate, Mg^{++}, and water. Dextrose and calcium are absorbed and serum pH rises. If more fluid removal is required, then a dialysate with 45 g/liter dextrose can be used. Peritoneal dialysis is usually performed for 36 to 48 hr 2 or 3 times per week as needed. Although this method can be done chronically in the home, close monitoring of fluid and electrolyte status is essential.

Although protein restriction is traditionally instituted in renal failure, with hemodialysis protein restriction is not required. In fact, catabolic patients should receive protein supplements. Potassium restriction is important in the management of renal failure before institution of hemodialysis, but may be liberalized after hemodialysis begins. Patients with acute renal failure generally receive too much fluid; overhydration may lead to both hypertension and edema formation. In addition to replacement of GI and urinary losses, patients should be restricted to 10 ml/kg per day. Additional fluid for excessive insensible loss should be provided with close monitoring of daily weights to help evaluate the level of hydration. Although overhydration may result in an elevation in central venous pressure, pulmonary edema, hypertension, or increase in heart size, cardiac output, tissue oxygenation, and circulation time are usually normal. Administration of digitalis will *not* correct the abnormalities of overhydration and should be reserved only for true congestive heart failure. Extreme caution is advised to avoid digitalis toxicity.

5.1.4. Electrolytes in Renal Failure

Urinary sodium losses should be measured and replaced. As many patients may develop hyponatremia secondary to overhydration, fluid restriction coupled with hemodialysis may be necessary.

Hyperkalemia is a major problem in acute renal failure and represents a potential emergency. Particularly in postoperative or trauma patients, serum potassium can climb rapidly in acute renal failure. Potassium should not be replaced in acute renal failure unless hypokalemia is present and, even then, replacement should be limited to identifiable losses. Potassium-containing drugs (particularly penicillin) should be avoided. Although the ECG changes of hyperkalemia may lag behind the serum K^+, they are predictive of toxicity and can be monitored. Peaked elevation of the T wave, prolonged Q-T interval, QRS widening, and prolonged P-R interval precede the development of a sine wave cardiac arrest in acute renal failure. Hyperkalemia can be treated in many ways: sodium polystyrene sulfonate (Kayexalate®) is an exchange resin that will bind K^+ in the GI tract. It may be given orally or as an enema. Fifteen to sixty grams in 3 to 4 ml/g fluid can be given 4 times per day. Sorbitol® 20% administered concomitantly will prevent the constipation caused by the oral Kayexalate, a particular problem to the elderly who may have preexisting bowel problems. Any serum K^+ above 6.5 meq/liter mandates immediate therapy. Besides the administration of Kayexalate, the patient should be given glucose and insulin. A rapid IV push of 25 g glucose and 8 to 10 units regular insulin will rapidly lower the serum K^+ due to a shift of potassium from the extracellular to the intracellular space. Administration of IV $NaHCO_3$ (45 meq) will also lower serum K^+ and should be combined with the glucose/insulin therapy. Hemodialysis should be started as soon as possible. If the serum K^+ reaches 7.5 meq/liter or if significant ECG changes are present, IV calcium (5 to 10 ml 10% $CaCl_2$) should be given slowly to antagonize the effect of K^+ on the myocardium. The treatment may need to be repeated every 30 to 120 min.

As renal function declines, problems can result from retained dietary phosphorus due to diminished excretion. A reduced dietary phosphorus intake and administration of phosphate-binding gels (antacids containing aluminum hydroxide) are indicated for an elevated serum phosphate. As magnesium intake must also be restricted in patients with renal failure, many common antacid preparations containing large amounts of magnesium are contraindicated (see Table I). An increase in the serum Mg^{++} level may result in neuromuscular weakness, loss of deep tendon reflexes, complete heart block, hypertension, and respiratory depression.

Table I. Indicated and Contraindicated Antacids

Indicated in renal failure	Contraindicated in renal failure
Amphogel®	Maalox®
Basalgel®	Riopan®
Alternagel®	Mylanta®
	Aludrox®
	Gaviscon®
	Gelusil®

5.1.5. Neurologic Manifestations of Renal Failure

Uremia may be associated with dysarthria, asterixis, tremors, myoclonus, and generalized sensorial clouding. As uremia worsens, symptoms of delirium with hallucinations, tetany, and frontal lobe depression may appear. Convulsions occur late in uremia and may be either focal or generalized motor seizures. Since elevated serum levels of penicillin can exacerbate any and all of these neurologic disorders in uremia, caution must be exercised in concomitant usage. Uremic convulsions are best treated acutely with 10 to 20 mg diazepam (Valium®) IV over 3 to 5 min. Since acute respiratory arrest can occur with such treatment, ventilatory assistance may be necessary. Diphenylhydantoin (Dilantin®) can acutely be given IV; however, 100 mg 2 to 4 times a day orally is the preferred dosage for the patient not in status epilepticus. Phenobarbitol 90 to 180 mg/day may be useful both acutely and chronically in preventing seizures; however, a paradoxical effect may result in the elderly. If these drugs fail to control uremic convulsions, an IV bolus injection of 10 mg lidocaine followed by an infusion of 30 μg/kg per min should prove effective in controlling the seizures.

After dialysis, either hemodialysis or peritoneal dialysis, a dysequilibrium syndrome commonly occurs. Patients complain of headache, nausea, or muscle cramps, and display agitation, irritability, and even delirium, obtundation, or convulsions. The signs and symptoms are directly related to the rapidity and completeness of the dialysis and are most common during the first few dialyses. It is thought that shifts of water into the brain cause this dysequilibrium syndrome. By using more gentle, less efficient early dialyses, the patient will better adapt to the fluid change occurring during dialysis.

5.1.6. Chronic Renal Failure

Chronic renal failure is not the lethal disease it once was. Remarkable advances have been made in the last three decades in slowing the progression of chronic renal failure and in managing patients with dialysis or renal transplantation after the end stage is reached. Renal transplantation is the preferred method of treatment for younger patients with approximately 3000 transplants performed annually in the United States. Although less than 10% of all renal transplants are performed in patients over 50 years of age,[4] 80% of patients with chronic renal failure are over age 50. Interestingly, renal transplant survival data show that kidney transplants function just as well in the older patient. The limiting factor, however, is the fact that the elderly do poorer with immunosuppression therapy, requiring more gentle immunosuppressive treatment.[5] After age 70, very few patients receive renal transplants.

The indications for dialysis are expanding and patients with systemic diseases, such as diabetes or cancer, are at present not necessarily excluded. There is an approximate 20% mortality rate in the first year on maintenance dialysis with a 10% annual mortality thereafter. Excessive delay in starting dialysis and allowing patients to enter with far advanced uremia is associated with even higher mortality. Patients should be managed conservatively until creatinine clearance falls to about 10 ml/min. At this time, preparation for dialysis is made and when symptoms of uremia begin to appear, dialysis treatment is initiated. Fatigue, nausea, vomiting, and/or neurological change are suggestive symptoms to start dialysis. In the elderly, dialysis is best initiated early before complications of uremia begin.

5.1.7. Hemodialysis

Once the decision to start dialysis has been made, the mode of dialysis must be determined. Numerous patient variables must be considered prior to this determination. Hemodialysis in a dialysis center is fastest; however, it is the most costly. In addition, it causes the most extreme systemic changes during therapy and requires transportation to the center three times a week. Patients awaiting renal transplantation are generally best handled by hemodialysis in a center.

Home hemodialysis has the advantage of considerable cost savings over center hemodialysis. In addition, survival of patients on home hemodialysis is probably better than center dialysis. In general, the patients on home dialysis are more intelligent, highly motivated, and well rehabilitated. Older patients ($>$ 50 years) or those with diabetes or hypertension do less well with home dialysis. Currently, there is no economic incentive for patients to select home dialysis.

5.1.8. Peritoneal Dialysis

Peritoneal dialysis is currently undergoing a resurgence in popularity. Indications for peritoneal dialysis include diabetes, advanced age, cardiovascular disease, or difficulty with vascular access. Peritoneal dialysis is slower, but gentler, making it more appropriate for the geriatric patient. Clearance rates across the peritoneal membrane are one-quarter to one-seventh of those obtained by hemodialysis. Diabetic retinopathy clearly progresses more slowly with peritoneal dialysis than with hemodialysis.[6]

Chronic peritoneal dialysis is delivered through a catheter in the abdominal wall. Infection of the peritoneal catheter is the major complication and limitation of the modality. Previous abdominal surgery may limit the freedom of fluid to diffuse within the peritoneal cavity. Continuous irrigation of the peritoneal membrane must be performed for about 40 hr/week.[6] The dialysis can be performed in two dialyses/week at the center or in four overnight dialyses at home. The requirements for self home peritoneal dialysis are the ability to perform the appropriate connections sterily, not beyond the capabilities of many geriatric patients. Because of the significant continued advantage of peritoneal dialysis and particularly in home dialysis, the Medicare's end-stage renal disease program is encouraging widespread use of these modalities. In the United States, Medicare pays for all end-stage renal disease care with more than 30,000 patients on maintenance hemodialysis at present.

5.1.9. Rehabilitation on Dialysis

Rehabilitation of the patient while on long-term maintenance dialysis is difficult. Life on dialysis can be very gloomy and dismal unless some patient independence is developed. Patients who can return to work or other purposeful activity appear to make a better psychological adjustment. Obviously, those who can perform home dialysis minimize their self-image as a sick person. Limited data suggest that patients over age 50 on dialysis are less rehabilitatible than those under age 50. In one study, 30% of patients over the age of 50 on dialysis had retired from working or housework as compared to only 2% in the under-50 age group. Interestingly, there were no differences noted between the age groups with regard to their estimates of life satisfaction and contributions to society.[7] Although attempts to maintain a high quality of life must be fostered regardless of age or health status, the elderly present a particular challenge in this regard due to more-often associated chronic illness and changes in lifestyle.

5.2. Bladder Physiology

5.2.1. Anatomy and Physiology of Micturition

The body of knowledge of neuroanatomy and neurophysiology of micturition has increased greatly during the past decade. Some of the traditional concepts of the innervation of the bladder and of the various neurological and muscular factors involved in micturition have changed substantially. Unfortunately, there is still no general agreement on the precise way in which all the factors involved in normal micturition interact. Although much discussion continues to take place, many of the points in dispute are of more importance to the neurophysiologist than to the clinician. The following description of the normal structure and function of the urinary bladder is an overview of the present data, emphasizing the features that are of particular value to the practicing clinician.

The bladder or detrusor muscle receives innervation from the parasympathetic efferent nerves from the S2 to S4 segments of the spinal cord which travel to the bladder in the pelvic nerve and supply both the detrusor (bladder body) and trigone (bladder base). The neurotransmitter for these parasympathetic motor nerves at the bladder is acetylcholine and large numbers of cholinergic receptors are present throughout the bladder, particularly in the bladder body. Stimulation of these cholinergic receptors causes contraction in all areas of the bladder. Parasympathetic afferent nerves from the bladder also travel in the pelvic nerve to the spinal cord where they synapse at the S2 to S4 levels.

Sympathetic efferent nerves from the T11 to L2 segments travel to the bladder in the hypogastric nerve. The sympathetic system neurotransmitter at the bladder is norepinephrine and there are two types of adrenergic receptors in the bladder: β (inhibitory) and α (excitatory). The β-receptors are located in the bladder body. Stimulation of these inhibitory β-receptors causes relaxation of the bladder body, whereas stimulation of the α-receptors, located in the bladder base and proximal urethra, causes contraction of the bladder outlet with increased resistance to voiding. Sympathetic stimulation also depresses bladder contractility in an indirect fashion by inhibiting parasympathetic discharge to the bladder body. Thus, sympathetic stimulation promotes the storage of urine in three ways. Sympathetic afferent nerves from the bladder and proximal urethra also run in the hypogastric nerve to the spinal cord.

The voluntary nerve supply to the external urethral sphincter is the pudendal nerve, from the S2 to S4 segments. Stimulation of this voluntary nerve causes increased contraction of the external urethral sphincter, increased bladder outlet resistance, and increased resistance to voiding. Afferent fibers from the external urethral sphincter reach the spinal cord through the pudendal nerve.

The overall function of the bladder can be divided into the two distinct functions of bladder filling and bladder emptying. During the early part of bladder filling, there is little increase in bladder pressure and little activity in the afferent nerves from the bladder. When a certain critical intravesical pressure is reached, the afferent fibers in the pelvic nerve are stimulated. Through a reflex in the spinal cord, the sympathetic efferent fibers in the hypogastric nerve are then stimulated, causing relaxation of the bladder and allowing further filling to occur. Filling is also aided by gradual stimulation of the pudendal nerve, increasing the contractility of the external urethral sphincter.

Bladder emptying, which is normally a voluntary act, is generally considered to be a sacral spinal cord reflex, further modified by many influences within the central nervous system. The afferent limb of this reflex is stimulated by the increasing pressure within the bladder; the efferent limb of the reflex is carried through the pelvic nerve. It appears the micturition center in normal voiding is located in the brainstem and that ascending and descending spinal cord pathways from this area to the sacral spinal cord act to modify voiding. The micturition center in the brainstem is itself subject to various facilitatory and inhibitory influences from other parts of the brain, including the cerebellum and the cerebral cortex. Although the central pathways are still poorly understood, normal bladder emptying involves the coordination of a number of actions. These include contraction of the bladder body (parasympathetic stimulation), depression of the sympathetic inhibitory effect on the bladder body (sympathetic β-receptor inhibition), funneling of the bladder base and urethra into an open bladder outlet (sympathetic α-receptor inhibition), and relaxation of the external urethral sphincter (voluntary muscle relaxation).[8,9,10]

5.2.2. Urodynamics

As with neuroanatomy and neurophysiology, controversy is widespread in the rapidly developing field of urodynamics. The term *urodynamics* itself is a confusing term for many people. Urodynamics is best considered as a group of investigations that are sometimes necessary in evaluating the patient with abnormal bladder or sphincter function. It should be stressed that the majority of patients will not need urodynamic investigation, but can be evaluated adequately by more standard methods. Standard (nonurodynamic) urological investigations in the patient with lower urinary tract symptoms include: urinalysis, urine culture, urine cytology, measurement of residual urine, intravenous pyelogram, and cystoscopy. Only those patients whose lower-tract symptoms remain unclear following this standard workup will require further urodynamic evaluation. At present, the urodynamic tests that are of value in clinical practice include measurement of urinary flow, the cystometrogram (CMG), the voiding cystourethrogram (VCUG), the sphincter electromyogram (EMG), and, to a lesser extent, the urethral pressure profile (UPP).

Urinary flow rate is defined as the volume of urine voided per unit time reported in ml/sec. A number of commercial flowmeters are now available, based on one of two types of measurement. Urine volume over a period of time can be measured and by differentiation with respect to time, urine flow can be derived. Alternatively, flow measurement over a period of time can be obtained and, by integration, urine volume can be derived. Measurement of urinary flow rate is a simple, repeatable, noninvasive procedure that is a good screening test for bladder outlet obstruction and can be used to monitor the patient's progress or response to treatment. Flow rates are accurate only at total voided volumes in excess of 200 ml and care must be taken to ensure an adequate total voided volume of urine in all patients. For men and women under 50, the normal value for maximum urine flow rate is 20 ml/sec or above. For women over the age of 50, this value decreases slightly and normal maximum flow rate is 18 ml/sec or above. For men over the age of 50, there is a greater decrease (reflecting the influence of benign prostatic enlargement) and the normal peak flow rate is approximately 14 ml/sec or above.[11]

The cystometrogram (performed with either water or carbon dioxide) is used to investigate the phase of bladder filling. Although it gives a permanent graphical representation of bladder pressure as a function of bladder volume, it has the disadvantages of requiring catheterization, of being somewhat poorly reproducible, and of providing little information about the phase of bladder emptying. These advantages are nevertheless well outweighed by the information that can be gained from a properly conducted study. During filling, bladder sensation can be assessed by recording the volume at which the first sensation of filling occurs and a rough approximation of bladder capacity can be assessed by measuring the volume at which discomfort occurs. The presence of voluntary or involuntary bladder contractions can be recorded as well as the ability of the patient to suppress these contractions. If necessary, provocative maneuvers (suprapubic tapping, rapid filling of the bladder, etc.) can be carried out in an attempt to provoke involuntary contractions. The effect of various pharmacological agents on bladder contraction can be measured. Some assessment of the phase of bladder emptying can also be made by the ability of the patient to void on command and to suppress this voiding voluntarily.[12]

The voiding cystourethrogram provides visual information on bladder function during bladder filling, storage, and emptying. It should always be performed under fluoroscopy to obtain the maximum amount of information from the study. A VCUG can now also be combined with other urodynamic tests (such as urinary flow-rate) to provide simultaneous information.[13] Bladder filling can be used to obtain similar information to that obtained from a cystometrogram. Bladder emptying is used to check for the presence of vesical–ureteral reflux and to localize the site of any bladder outlet obstruction. An incompetent sphincteric mechanism may be identified by leakage of contrast from the bladder or by failure to voluntarily close the sphincter during voiding.

Electromyography (EMG of the external urethral sphincter) is rarely performed alone and most information is obtained when it is carried out in conjunction with a cystometrogram.[14] In theory, recording from needle electrodes placed through the perineum directly into the external urethral sphincter gives the most precise information. Needle electrodes should probably be used in cases of suspected neuropathy (alcoholism, diabetes, trauma of the cauda equina) because the neuropathy may not involve the urethral sphincter and the anal sphincter to the same degree. In practice, adequate information can usually be obtained by indirect recording from surface electrodes placed either in the perianal region or as an anal plug. The sphincter EMG and the cystometrogram are recorded simultaneously and the two are then correlated to see if the bladder and sphincter are working in a coordinated or uncoordinated manner. Normally, the sphincter relaxes (and so sphincter EMG activity stops) just before bladder contraction occurs. If sphincter EMG activity persists during detrusor contraction, this type of uncoordinated activity is known as *detrusor sphincter dyssynergia*.

The urethral pressure profile measures and records the competence of the urethral sphincter. A special catheter with side holes is introduced into the bladder and saline or carbon dioxide is infused through the side holes at a steady flow-rate. The pressure changes within the urethra, and the urethral length over which these changes occur is then recorded as the catheter is withdrawn from the bladder at a known rate. The resistance of the urethra is expressed in terms of the pressure necessary to maintain a steady flow of saline or carbon dioxide through the catheter. In normal men, representative values would be a maximum urethral pressure of approximately 100 cm of water over a functional urethral length of 4 cm. In normal women, the corresponding representative values would be a maximum urethral pressure of 70 cm of water over a functional urethral length of 2.5 cm.[15] The UPP is not performed as commonly as the other tests above, but it is often of value in the assessment of such problems as bladder outlet obstruction, incontinence, spinal cord trauma, and the investigation of drugs acting on the urethra.

A full battery of urodynamic investigations may not be indicated in an individual patient and a single test such as a cystometrogram may provide all the information necessary. If required, tests can be combined in various ways (such as simultaneous flow rate and sphincter EMG) to obtain the correct diagnosis.

5.2.3. Neurogenic Bladder

A large number of systems, none of them ideal, exist for the classification on the neurogenic bladder. The three most common classifications are those devised by Bors and Comarr,[16] by Lapides,[17] and more recently by Wein.[18] The first two rather complex classifications have been widely used in the past, though each system has a number of drawbacks. The omission of any reference to treatment is a disadvantage shared by both the Lapides and Bors and Comarr classifications. For this reason, the most valuable guide to clinical management of a patient with bladder dysfunction is Wein's simple classification that is both new and controversial.

The Wein classification is based on the premise that the bladder has two principal functions (storage of urine and emptying of urine) and divides all voiding dysfunction into failure to store or failure to empty.[19] Storage of urine requires accommodation of increasing volumes of urine at a low bladder pressure, absence of inappropriate detrusor contraction, and a closed bladder outlet. Failure to store urine may be due to bladder problems (abnormally high bladder pressures or abnormal bladder contractions) or outlet problems (permanent or intermittent decrease in outlet resistance). Emptying of urine requires bladder contraction and a simultaneous lowering of the outlet resistance provided by the bladder neck, urethra, and external sphincter. Failure to empty urine may also be due to either bladder (decreased bladder contractility) or outlet problems (increased outlet resistance). Usually, both failure to store and failure to empty are due to a combination of bladder and outlet problems rather than to a single factor. Besides its simplicity, the great advantage of this classification is that effective treatment can be given without an exact diagnosis.

5.2.4. Treatment of Neurogenic Bladder

Drugs used in the treatment of urinary incontinence (failure to store) can be divided into drugs that inhibit bladder contractility and drugs that increase outlet resistance. The drug most commonly used to inhibit bladder contractility is the anticholinergic agent propantheline (Probanthine®). It is supplied in 7.5-mg and 15-mg tablets, and the usual starting geriatric dose is 7.5 mg 4 times daily. The dose can subsequently be adjusted according to the individual patient's response and associated side effects. Many patients become resistant to the drug over a period of months and progressively larger doses may be required. This increase in dosage may be limited by the atropinelike side effects of blurred vision, dry mouth, decreased sweating, constipation, and occasional mental confusion, all of which are particularly poorly tolerated by the elderly. Patients who develop resistance to Probanthine may occasionally respond to hyoscyamine (Cystospaz®), a natural belladona alkaloid that has similar anticholinergic actions and side effects to those of Probanthine.

Imipramine hydrochloride (Tofranil®) has proved useful in facilitating urine storage in adults.[20] Although the exact mechanism of action is unclear, it probably acts by stimulating both the β-adrenergic receptors in the bladder body (causing inhibition of bladder contractility) and the α-adrenergic receptors in the bladder base (causing increased bladder outlet resistance). If necessary, imipramine and propantheline may be given together to obtain a reduction in both bladder pressure and bladder contractility. The usual dose of imipramine in adults is 25 mg 4 times daily. At this dosage, the side effects of blurred vision, dry mouth, excessive sweating, tachycardia, and tremor are rarely seen, though extreme caution is advised in the elderly, especially those with preexisting cardiovascular disease.

Drugs such as flavoxate hydrochloride (Urispas®) and oxybutynin chloride (Ditropan®) are musculotropic relaxants, having a direct antispasmotic action on smooth muscle.[21] The site of action is believed to be at some intracellular location separate from the cholinergic receptor site.[15] In addition to the direct antispasmodic effect, Ditropan also has weak anticholinergic action which makes it the more effective of the two agents. The usual adult dose of Ditropan is 5 mg twice daily with the usual side effects of any anticholinergic drug. Drugs that facilitate the storage of urine by their actions on the bladder base all act by stimulating the α receptors, thus increasing bladder outlet resistance. The action of imipramine in this regard has been previously described. Somewhat variable results have been obtained with a number of other drugs including ephedrine, pseudoephedrine (Sudafed®), and phenylpropanolamine (Ornade®). None of these agents has been shown to be consistently effective although ephedrine may be useful on a short-term basis. The external urethral sphincter cannot be manipulated pharmacologically to increase bladder outlet resistance as there is no drug available which will selectively increase the contractility of striated muscle.

Drugs that act to facilitate emptying of urine act by increasing bladder contractility or decreasing bladder outlet resistance. The standard cholinergic drug to increase bladder contractility is bethanechol chloride (Urecholine®). The usual adult starting dose is 10 mg 4 times daily, but this may need to be increased up to 50 mg 4 times daily before a satisfactory response is seen. The long-term effectiveness is unpredictable[22] and many patients become resistant to the drug or cannot tolerate associated side effects.

Bladder outlet resistance can be decreased by the use of α-adrenergic blocking agents. The most commonly used α blocker is phenoxybenzamine (Dibenzyline®) which has been used successfully in combination with bethanechol.[23] Phenoxybenzamine may be given in an initial dose of 10 mg twice daily, but special care must be taken in the geriatric patient because of the potentially dangerous side effect of postural hypotension.

There is no drug available to selectively treat spasticity of the pelvic floor and any relaxation of the external urethral sphincter can only be achieved by agents that cause generalized skeletal muscle relaxation. Centrally acting muscle relaxants include diazepam (Valium®) and lioresal (Baclofen®), both of which require large doses to produce effective relaxation, making their usefulness limited in the elderly. Dantroline sodium (Dantrium®) has a direct relaxant action on all skeletal muscles, again commonly requiring high dosage levels. As well as severe potential hepatotoxicity, dantroline sodium also has the disadvantage of commonly producing diffuse muscle weakness and hypotonicity at a dosage needed for good sphincteric relaxation.[24] These skeletal muscle relaxants are of some value in patients with spastic lower extremities where attempt to void may trigger spasm of the lower limbs as well as the urethral sphincter. Apart from this, they have limited use in lowering of bladder outlet resistance.

Apart from the pharmacological treatment, there are three other common approaches to the problem of impaired bladder emptying. First, an attempt may be made to increase the bladder pressure during voiding by one of a series of maneuvers (abdominal straining, credé, triggering of bladder function). Second, bladder outlet resistance may be lowered or destroyed by one of a series of surgical procedures (transurethral resection of the bladder neck, open surgical widening of the bladder neck, external sphincterotomy). Last, the problem may be circumvented by intermittent catheterization or urinary diversion.[19]

External pressure, generated by abdominal straining or abdominal compression in the credé method, can increase bladder pressure during voiding. These techniques are sometimes useful in the patient with a flaccid bladder due to sacral spinal cord trauma, diabetes, or a longer-term overdistention of the bladder. In most cases, however, the bladder will empty completely only if the bladder outlet resistance is lowered by some other means. Otherwise, unphysiologically high pressures have to be generated within the bladder to overcome the normal bladder outlet resistance. Reflex bladder contraction can sometimes be provoked by suprapubic tapping, pinching the abdominal skin, etc. Use of this technique is limited to patients with lesions above the level of the sacral spinal cord. It is sometimes sufficient to empty the bladder completely, but more often procedures to lower the bladder outlet resistance must be added.

In elderly men, transurethral resection of the prostate is the most common surgical procedure done to reduce bladder outlet resistance. Other endoscopic procedures, such as bladder neck resection or external sphincterotomy, are of most use in patients with spinal cord injuries and are rarely indicated in the geriatric patient.

In addition to drug treatment, there are also three other main approaches to the problem of failure to store urine. First, bladder contractility can be lowered by interrupting bladder innervation (subarachnoid block, sacral rhizotomy). Second, bladder outlet resistance can be replaced by some form of mechanical compression (e.g., an artificial sphincter device). Last, the problem can be circumvented by intermittent catheterization or a urinary diversion.

The use of implantable compression devices to treat urinary incontinence has developed greatly in recent years. The two most common devices currently used are the Kaufman silicone gel prosthesis[25] and the Scott artificial sphincter,[26] both first reported in 1973. The Kaufman prosthesis is implanted in the perineum and applies constant passive compression to a portion of the urethra. The Scott artificial sphincter is a hydraulic device consisting of three components connected by tubing: an inflatable cuff placed around the urethra, a two-way pump placed in the scrotum or labium, and a retropubically placed fluid reservoir. The cuff around the urethra is normally inflated to mimic the action of the true external urethral sphincter. When the patient wants to void, the cuff is deflated by pumping the fluid from the cuff to the reservoir. The bladder is then emptied and the patient then reinflates the urethral cuff by pumping fluid in the reverse direction from the reservoir to the cuff. Both of these devices have proved valuable in the treatment of many types of incontinence, particularly postprostatectomy incontinence. The Kaufman device, as it applies continuous pressure to the urethra, suffers from the disadvantage of urethral erosion, but is considerably simpler and less liable to mechanical failure. The Scott device, applying intermittent pressure to the urethra, is more physiological; however, it can only be implanted in those patients who are capable of understanding and using the device. The best results with both devices have been obtained in low or normal pressure bladders because the urethra can then be compressed at a pressure high enough to maintain continence, but not sufficiently high to cause urethral erosion. Many patients, for reasons such as dementia, lack of cooperation, or lack of manual dexterity, will not be good candidates for a Scott artificial sphincter.

5.2.5. Intermittent Catheterization and Diversion

Drainage of urine must be provided for patients who failed to respond to the treatment outlined above. This is obviously so in cases of urine retention, but may be equally important in cases of incontinence for management and social reasons. Drainage, in order of preference, can be accomplished by intermittent catheterization, continuous catheterization, or surgical urinary diversion.

Intermittent catheterization, if feasible, is an excellent means of providing urinary drainage. Drug treatment can often convert the problem of incontinence to one of retention and the bladder can then be drained by intermittent catheterization. This technique can only be used with a reliable, cooperative, well-motivated patient (if self-catheterization), or family. It is time-consuming because it needs to be done often enough to prevent overdistention of the bladder, usually every 4 to 6 hr. Sterile catheterization is necessary in the hospital setting while the patient is learning the technique; however, clean, but unsterile catheterization, has proven perfectly adequate in the home setting.[27] Long-term, low-dose suppressive antibiotics (such as Bactrim® or Nitrofurantoin®) are usually given, but the significance of asymptomatic bacteriuria in these patients is debatable. Long-term follow-up, however, is important and any symptomatic urinary tract infections should be treated with a full course of antibiotics.

Use of indwelling catheters, either urethral or suprapubic, is undesirable and ideally should only be employed as a last resort. This is unfortunately often unrealistic, especially outside the hospital setting. There are, however, definite indications for indwelling catheter drainage, most important, damage to the upper urinary tracts progressing on other treatment. Patients with bladder dysfunction due to progressive malignant disease are often best treated with an indwelling catheter. However, it should be realized that all patients with chronic indwelling catheters invariably have bacteriuria and that complications related to this chronic bacteriuria are common. These well-documented complications include acute and chronic pyelonephritis; bacteremia; perinephric, vesical, and urethral abscess; bladder and renal stones; renal failure; and death.[28] Many different approaches have been used in an attempt to lower this instance of urinary infection. Strict sterile technique in catheterization is essential. Although the use of closed catheter drainage systems has clearly postponed the onset of bacteriuria, catheter irrigation with saline or antibiotic solutions, although commonly performed, is of doubtful value. Breaking the closed catheter system to irrigate the bladder may actually result in an increased incidence of infection.[29] As currently used, routine bladder irrigation is not recommended. Antibacterial and disinfectant ointments have been applied to the meatus in an attempt to prevent ascending infection although it has been shown that the major path of entry into the bladder in closed drainage systems is ascent of organisms along the outside of the catheter.[30] Long-term application of these antibiotic or antiseptic ointments to the meatus appear not to reduce the infection rate and is not recommended as a clinical routine. Simple washing of the meatus with saline to remove encrusted secretions is all that is necessary. The time interval between catheter change is debatable (commonly 4 to 6 weeks). Data from a preliminary study suggest that changing catheters less often than this may predispose to a higher rate of infection.[31] How often a catheter needs to be changed in any individual patient depends on how quickly encrustations build up on the catheter to interfere with drainage of urine. Some patients will develop troublesome encrustations in a matter of weeks while others will remain completely free of encrustations for many months. Although controversial, it is reasonable to pick a compromise time (such as every 4 weeks) for catheter changes and modify this time schedule as needed in the individual patient. Antibiotic prophylaxis and antibiotic treatment in long-term catheterized patients are also both controversial areas. On theoretical grounds, long-term elimination of infection is not likely in the presence of a chronic foreign body in the bladder and treatment may encourage the selection of resistant organisms. Additional disadvantages include allergic reactions to the antibiotic and increased cost of long-term treatment. The use of long-term antibiotics is based on the assumption that chronic infection is harmful to the patient, but there is no agreement on the significance of asymptomatic bacteriuria.[28] Although conflicting evidence exists, routine prophylactic antibiotics or routine antibiotic treatment of asymptomatic bacteriuria cannot be recommended. Antibiotics should be reserved for the specific treatment of acute febrile episodes, symptomatic urinary tract infections or complications such as epididymitis. The acidification of the urine with vitamin C is of limited use because of the high doses (1 to 2 g every 6 hr) needed to lower urine pH sufficiently. Although frequently used, methenamine mandelate (Mandelamine®) has no place in the management of patients with chronic indwelling catheters. Methenamine must be present in the urine for a period of 90 min before the active agent, formaldehyde, is released,[32] obviously not the case in the patient with continuous bladder drainage.[33]

A small percentage of adults with neurogenic bladders, ranging from 1 to 3%, will eventually require surgical urinary diversion.[19] Cutaneous ureterostomies may be possible in the patient with dilated ureters. Otherwise, urinary diversion is usually performed by creating either an ileal or a colon conduit. Both types of conduit have been satisfactory in stabilizing upper tract function. Long-term follow-up of ileal conduits shows that the incidence of complication depends chiefly on the length of postoperative follow-up with the complication rate remaining low for a period of 10 to 15 years postoperatively before it begins to rise. The ileal conduit is, therefore, the standard diversion procedure in the geriatric population as a stable period of approximately 15 years can be anticipated.

5.3. Carcinoma of the Bladder

5.3.1. Etiology and Natural History of Bladder Cancer

Although cancer of the bladder can occur at all ages, it is primarily a disease of the aged population. Age–incidence curves for both men and women in the United States show an increase in incidence throughout adult life. Approximately 30,000 new cases of bladder cancer occur annually in the United States, with a male to female ratio of occurrence of approximately 3:1.[34] Approximately 10,000 people die annually from bladder cancer in the United States and it is the fifth leading cause of death in men 75 years of age or older. The incidence of bladder cancer varies widely throughout the world. Certain countries such as Japan and Sweden have a very low age-specific incidence, whereas countries such as England and Denmark have a high age-specific incidence. Epidemiological studies, in the United States and worldwide, have shown a striking variation in the incidence of bladder cancer in different geographical regions. The highest incidence of bladder cancer occurs in highly industrialized areas.[35] As mentioned above, men are affected three times more commonly than women and whites are affected four times more commonly than nonwhites. Geographical, sex, and racial differences in incidence are thought to be due to differences in exposure to known or suspected risk factors such as occupational bladder carcinogens, tobacco, coffee, and dietary sweeteners.

In Britain, up to one-third of bladder cancers have been attributed to occupational exposure.[36] In the United States, the association of occupation and bladder cancer has been less pronounced, although many specific occupations have been shown to be associated with increased risk of bladder cancer. Occupations known to be associated with increased risk include: aniline dye workers, rubber and cable workers, textile weavers, petroleum workers, spray painters, hairdressers, and leather workers.[37] Aniline dye derivatives such as β-naphthylamine and benzidine are well-documented carcinogens, but in many occupations the specific carcinogen has not yet been identified. The latent period between exposure to a weak carcinogen and clinical development of bladder cancer can be as long as 40 years, and for this reason, identification of the specific carcinogen can be impossible. Cigarette smoking (but not cigar or pipe smoking) has also been associated with an increased incidence of bladder cancer.[38] However, these data have not been reproduced in all studies and the importance of cigarette smoking in inducing bladder cancer is still unclear. Similarly, there are many conflicting reports on the association of bladder cancer with such possible risk factors as coffee drinking, tryptophan metabolites, and use of artificial sweeteners such as saccharin. Current evidence suggests that cocarcinogenesis can occur when a number of weak carcinogens act together in a synergistic manner to induce bladder cancer. Widespread exposure to many known or possible bladder carcinogens has increased together with the increased industrial production and synthesis of these compounds. Given the long latent period in humans between exposure and clinical presentation, it is possible that a dramatic increase in the incidence of bladder cancer may be seen in the future.

As increased risk of transitional cell carcinoma is associated with excretion of carcinogens, increased risk of squamous carcinoma of the bladder is associated with chronic infection and irritation. In areas of the world where *Schistosoma haematobium* infestation is epidemic, up to 20% of these patients will develop squamous carcinoma of the bladder.[39] In the United States, chronic indwelling Foley catheters[40] and cyclophosphamide cystitis[41] have been clearly shown to be associated with an increased incidence of squamous carcinoma of the bladder. Squamous carcinoma of the bladder is a rare cancer, accounting for approximately 5% of all bladder cancer.

5.3.2. Staging of Bladder Cancer

Both the histologic grading and the pathologic staging of bladder cancer are important in determining the prognosis and treatment. Histologic grading is based on the degree of cellular differentiation or dedifferentiation within a given tumor, ranging from Grade 1 or well-differentiated carcinoma to Grade 3 or dedifferentiated carcinoma. A general rule is that well-differentiated cancers tend to be slow-growing and noninfiltrating or only superficially infiltrating, whereas poorly differentiated cancers tend to be rapidly growing and are often deeply infiltrating. There are many exceptions to this rule and different portions of the given tumor may show wide variations of histologic grading within the tumor. However, the 5-year survival figures for patients with Grade 1 tumors based on histologic grading alone are 80% and are 20% for patients with Grade 3 tumors.[42] Histologic grading is thus of real value in estimating the prognosis in a given patient.

Pathologic staging of bladder cancer is based on the degree of infiltration of the tumor into the bladder wall and on the extent of metastatic spread. This is the single most important factor in determining prognosis and treatment of any individual patient. The most commonly used classification of tumor staging in the United States divides tumors into Stage 0 through Stage D. Stage 0 tumors are tumors confined to the mucosa that have not infiltrated the lamina propria. This is the noninvasive stage of bladder cancer where the tumor has not infiltrated into the muscle of the bladder wall. In general, these tumors tend to be well differentiated, are slow growing, and have a low incidence of metastatic spread. These tumors can be adequately treated with such low-morbidity procedures as repeated transurethral resection and topical chemotherapy. Stages B through D, in contrast, refer to different degrees of tumor invasion. Stage B1 cancer is a tumor that shows superficial invasion of the bladder muscle, Stage B2 shows deep invasion of the bladder muscle, and Stage C shows invasion through the entire bladder muscle wall to involve the surrounding fat. Such tumors cannot be controlled or cured by local means and require treatment such as cystectomy or definitive radiation therapy. Metastatic spread is defined by Stage D disease where D1 disease implies spread of the tumor to the regional lymph nodes and Stage D2 disease implies distant metastases. Such tumors are generally felt to be outside the range of surgical curability and are best treated with systemic chemotherapy.

Given the wide range of treatment modalities, accurate staging of the disease is essential before deciding on the best therapy. All patients should have excretory urography, cystoscopy, transurethral biopsy of the bladder tumor, and bimanual examination under anesthesia. The extent of local spread is best assessed by computerized tomography (CT) scanning of the bladder.[43] Distant spread should be assessed by routine liver function tests, chest X ray, and bone scan. The value of lymphangiography in detecting pelvic metastases is debatable, and its overall use has decreased as CT scanning of the pelvis has become more common. The above information represents the minimum amount of data necessary to accurately stage a patient with bladder carcinoma.

5.3.3. Treatment of Bladder Cancer

There is general agreement that low-stage (Stages 0 and A) tumors are best managed by transurethral resection. Excellent control of these tumors is possible by endoscopic resection and regular follow-up cystoscopy.[44] Some tumors with superficial muscle invasion (Stage B1 tumors) are also managed by transurethral resection, but the majority of urologists feel that these tumors are not amenable to endoscopic surgery alone.

An individual decision must be made in the case of the patient who has an uncomplicated transurethral resection of a bladder tumor that then demonstrates superficial muscle invasion on histologic examination. In this case, transurethral removal alone is a perfectly acceptable treatment for a poor-risk patient with a low-grade (well-differentiated) tumor. Periodic cystoscopy is essential in all cases during the lifetime of all patients as transurethral removal of a tumor does not control the tendency of the bladder mucosa to form new neoplasms in other areas of the bladder. Approximately 80% of all patients treated with transurethral resection will develop recurrent bladder tumors within 5 years of their initial presentation.[45,46] The majority of these recurrences will be similar in stage and grade to that of the original tumor (that is, low stage, low grade) and can thus be managed by repeated transurethral resection.

Open surgical treatment of invasive bladder cancer involves one of three operations: partial cystectomy, simple total cystectomy with ileal loop diversion, and radical cystectomy (cystectomy combined with removal of the pelvic lymph nodes). Partial cystectomy, with a low morbidity and mortality, would seem to be an ideal choice of operation for the older patient. Good results with partial cystectomy have been reported from many institutions.[47,48] However, partial cystectomy is best reserved for small, single, primary tumors located high on the bladder and few bladder cancers fulfill these criteria. The second disadvantage of partial cystectomy in many series has been the problem of local recurrence and seeding of the wound with tumor. For these reasons, partial cystectomy should only be performed in a highly selected group of patients.

Simple total cystectomy with ileal loop diversion is adequate treatment for the occasional patient with multiple superficial tumor recurrences. Normally, these recurrences can be treated by repeated cystoscopy and repeated transurethral resection. Occasionally, transurethral resection becomes impractical because the tumors recur too rapidly, in too diffuse a pattern, or in the area of the vesical neck or the urethral orifices. In these cases, adequate removal of the tumor can be achieved by simple cystoprostatectomy without pelvic lymph node dissection.

The majority of patients with locally invasive bladder cancer (Stages B1 through C) are best treated by preoperative irradiation followed by radical cystectomy. Definitive radiation therapy for invasive bladder cancer has waned in popularity and the results of radiation treatment alone have been disappointing.[49] Likewise, poor 5-year survival figures have been reported from many centers with radical surgery alone,[50] and most centers have discontinued the use of radical cystoprostatectomy alone. For Stage B2 and C bladder cancers, the 5-year survival with either definitive radiotherapy alone or radical cystectomy alone is only about 20%. Doubling of the 5-year survival rate to approximately 40% has been achieved by the integration of preoperative radiotherapy with radical cystectomy and this combined therapy is the treatment of choice for invasive bladder cancers in most centers. The optimal combination of preoperative radiation and cystectomy is still a matter of controversy, and radiation protocols differ widely from institution to institution. A reasonable middle road would be a total dose of 2000 to 4000 rads delivered over a time period of 1 to 4 weeks, followed by radical cystectomy 1 to 2 weeks after the end of radiation. Although radical cystectomy remains a major operation with significant morbidity and mortality, it is no longer a procedure carrying a mortality rate of some 20% as it was 20 years ago. Most centers now report mortality rates for a one-stage cystectomy (ileal loop diversion combined with cystectomy in a single procedure) in the order of 4%.[51] Two-stage cystectomy (ileal loop diversion at the first operation followed some weeks later by radical cystectomy) is now usually performed only for specific indications, such as the poor-risk patient, the particularly obese patient, or the patient who has had previous high-dosage (6500-rad) radiation therapy. With current methods of perioperative support and current surgical techniques, cystectomy can be performed safely in the great majority of patients. There is no higher incidence of morbidity and mortality in cystectomies performed on the elderly patient.[52] Age, per se, is not therefore a contraindication to cystectomy in the elderly patient who is otherwise in reasonable general health.

5.3.4. Topical Chemotherapy of Bladder Cancer

Topical chemotherapy (direct instillation of chemotherapeutic agents into the bladder) was first described with use of Thiotepa® in 1961.[53] Since then, many other agents have been used including doxorubicin (Adriamycin®), mitomycin-C, epodyl, and cis-platinum. As direct contact with the tumor cells is necessary, these chemotherapeutic agents are only suitable for use in superficial (Stages 0 and A) bladder cancers. Most clinical experience has been gained with Thiotepa and this has proved effective in two ways—destroying incompletely resected tumor and prolonging the onset of tumor recurrence. This is a particularly attractive method of treatment in the older patient as it does not require hospital admission and carries only a slight risk of white blood count depression due to systemic absorption. The usual method is to have the patient fast overnight to ensure concentration of the Thiotepa in the bladder. Thirty milligrams of Thiotepa in 30 cm³ of distilled water (many centers use 60 mg in 60 cm³ of distilled water) are then instilled into the bladder through a catheter and the patient is instructed to retain the solution for 2 hr and then to void. The treatment is repeated at weekly intervals for a 4-week rest period. If residual tumor is still present, a further 4-week period of treatment is given. The white blood cell count must be monitored in all patients and treatment will need to be stopped in a small percentage of patients due to significant, but completely reversible, depression of the white blood cell count.[54] It should be stressed that Thiotepa itself is not curative and all patients must still be followed up with periodic cystoscopy to check for tumor recurrences. However,

Thiotepa will benefit practically all patients in terms of fewer recurrences, increase in intervals free of tumor, and diminished frequency of new tumor formation.[55]

Good clinical responses have also been obtained with intravesical instillation of a number of other drugs, the most promising of which appears to be mitomycin-C. Clinical trials of intravesical mitomycin-C in the United States have demonstrated complete clinical response rates of between 50 and 70%, using a range of doses and schedules.[56,57] Further information, including longer follow-up, is needed, but the excellent early results hold promise that this may prove more effective in intravesical control of bladder tumor than Thiotepa.

5.3.5. Systemic Chemotherapy for Bladder Cancer

Historically, systemic chemotherapy for bladder cancer has largely focused on the use of single agents in patients with symptomatic Stage D carcinoma. Multiple single agents have been used, including 5-fluorouracil, cyclophosphamide, doxorubicin (Adriamycin), methotrexate, mitomycin-C, and *cis*-platinum. Single-agent chemotherapy produced a documented response in many patients with metastatic bladder cancer,[58] but no consistent pattern of response was seen. It should be emphasized that many reports are not comparable because of differences in size and location of metastases and differences in criteria for response. The overall results of single-agent chemotherapy and bladder cancer have been disappointing. However, the knowledge gained from the effect of single agents has aided greatly in the design and development of present combination regimens.

In contrast to the older concept of single-agent chemotherapy for measurable and advanced metastatic bladder cancer, present work is aimed at the development of combination chemotherapy for the treatment of micrometastatic disease. The main stimulus in the development of effective chemotherapy has been the introduction and development of *cis*-platinum. This is presently the most effective drug against urothelial tumors both singly and in combination and appears certain to be the drug around which combinations of chemotherapeutic agents will be based. Used alone, *cis*-platinum has achieved an objective response rate of between 45 and 75% in a number of series.[59,60,61] In particular, a number of patients had a complete response with complete disappearance of all tumor. Response, if it occurs, will occur early in the course of treatment (1 or 2 doses) and an increase in response is not likely to be achieved by increasing the number of doses. The most effective role for *cis*-platinum may thus be as an induction agent and other agents can then be combined to maintain remission. If so, the high toxicity of *cis*-platinum (especially severe vomiting and nephrotoxicity) which limits its long-term administration become relatively unimportant.

Most current studies on combination chemotherapy and bladder cancer utilize *cis*-platinum in combination with Adriamycin and either 5-fluorouracil or cyclophosphamide. Using these agents, encouraging early response rates have been reported.[62,63] No ideal regimen has been identified as yet but the introduction of *cis*-platinum has clearly altered the poor outlook for patients with late disseminated bladder cancer. Hopefully, combination chemotherapy will be refined enough so that it may be applied in the future to patients with early micrometastatic disease.

5.4. Physiology of the Prostate Gland

5.4.1. The Normal Prostate

The embryologic development of the human prostate just distal to the bladder neck is characterized by a diverse number of tissue interactions at different levels of the urethra. Most of the prostatic ducts develop in the lower half of urethra under the influence of fetal testosterone. The ducts are induced to grow into surrounding stroma, but the stroma has a powerful influence on the differentiation of the ducts and the formation of the prostate gland. About 25% of the glandular tissue develops around the ejaculatory ducts and is different morphologically.[64] These periurethral ducts are the ones that will develop into benign prostatic hyperplasia (BPH) while the outer glands are prone to develop carcinoma in the aged prostate.

At puberty, the prostate gland grows to its normal adult size under the influence again of androgens. Prostatic enzymes readily convert the circulatory testosterone to 5-dihydrotestosterone (5-DHT), the active form of testosterone for male accessory sex organs. There are specific androgen–receptor proteins that are responsible for retaining androgens within prostatic cell nuclei. Estrogens can affect the production of testosterone by the testes, but can only very weakly affect the prostate directly.

The epithelial cells of the adult prostate produce approximately 1 cm^3/day of prostatic fluid that is very rich in proteolytic enzymes, zinc, and the polyamines (spermine, spermidine, putrescine). The proteolytic enzymes are involved in the liquefaction of normal human semen and the negotiation of cervical mucus by spermatozoa. The exact role of zinc is unknown, but zinc is a major antibacterial element in prostatic fluid.

5.4.2. The Aging Prostate

As the prostate gland ages in animals, the epithelial cells change their shape and activity rate; they shrivel and atrophy. In contrast, man's epithelial cells from acini periurethrally become hyperplastic and the gland becomes swollen. As nodules of BPH arise, the epithelial cells become cuboidal or tall and columnar. Qualitatively, the secretions into the lumen are the same, but, quantitatively, fluid production decreases. Stromal nodules are induced that are fibrous or fibromuscular in nature and the epithelial cells appear to grow into them. Although the changes occurring in the prostate are thought to begin in adult life, roughly 15 to 20 years are required before the disease manifests significant clinical symptoms.

Currently, very little research is going on in the areas of epidemiology and natural history of BPH. The belief is widespread that BPH causes little morbidity and mortality. Actually, there is a considerable morbidity and mortality due to clinical problems after age 60. Annual mortality rates due to BPH in European countries is 50 to 80/100,000 population; lowest mortality rates due to BPH are in the Orient, 1 to 7/100,000/year.[65] Mortality in the United States is moderately low. Risk of developing BPH appears to be unrelated to social class, marital status, celibacy, sexual drive, or blood group. Black men present with clinical disease approximately 5 years earlier than white men. Any hypothesized relationship to prostatic cancer is suspect as both diseases occur in the same elderly population.

5.4.3. Relief of Prostatic Obstruction

When a patient presents with symptoms of urinary retention (slow stream, dribbling, nocturia, double-voiding), evaluation should be done early to provide the opportunity for relief of obstruction before bladder deterioration progresses. When bladder decompensation occurs, relief of obstruction may not help the symptoms. Prostatectomy, an operation of low mortality, may be done by either a transurethral or open surgical approach. The transurethral prostatectomy (TURP) is best for small to moderately sized prostatic adenomas. For larger glands, however, suprapubic or retropubic prostatectomy provides a safer means of relieving outlet obstruction. Trying to remove a large prostate by TURP is associated with a significant risk of excessive bleeding and hyponatremia.

Potential complications of prostatectomy include bleeding and incontinence, fortunately both uncommon. Impotence is not a complication of simple prostatectomy and mortality of the surgical procedures are now less than 1%. Potential complications must always be weighed against the complication of no treatment, i.e., bladder decompensation, urinary infection, and renal failure.

Medical treatment of BPH to date has been disappointing. Administration of estrogens of the antiandrogen cyproterone acetate will result in a decreased epithelial, but not stromal, component of BPH. Changes in obstruction by the gland are not demonstrable. The side effects of the drugs and potential cardiovascular complications make such treatment inadvisable at this time.

5.4.4. Infection of the Prostate Gland

Prostatitis is a common clinical problem for the urologist and the general practitioner. In the younger age groups, infections are often caused by *Chlamydia*, *Mycoplasma*, or herpes virus. Middle-aged or elderly symptomatic patients are more likely to have acute or chronic bacterial prostatitis. Often elderly patients will have the same prostatitis as an inciting cause for the appearance of obstructive symptoms due to BPH. Prostatitis in the elderly is most commonly due to *Escherichia coli, Enterobacter, Pseudomonas,* or the enterococci. The placement of urethral catheters can initiate or exacerbate such infection. Whereas acute infections present with initiative voiding symptoms (urgency, dysuria, frequency), chronic infections lead to scarring and the formation of calculi and nodules within the prostate.

The diagnosis of prostatitis is made by culturing and examining the prostatic fluid for white blood cells and bacteria. Patients with prostatic infection must be treated with antibiotics for a relatively long period of time (4 to 12 weeks). Since few drugs given orally will enter the prostatic fluid, the tetracyclines and trimethoprim/sulfamethoxasole are currently the drugs of choice. When prostatic calculi are present, total eradication of the infection is not possible and chronic suppression with antibiotics is necessary. Although prostatectomy will aid those patients in whom prostatitis is superimposed on BPH, it will markedly worsen those patients with prostatitis alone and therefore should be avoided in these cases.

5.5. Prostatic Carcinoma

5.5.1. Etiology and Natural History of Prostatic Carcinoma

After the age of 75, prostatic carcinoma is the leading cancer in terms of incidence and the second leading cause of cancer mortality in men. Approximately 54,000 new cases are diagnosed annually in the United States and approximately 18,000 men die from their cancer. Cancer of the prostate dramatically increases in incidence and mortality with age. After age 70, the death rate approaches 400/100,000 population per year.[66] The incidence of at least latent carcinoma of the prostate approaches 80% in men in their tenth decade of life. The incidence of clinically aggressive carcinoma of the prostate does vary between racial and geographic groups. For example, in the Orient, clinical disease is rare, whereas nonwhite men in the United States have a high incidence of advanced clinical disease.

Although the etiology of carcinoma of the prostate is unknown, a number of epidemiologic factors have provoked hypotheses. Differences in mortality rates in patients have been found according to race, age, blood group, martial status, and presence of BPH. Environmental agents suspected of causing prostatic carcinoma include herpes virus and cadmium. Clearly androgens are required to maintain prostatic epithelium so that malignant transformation of the epithelial cells can occur,[67] but there is no evidence that androgens actually cause prostatic cancer.

Prostatic cancer has a peculiar natural history.[68] A small focus or several foci of cancer develop in the peripheral portion of the prostate gland, known as Stage A carcinoma of the prostate. In most patients, this small cancer remains dormant for years. The length of dormancy is probably related to tumor grade with well-differentiated tumors displaying longer dormancy periods. This dormant preclinical stage explains why so many carcinomas are found incidentally at prostatectomy or at autopsy. For some unknown reason, the dormant focus of cancer may be activated and grows into a prostatic nodule. At this point, the cancer is considered to be Stage B and is eminently curable. Current estimates are that only about 25% of men presenting with a palpable prostatic nodule are then referred for proper therapy.[66] This means that approximately 75% of men presenting with a prostatic nodule are being treated by inappropriate modalities such as hormonal manipulation.

As the prostatic nodule grows, it perforates the prostatic capsule but still may be localized in the periprostatic area (Stage C carcinoma). This disease may become a local problem with obstruction of the urethra or both ureters. Though protrusion into the rectum occurs, actual rectal obstruction is extremely rare.

At some point, while a tumor is a Stage B or C, the propensity for metastasis occurs and pelvic lymph nodes become involved (Stage D1), implying that therapy must be directed at both the primary and the metastases. Stage D2 signifies the involvement of distal organ sites, usually bone.

5.5.2. Current Treatment of Prostatic Carcinoma

The appropriate treatment for Stage A1 prostatic carcinoma is regular observation of geriatric patient. In younger patients with multifocal or poorly differentiated Stage A disease, a more aggressive approach should be taken since these patients progress, whereas the elderly patients do not.

Appropriate treatment for Stage B prostatic carcinoma includes radical prostatectomy, external beam radiotherapy, or interstitial implants of radioactive seeds in the prostate. Complications of implantation of radioactive seeds, usually ^{125}I, into the prostate are minimal and both continence and potency are preserved. However, this treatment requires a radiotherapist familiar with interstitial techniques to be present at the open surgical placement of the seeds, somewhat limiting the popularity of this approach. External beam radiotherapy can be employed to treat both the primary prostatic nodule as well as the draining pelvic lymph nodes. The complications of this radiotherapy are primarily diarrhea and urinary urgency with a modest production of impotence. Other side effects include ablation of the pelvic bone marrow.

The appropriate treatment for Stage C carcinoma of the prostate is external beam radiotherapy. Because 50% of patients with clinical Stage C disease actually have metastatic involvement of the pelvic lymph nodes, the radiotherapy should include the whole pelvis.

Once disease reaches the Stage D2 level involving distant organs such as bone, lungs, or liver, treatment becomes palliative only. Since the report by Huggins and Hodges of the androgen sensitivity of prostatic adenocarcinoma, treatment by hormonal manipulation has been the first line of treatment. At least 40%

of patients with clinical carcinoma of the prostate will present as Stage D2. Whether to treat asymptomatic patients is open to debate. Much of the debate revolves around the complications of the hormonal manipulation. The most direct method of removal of androgen and induction of remission is bilateral orchiectomy. This is a simple procedure that can even be performed under local anesthesia. The complications of the procedure are almost exclusively psychologic; however, most patients tolerate the loss of their testes extremely well. With the reduction of circulating testosterone, most, but not all, patients will have diminished erections. Many physicians do not use bilateral orchiectomy as a treatment option because of unfamiliarity with the procedure and how to approach the patient. For the geriatric patient, bilateral orchiectomy is very frequently the treatment of choice.

Administration of exogenous estrogen will also decrease circulating androgen by causing the pituitary to reduce luteinizing hormone (LH) production. This will also necessarily reduce erections and libido. However, the exogenous estrogens also cause heart enlargement and tremendous fluid retention and a propensity for cardiovascular complications, notably myocardial infarction and venous thrombosis. In the Veterans Administration cooperative study, estrogen increased deaths due to cardiovascular cancer when compared to placebo.[69] Besides a potential for greater complications, choosing to administer estrogens to the geriatric patient also leaves open the possibility of inadequate dosage or noncompliance. Proper monitoring of the estrogen dose should be done with periodic serum testosterone levels to make sure this stays in the castrate range (< 300 ng%). Patients should all have irradiation of the breasts prior to estrogen therapy to prevent gynecomastia. Low-dose estrogen therapy provides no benefit but can cause complications. The minimum recommended dosage of diethylstilbesterol is 3 mg daily.

5.5.3. Screening for Prostatic Cancer

Screening tests should be sensitive, specific, and cost effective. The serum enzyme acid phosphatase is a known marker to detect and evaluate prostatic carcinoma and has been in use for over 40 years. The test is performed by making use of the enzymatic activity of acid phosphatase that is actually a series of isoenzymes, not all of prostatic origin. This led to some false-positives and false-negatives in the past. Recent technologic advances have resulted in the availability of a radioimmunoassay (RIA) specifically for human prostatic acid phosphatase (PAP). Determination of PAP by RIA has proven to be an effective research tool, but of little importance as a clinical test. Several commercial firms, however, are marketing the test and making rather extravagant claims for its usefulness. Watson and Tang[70] performed an extensive analysis of the utility of employing RIA for PAP as a screening tool. They concluded that as a screening tool RIA for PAP has no usefulness for the male population in general or even for populations at high risk, such as older men. Even for use in patients with a known palpable nodule, the test is of limited use in determining whether cancer is present.

Ultrasound of the prostate via a rectal ultrasound probe is being advocated as a screening test for prostatic cancer. It has been popularized by the Japanese who have found that regimented populations will accept routinely sitting on the rectal probe. Differentiating carcinoma from chronic inflammation or calculi is often difficult, however. Ultrasonography is more likely to be useful in determining the extent of disease in patients with known carcinoma than as a screening agent for asymptomatic patients.[71]

The most reliable and economical means for detecting prostatic carcinoma remains the rectal examination. Guinan et al.[72] compared 10 diagnostic screening tests on 30 elderly men. They compared the rectal exam to three different methods of acid phosphatase determination, four different cytology preparations, lactic dehydrogenase isozyme V:I ratio, and leukocyte adherence inhibition. Rectal examination proved to be the most sensitive, the most specific, and the most efficient test. Incidentally, rectal examination proved to be the least costly. The test is universally available and should be routinely performed as part of the physical examination in every patient over 40 years of age. When a prostatic nodule is detected, then transperineal biopsy will result in the diagnosis of prostatic carcinoma in about half of the cases with nodules.

5.5.4. Spread of Prostatic Cancer to Bone

Clearly, prostatic carcinoma selectively spreads to bone. The predilection of prostatic cancer to metastasize to bone has been recognized since Sir Henry Thompson reported the first case in 1854. The reason for specific organ localization has not been established.

Staging of carcinoma of the prostate is difficult because of a lack of absoluteness in clinical staging, surgical staging, and autopsy staging. Still, the concept is widespread that prostatic carcinoma begins as a small focus (Stage A) which, after some dormant period, enlarges to a palpable nodule (Stage B). After growing through the prostatic capsule (Stage C), the tumor spreads in an orderly manner through the pelvic lymph nodes (Stage D1), up the periaortic nodes, and then to bone. Whitmore,[68] however, has pointed out that the natural history of prostatic carcinoma is unpredictable, which certainly confounds treatment regimens. Approximately 40% of patients, however, do present with Stage D disease with most of these having bone metastases. Although metastases to bone occurs late in the natural history of each particular tumor, 20% of cases of Stage D carcinoma of the prostate survive at least 5 years.[69] Patients with prostatic carcinoma die from their tumor, but it takes them a long time to do so compared to patients with other tumors. This might account for some of the increase in the number of bone metastases; that is, patients with other carcinomas may die before clinical bone metastases become apparent.

5.5.5. Pattern of Metastatic Spread of Prostatic Cancer

Prostatic cancer most commonly metastasizes to lymph nodes. Bone is the second most common metastatic site, with up to 84% of patients with metastatic disease having bone metastases at autopsy. Bone may be underestimated as a metastatic site because pathologists do only a cursory examination of the skeleton at autopsy. Many other carcinomas metastasize to bone: breast cancer up to 74% of cases; thyroid cancer up to 60% of cases; renal adenocarcinoma up to 50% of cases; carcinoma of esophagus, colon, stomach, pancreas, testis, and uterus in 5 to 20% of cases.[73,74,75] Overall, the skeleton is the third most common site of cancer metastasis, surpassed only by lung and liver.

Metastases to bone appear first in the bone marrow within the cancellous portion of bone. Subperiosteal tumor appears mainly at bone sites where main foramina cross the hard cortical bone, the latter of which is involved primarily only by expansion or invasion from marrow metastases. Bone metastases are almost always multiple. The distribution of the metastases in the spine usually involves the vertebral bodies, only rarely the arches or processes. Metastases to the skull appear in the calvaria rather than the mandible. If bone marrow is compromised by tumor infiltration (or potentially radiation), then secondary sites of hematopoiesis are stimulated and prostatic carcinoma can metastasize to such sites (e.g., distal limb bones).

The bones most commonly involved by metastatic prostatic carcinoma at autopsy are in order: spine, femur, pelvis, ribs, sternum, skull, and humerus, essentially the same distribution of bone involvement by metastatic breast carcinoma, thyroid carcinoma, and rectal carcinoma following the same distribution as active red marrow in the adult. Renal carcinoma has a predilection for the humerus,[75] but otherwise follows a similar distribution of bone metastases. Dodds, Caride, and Lytton[76] have shown that when bone scanning is used for evidence of metastatic disease, the rank order of sites for both prostatic and nonprostatic cancer changes slightly to spine, ribs, pelvis, femur, shoulder, skull, sternum, and humerus. The order is probably affected by the difference in the detection methods: autopsy versus bone scan.

5.5.6. Host Response to Metastatic Prostatic Cancer

The dissemination of prostatic cancer depends on some as yet undefined host factors causing susceptibility. Epidemiologic studies show differences in incidence and mortality according to age, race, and possibly blood group. There are, however, a number of host responses to prostatic cancer that are known.

Human prostatic cancer is the only cancer that consistently produces osteoblastic, rather than osteolytic, bony metastases. More than 90% of bone lesions due to prostatic cancer are osteoblastic; breast cancer is the second most common cause of osteoblastic metastases (8%).[77] Histologic sections of bony metastases from prostatic carcinoma show a proliferation of osteoblasts with new bone formation within the cancellous bone of the marrow space. The trabeculae show increased remodeling activity and become broader and irregular. Osteoblasts are more numerous, particularly on the trabecular surface. Valentin-Opran et al.[78] have shown that new bone is laid down by the osteoblasts in the vicinity of the malignant prostatic cells. In normal bone remodeling, osteoblastic bone resorption must precede osteoblast activity. In this "juxta-metastatic modeling," osteoblastic resorption does not precede osteoblastic differentiation.[78] It appears that malignant prostatic cells directly stimulate the osteoblasts. Jacobs et al.[79,80] have described a prostatic osteoblastic factor (POF) in prostatic tissue that causes DNA synthesis and proliferation of osteoblasts and fibroblasts. This growth-stimulating protein may explain the response of bone to prostatic carcinoma.

Metastatic prostatic carcinoma is associated with elevations of α-globulin, fibrinogen, and hepatoglobin. Bone metastases are associated with elevations of haptoglobin, α_1 acid glycoprotein, and ceruloplasmin. To date, none of these has proven to be an effective tumor marker. Treatment of the prostatic cancer apparently does not influence these elevations.[81] Other steroid-binding proteins rise when estrogen is given in the treatment of prostatic cancer.

The immune response to metastatic prostatic cancer in bone is obviously important in determining the outcome of the cancer metastases, but is very complex. Host immune defense mechanisms involve both possible stimulation and inhibition of tumor growth. The reader is referred to a recent review by Catalona for a complete picture.[82]

5.5.7. Calcium Metabolism in Patients with Metastatic Prostatic Cancer

With extensive involvement by prostatic cancer bone metastases, total body calcium and phosphorus metabolism may become deranged. With osteolytic skeletal metastases, hypercalcemia is frequently a problem generally caused by mobilization of the calcium of the destroyed bone. Although tumors without extensive bone involvement can also cause hypercalcemia by: (1) ectopic production of parathyroid hormone (PTH) or PTHlike substance, (2) tumor production of prostaglandins, or possibly (3) tumor secretion of osteoclast activating factor or other bone resorbing humoral substances. Carcinoma of the prostate has never been associated with any of these.

The extensive osteoblastic bone growth occurring near the metastatic prostatic cancer cells is generally incompletely calcified. This newly elaborated woven bone is essentially calcium deprived. Valentin-Opran et al.[78] showed that in bone containing metastatic prostatic cancer there is an average 200% increase in osteoid surface to complete for the available serum calcium. Interestingly, with estrogen therapy of the prostatic cancer, there is even more osteoid laid down initially and calcium deprivation worsens. As new bone continues to be laid down, there is a redistribution of skeletal calcium. Uninvolved bones become rarified as involved bones become denser.

The most common metabolic alterations in patients with metastatic prostatic cancer are hypophosphatemia, hypocalcemia, and hypomagnesemia. Raskin, McClain, and Medsger found 36% of patients to be affected.[83] In fact, carcinoma of the prostate is probably the single most common malignant cause of hypocalcemia. Balance studies show an increased gastrointestinal absorption and decreased renal excretion of calcium, phosphorus, and magnesium. The tubular resorption of phosphorus, for example, is elevated to 91 to 98%.[84,85] Calcium replacement will increase the TRP further as more bone is calcified. Alkaline phosphatase activity is elevated in these patients, even when acid phosphatase activity is near normal. In general, the lower the serum phosphorus and calcium values, the higher the alkaline-phosphatase level.

Lyles et al.[86] recently described a second syndrome of low serum phosphorus and calcium in prostatic cancer patients, now known as hypophosphatemic osteomalcemia. Here the patients are in positive calcium balance with a low serum calcium, but have a malabsorption and renal wasting of phosphate; serum PTH and vitamin D levels are normal. It is postulated that the prostate cancer secretes a factor(s) that directly affects renal tubular function or vitamin D metabolism, resulting in phosphate loss.[86]

5.5.8. Assessment of Bone Metastases

Plain X rays of the skeleton are not accurate in telling whether a metastasis from prostatic cancer is present. An osteolytic metastasis in a vertebral body may have to destroy 67% or more of the spongy bone before it can be detected by a radiologist on an AP film. A lateral view of the vertebral body, a much better view for looking for metastases, may still require a 50% loss of cancellous bone before it is detected. However, the osteoblastic response of bone to prostatic cancer makes plain X-ray detection somewhat easier. Still, in a postmortem study by Bachman and Sproul, plain X-ray diagnosis of metastases was only made in 42% of spines with extensive osteoblastic metastatic carcinoma.[87]

If the metastasis changes the contour of the vertebral body, however, then it is quite easily distinguished. Hence, careful examination of the contours of a vertebral body for breaks in the cortex, blurring on margins, or an osteoblastic response on the margin is the most effective way to detect an early bony metastasis from prostatic cancer.

Radionucleide scanning of the skeleton using ^{99M}Tc-phosphate or phosphonate compounds (e.g., technetium methylene diphosphonate) is an accurate method of detecting bone metastases from prostatic cancer.[88] This technique is particularly sensitive in detecting occult bone metastases and is currently the method of choice in the staging evaluation of a patient with prostatic carcinoma. For a variety of technical reasons, other bone-seeking radiopharmaceuticals like $^{32}P^{18}F^{87}Sr$, ^{85}Sr, ^{45}Ca, ^{47}Ca, or ^{87M}Sr have not become popular clinically. The physical half-life of ^{99M}Tc is long enough to permit in-vitro-labeling of a variety of radiopharmaceuticals and to allow organ localization and imaging after administration, but is short enough to minimize unnecessary radiation exposure to the patient.[89] After IV injection of ^{99M}Tc methylene diphosphonate, bone uptake is rapid. By 1 to 2 hr, 40 to 50% of the administered dose is taken up by the skeleton. There are numerous hypotheses to explain the mechanism of localization of the ^{99M}Tc phosphate and phosphonate complexes in the skeleton—none established with certainty.[90,91] Focal increased uptake occurs in areas of the skeleton with increased metabolic activity. Although increased activity is quite easily detected and sensitivity of the test is great, bone scanning can also be affected by a large variety of benign lesions, so that specificity is not great.[88] Scanning can be done qualitatively for detection or quantitatively by interfacing the scanner with a computer for accurate following of the progress of lesions.

Galasko[92] has shown that radiolabeled bone-scanning agents accumulate best in early focal bone lesions when the immature osteoid is being formed or is only partially calcified. When mineralization of the new reactive bone is complete and stable (for example, after successful hormonal treatment of prostatic cancer), then bone scans may be normal even with extensive osteoblastic lesions seen on plain X ray. Conversely, during active healing in response to chemotherapy or hormonal therapy, the intensity of radionucleide uptake at the sites of known metastases may increase transiently.

If skeletal X rays or scans show a lesion, then in certain clinical settings biopsies of the specific bone(s) may be required. Biopsy can be performed by an open surgical approach or a percutaneous approach using a biopsy needle. Random or blind sampling of the bone marrow is another way of assessing whether prostatic cancer has metastasized to the bone. As pointed out earlier, the lumbar vertebral bodies would be the bones most likely to be positive for metastases. Clinically, however, bone biopsy or aspiration of the iliac crest or sternum is most often performed because of their accessibility. The specimen obtained is examined for prostatic cancer cells on a smear or a section.

In the early 1970s, there was a certain enthusiasm for determining the acid phosphatase on the serum from bone marrow, under the assumption that this would more likely be elevated if the metastases were present in the marrow space. Currently, enzymatic determination of bone marrow acid phosphatase is not useful clinically due to many false-positives.[93] Use of the RIA for acid phosphatase may, however, improve the specificity of the test. The reader is referred to the review by Henneberry, Engel, and Grayhack[94] for a succinct, but comprehensive review of the subject.

5.5.9. Treatment of Bone Metastases

The detection of prostatic cancer metastases to bone is important clinically so that patients may receive the appropriate therapy and be spared potentially morbid modalities that offer no hope for cure. Once bone metastases are detected, then treatment of the metastases is aimed at: (1) relief of pain, (2) prevention of pathologic fracture, and (3) prevention of neurologic sequelae.

Since the demonstration by Huggins and Hodges that many prostatic cancers are hormonally responsive,[95] manipulation of the endocrine system has usually been the first treatment modality employed. After hormonal resistance is established, treatment of generalized bone pain can be with: (1) chemotherapy,[96] (2) systemic bone-seeking radioactive materials, (3) hypophysectomy, or (4) wide-field radiation therapy. Although remissions caused by chemotherapy are reported enthusiastically by various research groups, clinical use of chemotherapeutic agents for prostatic carcinoma is frequently limited by its use only late in the disease. The low bone marrow, renal, nutritional, and cardiac reserve of the patients usually preclude use of aggressive meaningful chemotherapy in clinical practice.

The bone-seeking radioactive agents have not gained widespread acceptance as clinical therapeutic tools. Both ^{82}strontium and ^{32}phosphorus with or without testosterone or parathyroid hormone priming have been used with modest morbidity but also a low therapeutic index.

Hypophysectomy is now performed primarily via the transsphenoidal approach.[97,98] Impressive palliation with very prompt pain relief has been attained in both metastatic prostatic and breast carcinoma with a low morbidity. The mechanism of action for pain relief is not entirely understood though it may not be a simple manipulation of systemic androgen. The procedure is currently limited by the need for a neurosurgeon skilled in performing the transsphenoidal approach and close medical supervision following surgery.

Wide-field or half-body irradiation of bone metastases can be used to palliate widespread painful metastases. A 24% complete and 48% partial relief of pain has been reported, with pain relief lasting an average of 4.7 months.[99] The side effects have been primarily nausea and vomiting which remits and bone marrow depression. This latter complication may well limit its application in prostatic cancer patients who have little marrow reserve.

For a few specific spots of bone pain, external beam radiation therapy is often effective with very little morbidity. In clinical practice, this is the most effective method of palliatively treating a specific painful spot from patient tolerance and economic standpoints.[100]

The propensity for prostatic carcinoma to lead to paraplegia is well-known. Any neurological changes in the lower extremities require consideration of the possibility of impending paraplegia. Rapid evaluation and decompressive laminectomy performed as an emergency procedure can lead to salvage of lower extremity function.[101,102] Pathologic fracture is less common with prostatic carcinoma than with tumors yielding osteolytic metastases. Occasionally, however, bony surgical fixation of the spine or femur is required.

References

1. Goldman, R., 1977, Aging of the excretory system, in: *Handbook of the Biology of Aging* (C. E. Finch and L. Hayflick, eds.), Van Nostrand-Reinhold Company, New York, pp. 409–431.
2. Rowe, J. W., Andres, R., Tobin, J. D., Norris, A. M., and Shock, N. W., 1976, The effect of age on creatinine clearance in man: A cross-sectional and longitudinal study, *J. Gerontol.* 31:155–163.
3. Appel, G. B. and Neu, H. C., 1977, The nephrotoxicity of antimicrobial agents, *N. Engl. J. Med.* 296:663–670, 722–728, 784–787.
4. Sommer, B., Ferguson, R., Davin, T., Kjellstrand, C., and Fryd, D., 1981, Renal transplantation in patients over 50 years of age, VIII International Congress of the Transplantation Society, Boston, Mass., 6/29/80–7/5/80.
5. Ost, L., Groth, C. G., Lindholm, B., Lundgren, G., Magnesson, G., and Tillegard, A., 1980, Cadaveric renal transplantation in patients of 60 years and above, *Transplantation* 30:339–341.
6. Oreopoulos, D. G., 1978, Maintenance peritoneal dialysis, in: *Strategy in Renal Failure* (E. A. Friedman, ed.), John Wiley & Sons, New York, pp. 393–414.
7. Blagg, C. R., 1978, Objective quantification of rehabilitation in dialysis and transplantation, in: *Strategy in Renal Failure* (E. A. Friedman, ed.), John Wiley & Sons, New York, pp. 415–433.
8. Tanagho, E. A., 1978, Neuropathic bladder disorders, in: *General Urology* (D. R. Smith, ed.), Lange Medical Publications, Los Altos, pp. 333–353.
9. DeGroat, W. C. and Booth, A. M., 1980, Physiology of the urinary bladder and urethra, *Ann. Intern. Med.* 92(Part 2):312–315.
10. Wein, A. J. and Raezer, D. M., 1979, Physiology of micturition, in: *Clinical Neurourology* (R. J. Krane and M. B. Siroky, eds.), Little Brown Company, Boston, pp. 1–33.
11. Abrams, P. H. and Torrens, M., 1979, Urine flow studies, *Urol. Clin. N. Am.* 6(1):71–79.
12. Torrens, M. and Abrams, P. H., 1979, Cystometry, *Urol. Clin. North. Am.* 6(1):79–85.
13. Blaivas, J. G. and Fisher, D. M., 1981, Combined radiographic and urodynamic monitoring: Advances in technique, *J. Urol.* 125:693–694.
14. Diokno, A. C., Koff, S. A., and Anderson, W., 1976, Combined cystometry and perineal electromyography in the diagnosis and treatment of urinary incontinence, *J. Urol.*, 115:161–163.
15. Abrams, P. H., 1979, Perfusion urethral profilometry, *Urol. Clin. North. Am.*, 6(1):103–110.
16. Bors, E. and Comarr, A. E., 1971, *Neurological Urology,* University Park Press, Baltimore, pp. 129–135.

17. Lapides, J., 1970, Neuromuscular vesical and ureteral dysfunction, in: *Urology* (M. F. Campbell and J. M. Harrison, eds.), 3rd ed., W. B. Saunders Company, Philadelphia, pp. 1343-1378.

18. Wein, A. J., 1981, Classification of neurogenic voiding dysfunction, *J. Urol.*, 125:605-609.

19. Wein, A. J., Raezer, D. M., and Benson, G. S., 1976, Management of neurogenic bladder dysfunction in the adult, *Urology* 8:432-443.

20. Cole, A. T. and Fried, F. A., 1972, Favorable experiences with imipramine in the treatment of neurogenic bladder, *J. Urol.* 107:44-45.

21. Benson, G. S., Sarshik, S. A., Raezer, D. M., and Wein, A. J., 1977, Comparative effects and mechanisms of action of atropine, propantheline, flavoxate, and imipramine on bladder muscle contractility, *Urology* 9:31-35.

22. Gibbon, N. O. K., 1965, Urinary incontinence in disorders of the nervous system, *Br. J. Urol.* 37:624-632.

23. Krane, R. J. and Olsson, C. A., 1973, Phenoxybenzamine in neurogenic bladder dysfunction—Clinical considerations, *J. Urol.* 110:653-656.

24. Murdock, M., Sax, D., and Krane, R. J., 1976, Use of dantrolene sodium in external sphincter spasm, *Urology* 8:133-137.

25. Kaufman, J. J., 1973, Treatment of post-prostatectomy incontinence using a silicone-gel prosthesis, *Br. J. Urol.*, 45:646-653.

26. Scott, F. B., 1973, Treatment of urinary incontinence by implantable prosthetic sphincter, *Urology* 1:252-259.

27. Lapides, J., Diokno, A. C., Lowe, B. S., and Kalish, M. D., 1974, Follow-up on unsterile, intermittent self-catheterization, *J. Urol.* 111:184-187.

28. Warren, J. W., Muncie, H. L., Jr., Bergquist, E. J., and Hoopes, J. M., 1981, Sequalae and management of urinary infection in the patient requiring chronic catheterization, *J. Urol.* 125:1-8.

29. Warren, J. W., Platt, R., Thomas, R. J., Rosner, B., and Kass, E. H., 1978, Antibiotic irrigation and catheter—Associated urinary-tract infections, *N. Engl. J. Med.* 299:570-573.

30. Gribaldi, R. A., Burke, J. P., Britt, M. R., Miller, W. A., and Smith, C. B., 1980, Meatal colonization and catheter—Associated bacteriuria, *N. Engl. J. Med.* 303:316-318.

31. Priefer, B., Duthie, E. H., Jr., and Gambert, S. R., Frequency of urinary catheter change and clinical urinary tract infection in a skilled nursing home, *Urology*, 20: 141-142, 1982.

32. Musher, D. M., Griffith, D. P., and Richie, Y., 1976, The generation of formaldehyde from methenamine: Effect of urinary flow and residual volume, *Invest. Urol.* 13:380-382.

33. Vainrub, B. and Musher, D. M., 1977, Lack of effect of methenamine in suppression of, or prophylaxis against, chronic urinary infection, *Antimicrob. Agents Chemother.* 12:625-629.

34. Silverberg, E., 1977, Cancer statistics, *Cancer* 27:26.

35. Hoover, R., Mason, T. J., McKay, F. W., and Fraumeni, J. F., Jr., 1975, Cancer by county: New resources for etiologic clues, *Science* 189:1005-1007.

36. Veys, C. A., 1974, Bladder tumours and occupation: A coroner's notification scheme, *Br. J. Ind. Med.* 31:65-71.

37. Cole, P., Hoover, R., and Friedell, G. H., 1972, Occupation and cancer of the lower urinary tract, *Cancer* 29:1250-1260.
38. Morgan, R. W. and Jain, M. G., 1974, Bladder cancer: Smoking, beverages, and artificial sweeteners, *Can. Med. Assoc. J.* 111:1067-1070.
39. Mustacchi, P. and Shimkin, M. B., 1958, Cancer of the bladder and infestation with *Schistosoma haematobium*, *J. Natl. Cancer Inst.* 20:825-842.
40. Kaufman, J. M., Fam, B., Jacobs, S. C., Gabilondo, F., Yalla, S., Kane, J. P., and Rossier, A. B., 1977, Bladder cancer of squamous metaplasia in spinal cord injury patients, *J. Urol.* 118:967-971.
41. Wall, R. L. and Clausen, K. P., 1975, Carcinoma of the urinary bladder in patients receiving cycloplosphamide, *N. Engl. J. Med.* 293:271-273.
42. Baker, R. and Maxted, W., 1971, Tumours of the urinary bladder, in: *Urology* (Karafin, L. and Kendall, A. R., eds.), Harper and Row, New York.
43. Hamlin, D. J. and Cockett, A. T. K., 1980, Modification for computerized tomographic staging of infiltrative bladder cancer, *J. Urol.* 123:489-491.
44. Barnes, R. W., Dick, A. L., Hadley, H. L. and Johnston, O. L., 1977, Survival following transurethral resection of bladder carcinoma, *Cancer Res.* 37:2895.
45. Greene, L. F., Hanash, K. A., and Farrow, G. M., 1973, Benign papilloma or papillary carcinoma of the bladder?, *J. Urol.*, 110:205-207.
46. Althausen, A. F., Prout, G. R., Jr., and Daly, J. J., 1976, Noninvasive papillary carcinoma of the bladder associated with carcinoma in situ, *J. Urol.* 116:575-580.
47. Utz, D. C., Schmitz, S. E., Fugelso, P. D., and Farrow, G. M., 1973, A clinocopathologic evaluation of partial cystectomy for carcinoma of the urinary bladder, *Cancer* 32:1075-1077.
48. Novick, A. C. and Stewart, B. H., 1976, Partial cystectomy in the treatment of primary and secondary carcinoma of the bladder, *J. Urol.* 116:570-574.
49. Caldwell, W. L., 1976, Radiotherapy: Definitive, integrated, and palliative therapy, *Urol. Clin. North. Am.* 3:129-148.
50. Whitmore, W. F., Batata, M. A., Ghoneim, M., Grabstald, H., and Unal, A., 1977, Radical cystectomy with or without prior irradiation in the treatment of bladder cancer, *J. Urol.* 118:184-187.
51. Brannan, W., Fuselier, H. A., Jr., Ochsner, M., and Randrup, E. R., 1981, Critical evaluation of 1-stage cystectomy—Reduced morbidity and mortality, *J. Urol.* 125:640-642.
52. Kursh, E. D., Rabin, R., and Persky, L., 1977, Is cystectomy a safe procedure in elderly patients with carcinoma of the bladder?, *J. Urol.* 118:40-42.
53. Jones, H. C. and Swinney, J., 1961, Thiotepa in the management of tumours of the bladder, *Lancet* ii:615.
54. Koontz, W. W., Jr., Prout, G. R., Jr., Smith, W., Frable, W. J., and Minnis, J. E., 1981, The use of intravesical thiotepa in the management of non-invasive carcinoma of the bladder, *J. Urol.* 125:307-312.
55. Nocks, B. N., Nieh, P. T., and Prout, G. R., Jr., 1979, A longitudinal study of patients with superficial bladder carcinoma successfully treated with weekly intravesical thio-tepa, *J. Urol.* 122:27-29.
56. Soloway, M. S., Murphy, W. M., DeFuria, D., Crooke, S., and Finebaum, P., 1981, The effect of mitomycin C on superficial bladder cancer, *J. Urol.* 126:646.
57. Bracken, R. B., Johnson, D. E., von Eschenbach, A. C., Swanson, D. A., DeFuria,

D., and Crooke, S., 1980, Role of intravesical mitomycin C in management of bladder tumours, *Urology* 16:11.

58. Carter, S. K., 1975, The chemotherapy of bladder cancer, in: *Chemotherapy of Urogenital Tumours* (G. P. Murphy and A. Mittleman, eds.), Charles C. Thomas, Springfield, pp. 105-127.
59. Herr, H. W., 1980, Cis-diamminedichloride platinum II in the treatment of advanced bladder cancer, *J. Urol.* 123:853.
60. Soloway, M. S., Ikard, M., and Ford, K., 1981, Cis-diamminedichloroplatinum (II) in locally advanced and metastatic urothelial cancer, *Cancer* 47:476.
61. Yagoda, A., Watson, R. C., Gonzalez-Vitale, J. C., Grabstald, H., Whitmore, W. F., 1976, Cis-dichlorodiammineplatinum (II) in advanced bladder cancer, *Cancer Treat. Rep.* 60:917.
62. Sternberg, J. J., Bracken, R. B., Handel, P. B., and Johnson, D. E., 1977, Combination chemotherapy (CISCA) for advanced urinary tract carcinoma. A preliminary report, *JAMA* 238:2282.
63. Williams, S. D., Rohn, R. H., Donohue, J. P., and Einhorn, L. H., 1978, Chemotherapy of bladder cancer with cis-diamminedichloroplatinum (DDP), adriamycin (ADR), and 5-fluorouracil (5-FU), *Proc. Am. Assoc. Cancer Res.,* 19:316 (abstract).
64. McNeal, J. E., Developmental and comparative anatomy of the prostate, in: *Benign Prostatic Hyperplasia,* DHEW Publication No. NIH 76-1113, pp. 1-9.
65. Rotkin, I. D., Epidemiology of benign prostatic hypertrophy: Review and speculations, in: *Benign Prostatic Hyperplasia,* DHEW Publication No. NIH 76-1113, pp. 105-117.
66. Klein, L. A., 1979, Prostatic carcinoma. *N. Engl. J. Med.* 300:824-833.
67. Catalona, W. J. and Scott, W. W., Carcinoma of the prostate: A review, *J. Urol.* 119:1-8.
68. Whitmore, W. F., Jr., 1973, The natural history of prosatic cancer, *Cancer* 32:1104-1112.
69. Veterans Administration Cooperative Urological Research Group, 1976, Treatment and survival of patients with cancer of the prostate, *Surg. Gynecol. Obstet.* 124:1011-1017.
70. Watson, R. A. and Tang, D. B., 1980, The predictive value of prostatic acid phosphatase as a screening test for prostatic cancer, *N. Engl. J. Med.* 303:497-498.
71. Resnick, M. I., 1980, Evaluation of prostatic carcinoma: Noninvasive and preoperative techniques, *The Prostate* 1:311-320.
72. Guinan, P., Bush, I., Ray, V., Veith, R., Rao, R., and Bhatti, R., 1980, The accuracy of the rectal examination in the diagnosis of prostate carcinoma, *N. Engl. J. Med.* 303:499-502.
72a. Thompson, H., 1854, *Trans. Path. Soc. London* 5:524.
73. Franks, L. M., 1956, The spread of prostatic carcinoma, *J. Pathol. Bact.* 72:603-611.
74. Drury, R. A. B., Palmer, P. H., and Highman, W. J., 1964, Carcinomatous metastatis to the vertebral bodies, *J. Clin. Pathol.* 17:448-457.
75. Willis, R. A., 1973, Secondary tumors of bones, in: *The Spread of Tumours in the Human Body,* 3rd ed., Butterworth and Company, London, pp. 229-250.

76. Dodds, P. R., Caride, V. J., and Lytton, B., 1981, The role of vertebral veins in the dissemination of prostatic cancer, *J. Urol.* 126:753–755.

77. Cook, G. B. and Watson, F. R., 1968, Events in the natural history of prostate cancer: Using salvage curve, mean age distributions, and contingency coefficients, *J. Urol.* 99:87–96.

78. Valentin-Opran, A., Edouard, C., Charhon, S., and Meunier, P., 1980, Histomorphometric analysis of iliac bone metastases of prosatic origin, in: *Symposium C.E.M.O. III Bone and Tumors,* Editions Medicine and Hygiene, Geneva, pp. 24–28.

79. Jacobs, S. C., Pikna, D., and Lawson, R. K., 1979, Prostatic osteoblastic factor, *Invest. Urol.* 17:195–198.

80. Jacobs, S. C. and Lawson, R. K., 1980, Mitogenic factor in human prostate extracts, *Urology* 14:488–491.

81. Cooper, E. H. and Stone, J., 1979, Acute phase reactant proteins in cancer, *Adv. Cancer Res.* 30:1–44.

82. Catalona, W. J., 1980, Immunobiology of carcinoma of the prostate, *Invest. Urol.* 17:373–377.

83. Raskin, P., McClain, C. J., and Medsger, T. A., Jr., 1973, Hypocalcemia associated with metastatic bone disease, *Arch. Intern. Med.* 132:538–543.

84. Erlich, M., Goldstein, M., and Heinemann, H. O., 1963, Hypocalcemia, hypoparathyroidism, and osteoblastic metastases, *Metabolism* 12:516–526.

85. Randall, R. E., Jr. and Lireman, D. S., 1964, Hypocalcemia and hypophosphatemia accompanying osteoblastic metastases, *J. Clin. Endocrinol. Metab.* 24:1331–1333.

86. Lyles, K. W., Berry, W. R., Haussler, M., Harrelson, J. M., Drenzer, M. K., 1980, Hypophosphatemic, osteomalacia: Association with prostatic carcinoma. *Ann. Intern. Med.* 93:275–278.

87. Bachman, A. L. and Sproul, E. E., 1955, Correlation of radiographic and autopsy findings in suspected metastases in the spine, *Bull. N.Y. Acad. Med.* 31:146–152.

88. O'Mara, R. E., 1976, Skeletal scanning in neoplastic disease, *Cancer* 37:480.

89. Marrar, A. G. and Siegel, B. A., 1979, Bone tracers: Radionucleide imaging in related techniques, in: *Skeletal Research* (Simmons, O. J. and Kunin, A. S., eds.), Academic Press, New York, pp. 456–486.

90. Jones, A. G., Francis, M. D., and Davis, M. A., 1976, Bone scanning: Radionuclidic reaction mechanisms, *Sem. Nucl. Med.* 6:3–18.

91. Davis, M. A. and Jones, A. G., 1976, Comparison of ^{99M}Tc-labeled phosphate and phosphonate agents for skeletal imaging, *Sem. Nucl. Med.* 6:19–31.

92. Galasko, C. S. B., 1975, The pathological basis for skeletal scintigraphy, *J. Bone Joint Surg.* 578:353–359.

93. Pontes, J. E., 1980, Clinical significance of serum and bone marrow acid phosphatase, *The Prostate* 1:465–470.

94. Henneberry, M. D., Engel, G., and Grayhack, S. T., 1979, Acid phosphatase, *Urol. Clin. North. Am.* 6:629–641.

95. Huggins, C. and Hodges, C. V., 1941, Studies on prostatic cancer. I. The effect of castration, estrogen, and androgen injection on serum phosphatases in metastatic carcinoma of the prostate, *Cancer Res.* 1:293–297.

96. Torti, F. M. and Carter, S. K., 1980, The chemotherapy of prostatic adenocarcinoma, *Ann. Intern. Med.* 92:681–689.

97. Tindall, G. T., Paume, N. S., and Nixon, D. W., 1979, Transsphenoidal hypophysectomy for disseminated carcinoma of the prostate gland, *J. Neurosurg.* 50:275–282.

98. Silverberg, G. D., 1977, Hypophysectomy in the treatment of disseminated prostate carcinoma, *Cancer* 39:1727–1731.

99. Fitzpatrick, P. J., 1981, Wide-field irradiation of bone metastases, in: *Bone Metastasis* (Weiss, L. and Gilbert, H. A., eds.), C. K. Hall, Boston, pp. 399–428.

100. Wizenberg, M. J., 1981, The philosophy and economics of palliative radiotherapy for bone metastases, in: *Bone Metastasis* (Weiss, L. and Gilbert, H. A., eds.), C. K. Hall, Boston, pp. 390–398.

101. Marshall, S., Tavel, F. R., and Schulte, J. W., 1963, Spinal cord compression secondary to metastatic carcinoma of the prostate treated by decompressive laminectomy, *J. Urol.* 88:667–673.

102. Rubin, H., Lome, L. G., and Presman, D., 1974, Neurological manifestations of metastatic prostatic carcinoma, *J. Urol.* 111:799–802.

Endocrinology and Metabolism in the Elderly

Uriel S. Barzel, Steven R. Gambert, and Panayiotis D. Tsitouras

6.1. Osteoporosis

6.1.1. Introduction

A widowed woman of 63 who had been living alone was visiting her daughter in the suburbs one day in the spring. She went out with her grandchild to jump rope. On her second jump, she developed severe back pain—collapse fracture of a vertebra—which immobilized her for some 3 weeks. She stayed in her daughter's house during this time, and later, when the pain began to subside, returned to her own apartment. Eventually, she was able to resume her previous way of life.

A slender, 95-pound, 70-year-old woman was on her way to answer the phone in the hall when she slipped on a throw rug that was placed on a shiny

URIEL S. BARZEL (Metabolic Bone Disease) • Endocrine Section, Department of Medicine, Montefiore Hospital and Medical Center, Albert Einstein College of Medicine, Bronx, New York, 10467.   STEVEN R. GAMBERT (Thyroid) • Section of Geriatrics and Gerontology, Department of Medicine, The Medical College of Wisconsin, Milwaukee, Wisconsin 53226; Milwaukee Long-Term Care Gerontology Center, Milwaukee, Wisconsin 53226; Geriatrics Section, Medical Service, Wood Veterans Administration Medical Center, Wood, Wisconsin 53193; and Geriatrics Service, Milwaukee County Medical Complex, Milwaukee, Wisconsin 53226.   PANAYIOTIS D. TSITOURAS (Gonadal Function, Menopause) • Sections of Geriatrics and Gerontology and of Endocrinology, Department of Medicine, The Medical College of Wisconsin, Milwaukee, Wisconsin 53226; and Geriatrics Section, Medical Service, Wood Veterans Administration Medical Center, Wood, Wisconsin 53193.

waxed floor. She was unable to prevent the fall. When she hit the floor, she developed an excruciating pain in her left hip. She tried to get up, but was unable to support the weight of her body on the injured hip. Her husband, a 72-year-old retired subway engineer, was in the living room tending to his stamp collection when she fell. He heard the thud of her fall and was already on his way to the hall when she called for help. He bent over her, put his arms around her upper back, and, very gently, tried to lift her up. They both heard the sound. It was like a snap of a taught wire, and it came from the man's back. He froze with the sudden surge of pain. The pain was unbearable and he was covered with cold sweat. With a gargantuan effort, he tried to return her to the floor without literally letting her drop.

The call for emergency help was very cryptic. There were two people injured in the apartment, but no violence had been reported. The members of the emergency squad who responded climbed the three flights of stairs in the well-kept, middle-class apartment house, and saw some stirring at the door of apartment 3D. Two older ladies, neighbors of the couple, beckoned to the uniformed men to hurry in. Inside, the men found the woman sprawled on the floor, her husband sitting, doubled up, next to her.

Using appropriate radiologic examinations, the emergency room staff had little difficulty in establishing the diagnosis: The woman had fractured her hip, the man had a collapse-fracture of a spinal vertebra. The woman was to go through a hip operation and a period of rehabilitation that would last 5 to 8 weeks. Her husband's period of confinement was to be shorter, approximately 3 weeks, but full recovery would take up to 10 weeks.

In reality, surgery was not successful for the woman, and hip function did not return in full. She remained confined to a walker for movement around the apartment and dependent on a cadre of two men to get her down and up the three flights of stairs to her apartment. To get about away from home, a wheelchair was necessary. She was unable to carry on those housekeeping chores which kept her home a shining jewel for many years. All shopping, cooking, and cleaning became the responsibility of the husband. He had helped in all of these in the past, but now that these became his exclusive responsibility, things had begun to slip. The apartment was not as clean, the clothes not as neatly pressed, the personal appearance not as well-kept. They rarely went out in the sun, and their diet was more monotonous and less nutritionally sound.

A second collapse-fracture of a vertebra in the husband led to the total disintegration of this family unit, thus completing a process in which a proud, independent, functioning aged family unit lost its posture and its independence and became a ward of society.

These cases illustrate the effects of osteoporosis on an individual and a family unit. The direct cost of osteoporosis to society can be calculated in part on the basis of the fact that yearly some 200,000 hip fractures require hospital care in the U.S. At an average cost of $5000 per case, this amounts to $1,000,000,000 per year.

This is only the direct cost of hospitalization of hip fracture patients. One can only guess at the costs of the wrist fractures, the rib fractures, the vertebral collapses, and the various social service costs which are generated by this disorder.

6.1.2. Definition ϫ

Osteoporosis[1-6] is a disorder characterized by paucity of bone in the axial skeleton as well as in the peripheral bones. This results in bones that are structurally weak and thus predisposes the patient to fracture from little or no trauma. Falling from standing level, lifting of a stuck window, or raising of a grandchild up in the air may create sufficient stress on the weakened bone to bring about its fracture or collapse.

6.1.3. Pathogenesis

The pathogenic mechanisms leading to the development of osteoporosis had been subject to intense investigation by a variety of techniques. Biochemical analyses of bone tissue from osteoporotic individuals have failed to discover any deficiency in the organic matrix or in the inorganic phase of the bone. The ratios of inorganic to organic matter and of calcium to phosphorus are normal. The bone in the osteoporotic individual appears normal histologically. Although it is accepted today that osteoporosis is the result of excessive resorption of bone, there is no gross evidence of a functional imbalance, such as increased osteoclastic activity or decreased osteoblastic activity, to account for the paucity of bone per unit volume which is the characteristic microscopic finding in this disorder.

Applying to osteoporosis more analytic methods of histomorphometry, methods in which tetracycline labeling is used to delineate rates of bone growth and turnover improved our understanding of the process involved somewhat. The majority of osteoporotics in such studies have "physiological" diminution of trabecular bone volume, one-third show depressed osteoblastic activity, and one-tenth show a high bone remodeling rate.[7] The emergent concept that osteoporosis is a heterogeneous collection of disorders is supported by findings of others. Some investigators find that 10% of the osteoporotic population have an inexplicable increase in the measured level of circulating immunoassayable parathyroid hormone without any clinical evidence of hyperparathyroidism.[8,9]

Insufficient calcium intake is a major mechanism for the development of osteoporosis: Osteoporosis can be produced experimentally in animals by the feeding of a diet low in calcium but adequate in vitamin D. In man, the data are less clear: There is a fall in efficiency of calcium absorption with age.[10-13] This may compound the effects of varying dietary calcium intake on skeletal metabolism. Low calcium intake can result in lower bone mineral content[14] and high calcium intake can result in lower rate of osteoporosis,[15] but the overall calcium intake alone did not correlate with osteoporosis in a very large population study.[16] A number of investigators observed, however, that adequate calcium intake alone (in the range of 1200 to 1400 mg of elemental calcium/day) improves bone metabolism in osteoporotics whose calcium intake previously had been deficient.[17-22]

Another metabolic mechanism for the development of osteoporosis was based on known observations that excess acid intake causes increased urinary calcium loss. It was postulated that since the average American diet is rich in acid ash, this acid intake, if excessive, could be responsible for the excessive resorption of bone and the development of osteoporosis. In the rat, the chronic ingestion of excess acid was demonstrated to cause bone loss and the development of osteoporosis without causing overt metabolic acidosis.[23-25] Human studies supporting this concept have been reported. It has been shown that calciuria is increased in direct proportion to the amount of ingested protein which is acid ash,[26-30] a conclusion disputed by one group of investigators.[31,32] More recent studies demonstrate a clear correlation between high-protein intake and the development of osteoporosis (B. E. C. Nordin, personal communication).[33]

A well-documented endocrinologic cause for osteoporosis in woman is deficiency or absence of estrogenic hormones. It is well established that osteoporosis develops rapidly after bilateral oophorectomy in menstruating women who are not given replacement estrogen therapy. Hormone replacement prevents the development of osteoporosis as long as the replacement is continued.[34-41] Inexplicably, however, no one had been able to demonstrate the presence of estrogen receptors in bone cells,[42,43] and it is hard to accept the notion that the estrogenic hormones can directly affect bone metabolism without, in some fashion, influencing bone cell function. This is all the more significant since bone cells have been shown to have cytosol receptors for adrenocortical steroid hormones, and to translocate these hormones from the cytosol receptor to the nucleus of these cells.[44] There is also evidence that bone cells can metabolize testosterone.[45] No such functions have been uncovered for estrogenic hormones.

Since a direct effect of estrogen on bone cell metabolism is unlikely, it is postulated that the estrogenic effect on bone metabolism may be indirect. There is some evidence for this possibility: A number of investigators have shown that calcium metabolism is influenced by estrogens. Specifically, a negative calcium balance with accelerated bone loss is seen early in the postmenopausal years, but the intake of large amounts of calcium will reverse this loss. The ingestion of estrogenic hormones significantly lowers the daily calcium requirement and the rate of bone loss.[46] There is also evidence that the urinary excretion of calcium in postmenopausal women is related to the endogenous peripheral production of estrogenic hormones. It has been suggested that the effect of estrogens on calcium metabolism is achieved by an estrogen-induced increase in the rate of synthesis of the derivative of vitamin D, 1,25-dihydroxyvitamin D, which has a powerful effect on the absorption of calcium from the gut.[47] It is the contention of some investigators that the osteoporosis of the aged may be secondary to calcium malabsorption due to insufficient production of this vitamin D derivative.

The ingestion of some diuretics, some antibiotics, antacids, and antacids combined with steroid hormones had been shown, in a younger population of male osteoporotics, to lead to the development of osteoporosis.[48] Other factors that may contribute to the development of osteoporosis include the ingestion of alcohol,[49,50] degree of adiposity,[51,52] smoking,[52-54] and caffeine intake.[55] Immobilization, relative or absolute, is a factor in the diminution of bone substance seen in osteoporotic individuals.[56,57]

6.1.4. Natural History

Fractures are the clinical expression of osteoporosis, but radiologically, osteoporosis can be suspected before fracture activity takes place. Fractures cause, of course, a very severe and very disabling pain. The pain slowly abates, and the disability lessens as the natural healing processes proceed and bone repair reaches completion. Eventually, the patient will have complete freedom from pain. The pain-free period may last months or years, and up to 10 years of symptom-free existence have been recorded. The next attack of pain will be due to a recurrence of fracture activity. (Continuous back or hip pain is not characteristic of osteoporosis, and, if present, should suggest a complete diagnostic work-up for other causes of such pain.) Evaluation of the response of individual patients to a given therapy and critical reading of reports of therapeutic trials that are published in the literature must take into consideration the fact that incidents of fracture activity can be separated by years of symptom-free existence: Since patients generally enjoy symptom-free periods, the assessment of any therapy in an individual patient becomes rather difficult. The patient is likely to believe that the current therapy is responsible for the relief from symptoms, but the physician should maintain a healthy state of skepticism. Very large and long-term studies will have to be performed before any therapy for osteoporosis can be said to be definitely effective.

6.1.5. Diagnosis (Table I)

For physicians dealing with osteoporosis as a clinical entity, it is important to recognize that the diagnosis of osteoporosis is one of exclusion,[58] since there is nothing specific or pathognomonic about this disorder (Table II). The serum calcium, phosphorus, alkaline phosphatase, urea nitrogen, and electrolytes are all normal, and urinary calcium excretion is within the normal limits.

The foremost diagnosis to be ruled out is osteomalacia,[59] which, as we will see, is due to a disorder of vitamin D metabolism. The most common cause in the geriatric population is simple deficiency of vitamin D. Such a state of affairs frequently prevails in the despondent and depressed elderly. In some special cases, the deficiency of vitamin D is a manifestation of a more serious underlying problem, such as occult malabsorption, or vitamin D resistance. Vitamin D resistance

Table I. Some Typical Differential Features of Metabolic Bone Disease

Condition	Symptoms	Serum[a]			Urine[a]			X-ray findings
		Calcium	Phosphate	Alkaline phosphatase	Calcium	Phosphate	Hydroxy-proline	
Osteoporosis	Vertebral compression fracture Hip fracture Wrist fracture all with little or no trauma	↔	↔	↔	↔	↔	↔	Generalized osteopenia Cortical thinning and endosteal resorption Accentuated vertical trabeculae in vertebrae and wedging
Osteomalacia	Generalized bone pain Proximal muscle weakness	↔↓	↔↓	↑	↓	↑	↑	Generalized osteopenia Pseudofractures
Hyperparathyroidism	Bone pain, generalized or local Kidney stones	↑	↓	↔↑	↓ + ↑	↑	↑	Subperiosteal resorption Absent lamina dura Bone cysts
Paget's disease	Localized areas of bone pain Deformity of bone Deafness	↔	↔	↑↑	↔	↔	↑↑	Adjacent areas of sclerosis and demineralization

[a](↔) Normal; (↓) low; (↑) high; (↑↑)very high.

Table II. Conditions to Consider
in the Differential Diagnosis
of Osteoporosis

Osteomalacia
Hyperparathyroidism
Hyperthyroidism
Hyperadrenocorticism
Achromegaly
Multiple myeloma
Immobilization
Heparin administration
Severe liver disease
Chronic anemia

is an extremely rare disorder in the adult, and is likely to be associated with hypophosphatemia and a tumor.[121,122,123]

Multiple myeloma frequently presents with bone pain, collapse of vertebrae, and a radiologic picture of osteopenia (diminution of the density of bone as seen on the X-ray picture) which is indistinguishable from osteoporosis. Generally, the diagnosis is easily made if blood protein electrophoresis and examination for urinary Bence Jones protein are made. A bone marrow examination will confirm the diagnosis of myeloma and lead to a therapeutic course that is radically different from that of osteoporosis.

Hyperparathyroidism[60,61] is associated with elevation of the serum calcium. This may be intermittent, and a number of determinations of this parameter are required to ensure that the osteoporosis is not a diffuse manifestation of excessive production of parathyroid hormone by an adenoma or hyperplastic glands. As previously noted,[9] 10% of patients with osteoporosis have elevation of the plasma parathyroid hormone level without hypercalcemia and, presumably, without hyperparathyroidism. Patients with achromegaly will develop osteoporosis, but the treatment here must be directed at the underlying disease.[62] Cushing's disease[63] and hyperthyroidism[64] can also be associated with osteoporotic changes of the bones. Similar osteoporotic changes are found in people on steroid therapy,[65,66] chronic heparin therapy,[67,68] in patients with severe liver disease,[69] and patients with chronic anemias.

6.1.6. Treatment

Management of the patient with collapse-fracture of a vertebra is quite difficult. The back pain causes complete immobilization and requires hospitalization. The immobilization, the kyphosis-induced protuberance of the abdomen, and the aggravation of pain when straining at stool, tend to produce constipation which will be accentuated by the administration of codeine for pain control. Therefore, patients should be given as little codeine as possible, and fed a diet high in fiber and fluid content. (It is reported that senna extract may correct narcotic-induced intestinal hypoactivity.) The patient will find it possible to begin to move by the tenth day. At about that time, measurements for a lightweight corset should be taken and one with two steel stays should be constructed. This will be used by the patient when out of bed. In the early stages of ambulation, the patient should not be required to sit "erect" since that will increase the pressure on the collapsed vertebrae, especially if there has been a partial, anterior collapse. Sitting semi-prone will be comfortable and physiologically sound.

When bone healing is complete, and the disorders previously listed have been ruled out, one can turn to the long-term treatment of the osteoporosis. The patient should engage in physical exercises[70-72] that will be directed to strengthening the abdominal and back muscles. If the facilities are available and the patient can swim, the patient will find swimming an enjoyable way of achieving this objective. The diet should contain 1500 mg of calcium. This is the calcium content of 1½ quarts of milk (regular or skim) and few older people are likely to drink that much milk. A capsule of 650 mg calcium carbonate contains approximately 250 mg calcium, which is also the content of commercially available ground shells tablets. Calcium carbonate preparations can be substituted for part or all of the recommended milk intake. Adequate vitamin D intake (400 units/day) should also be assured. It will be prudent to examine in patients on this regimen serum calcium and 24-hr urinary calcium in order to identify deviations from normal (i.e., hypercalciuria) and take appropriate corrective actions early.

It is important to recognize that healing proceeds in the fractured osteoporotic bone in the same way as in any other fracture. The broken bone develops a callus that calcifies normally and reestablishes the continuity of the bone. The actual management of the osteoporotic fracture varies, of course, with the involved site. Vertebrae and ribs are allowed to heal spontaneously. Wrist fractures are generally set in a cast, and hip fractures require pinning or total hip replacement. The recommendations for diet and exercise previously given are not limited to patients with collapse fracture of the vertebrae, but are applicable to all those in whom the diagnosis of osteoporosis had been made, even before any fracture had occurred.

Although we know that osteoporosis is rare in blacks,[73,74] frequent in people of nordic extraction, and less frequent in people of Mediterranean extraction, we do not yet have a method of predicting which individual or group is at risk of developing osteoporosis, and therefore, no mass preventive measures can be recommended. It is the concensus of the physicians and investigators who deal with osteoporosis that in order to maintain calcium balance, the calcium intake of premenopausal white women should be at least 800 mg/day (the reported national average at present is 500 mg daily). Postmenopausal women should be encouraged to take adequate vitamin D and up to 1500 mg calcium/day under proper supervision.

A number of agents are being assessed for the possible beneficial effect that they may have on the osteoporotic state. These include estrogens,[75-79] anabolic steroids,[80,81] calcitonin,[82–86] parathyroid hormone fragments,[87] 1,25-dihydroxyvitamin D and other vitamin D metabolites,[88–92] diphosphonates,[93] and fluoride.[94–97] Some of these agents, such as methandrostenolone (an anabolic agent), and calcitonin have given promising preliminary results when assessed by measurement of total body calcium, but their efficacy in preventing fractures has not been proven as yet. It is important for the critical reader to recognize that the investigations of all the therapeutic agents and regimens mentioned thus far have been assessed by quantitative radiology,[98] densitometry,[99] computed tomography,[100] histomorphometry,[101,102] and other measurements such as total body calcium,[103–106] but that almost none has been shown to definitely diminish fracture rate. The natural history of the disease, as previously described, makes a definitive study of prevention of fractures and collapses most difficult and expensive.

An effort at such an evaluation has been recently reported.[107] One hundred sixty-five patients were recruited over a 12-year period. They were placed on a variety of treatments: Almost one-third received no treatment or placebo and smaller numbers received either calcium carbonate, fluoride and calcium, cyclic estrogen and calcium, or fluoride, calcium carbonate, and cyclic estrogen therapy. Some patients in each of the last four groups received, in addition, pharmacologic doses of vitamin D. There were approximately 30 patients in each of the treatment groups, and the follow-up period averaged 3 to 4 years in all. Overall fracture rate in the untreated group (with average follow-up of 2 years) was calculated to be 834 per 1000 patient-years. Calcium carbonate therapy (1500 to 2500 mg of calcium) lowered the fracture rate in half, to 419. The combination of fluoride (50 to 60 mg/day) and calcium therapy reduced fracture rates in half again to 210. (Fluoride had no effect at all in 40% of patients.) A similar degree of rate reduction, to 205, was seen when estrogen (0.625 to 2.5 mg conjugated estrogen/day) was combined with calcium therapy. The group of patients receiving a combination of calcium, fluoride, and estrogen had a fracture rate of 35 per 1000 patient-years. The study reported, however, a significant prevalence of side effects: 38% of patients receiving fluoride had rheumatic and/or gastric complications, and 13% of patients receiving estrogens required a dilation and curettage or hysterectomy. Furthermore, vitamin D therapy (50,000 units once or twice weekly), which was useful only in the group receiving fluoride, had to be discontinued in 24% of the cases because of hypercalcemia or hypercalciuria. No complications were reported in the patients given calcium carbonate therapy alone.

6.1.7. Summary

One can look into the future with the hope that increased calcium intake and increased physical activity will retard the emergence of osteoporosis in the aging population, and that ongoing studies will define populations at risk and definitive preventive measures that would eliminate this disorder from the gerontological practice.

6.2. Osteomalacia

6.2.1. Pathophysiology and Natural History

Vitamin D deficiency causes rickets in the child and osteomalacia in the adult.[108-111] The pathophysiology in vitamin D deficiency is related to the two known functions of vitamin D: (1) the promotion of calcium absorption from the gut, and (2) the promotion of calcification of osteoid in the bone. In vitamin D deficiency, the lack of calcium absorption results in a stress on calcium metabolism: Serum calcium tends to fall and, as a response, parathyroid secretion increases with resultant increase in bone resorption, decreased phosphorus reabsorption, and increased reabsorption of calcium by the kidney. This mechanism is responsible for the muscular weakness,[112,113] the increase in alkaline phosphatase, and the fall in serum phosphorus. As the disease progresses, this compensatory response fails and serum calcium falls below normal as well. The effect of vitamin D lack on mineralization of osteoid is manifested by the development of widened uncalcified osteoid seams which are the histological hallmark of osteomalacia. This contributes to the malaise and the bone pain and appears as pseudofractures on roentgenograms late in the natural history of the disease. Repletion of vitamin D corrects all the pathologic lesions.

Since the adoption of the legal requirement to fortify milk with vitamin D, deficiency of this vitamin in the pediatric population and the general population in the U.S. has become a rarity. In the elderly, however, osteomalacia is common[114] and its most common cause is simple deficiency of vitamin D.

Vitamin D is added to milk in a concentration of 400 units per quart, is found in some multivitamin preparations, and is formed in the skin upon exposure to sunlight.[115] In spite of these multiple potential sources of the vitamin, it is common for people in the geriatric population to avoid sun exposure, to exclude milk from their diet, and to shun appropriate supplementary vitamin preparations. Under such circumstances, the older person will sooner or later develop vitamin D deficiency and osteomalacia (which may be superimposed on preexisting osteoporosis). This state of affairs frequently prevails in the despondent and elderly. Patients on Dilantin® and/or phenobarbital therapy, whose intake of vitamin D is marginal, are particularly prone to the development of osteomalacia.

6.2.2. Diagnosis (Table I)

The full-blown syndrome of osteomalacia is seen only very late in the natural history of the disease, at a time in which severe disability has been present for quite some time. The early findings of osteomalacia are very subtle, and physicians who do not consider their patients' habits and do not obtain dietary histories tend to consider diffuse neoplasia rather than vitamin deficiency in cases where patients complain of feeling poorly, having bone pain, and losing weight. Laboratory tests at this early stage may show no abnormality, or only an elevation of the serum alkaline phosphatase, a sign so nonspecific as to be frequently misinterpreted by the physician to represent liver disease or to support the possibility of metastatic neoplasia. In spite of the diffuse bone pain and the generalized weakness, the radiograms may reveal no abnormality other than diffuse undermineralization (indistinguishable from osteoporosis which may precede or coexist with the osteomalacia), and a bone scan may show multiple areas of increased activity. The radiologist who sees an osteopenic bone cannot differentiate osteomalacia from osteoporosis at the early stages of the osteomalacic process.

In the late phase, the radiologic diagnosis is specific as the radiograms will display the pathognomonic picture of pseudofractures (Looser's lines or Milkman's fractures). The blood chemistries may reveal an elevation of the alkaline phosphatase, a depression of the phosphorus, and a fall in the serum calcium. Blood parathyroid hormone level is elevated. Vitamin D and 25-hydroxyvitamin D blood levels are low, whereas the 1,25-dihydroxyvitamin D level may be normal or low. Urinary calcium excretion will be very small. In some cases, only bone biopsy allows for the correct diagnosis, but this is not common.

Patients on Dilantin® and/or phenobarbital therapy whose intake of vitamin D is marginal are particularly prone to the development of osteomalacia.[116] Also at risk are patients who are receiving cholestyramine,[117] diphosphonates,[118] corticosteroids,[66] and aluminum hydroxide gels.[49]

In some special cases, the deficiency of vitamin D is a manifestation of another underlying problem, such as malabsorption, which may be occult, or vitamin D resistance. Chronic liver disease is associated with faulty absorption and metabolism of vitamin D may cause florid osteomalacia.[119] In chronic renal failure, abnormality of vitamin D metabolism is a prominent part of the syndrome of uremic osteodystrophy. The diagnosis of liver and renal failure need not be discussed in this context. Malabsorption is accompanied by elevation of the prothrombin time and depression of the blood carotene level due to the failure of absorption of the other oil-soluble vitamins (vitamins K and A, respectively). Definitive diagnosis can be reached by the measurement of the fat content of 72 hr of stool collection. Vitamin D resistance is an extremely rare disorder in the adult, and is likely to be associated with hypophosphatemia with or without a tumor.[120-122]

6.2.3. Treatment

The recommended daily dose of vitamin D is 400 units/day, although some authorities believe that the adult can make do with 100 units daily. When the diagnosis of vitamin D deficiency is entertained, a trial of therapy with 2000 units vitamin D/day for 2 weeks will return some biochemical parameters to normal and will result in a dramatic clinical improvement. Thereafter, maintenance therapy with 400 units daily should be prescribed. If the osteomalacia is the result of steatorrhea, the dosage of vitamin D required falls into the pharmacologic range of 50,000 to 500,000 units/day. In vitamin D resistance and hypophosphatemia, where a soft-tissue tumor cannot be found and removed, the treatment of choice is phosphate therapy and calcitriol (1,25-dihydroxyvitamin D) in dose of 0.5 to 1.0 μg/day.

6.2.4. Summary

Osteomalacia is frequently an easily treatable condition that should be considered in the aged patient who presents with vague symptoms of malaise and bone pain. The presumptive diagnosis can be established by taking an appropriate history and can be substantiated by the demonstration of a rising alkaline phosphatase and a falling serum calcium. Vitamin D repletion quickly corrects the clinical abnormality in most cases.

6.3. Paget's Disease of Bone

6.3.1. Definition

The primary anatomical lesion of Paget's disease is focal excessive and abnormal remodeling of bone. This may lead to deformity and fracture of the involved bone(s) and to neurological and other complications. Paget's disease, which is more common in men than in women, is first seen after the age of 40 and increases in frequency in subsequent decades. First described by Sir James Paget, a British physician, the disease is seen primarily in Britain, in countries to which Anglo-Saxons have migrated, such as the USA, Australia, and New Zealand, as well as in Western Europe. It is extremely rare in Japan, China, the Middle East, and Africa. Epidemiologic studies reveal variable rates, with marked local variations, and some familial clustering.[123]

6.3.2. Pathophysiology

Recent investigations suggest that Paget's disease may be caused by a "slow" virus that infects osteoclasts selectively. Viruslike particles were found in the cytoplasm and the nuclei of osteoclasts from lesions of Paget's disease, but not in any other bone cells in patients with Paget's, nor in osteoclasts or other bone cells from patients with other disorders of the skeleton.[124,125] These particles will have to be identified and Koch's postulate will have to be satisfied before viral etiology for this disorder is secure.

Histologically, it appears that the primary lesion is excessive resorption of bone by abnormal multinucleated osteoclasts. The resorption is followed by an intense bone-forming activity, but the resultant bone is disorganized and abnormal in structure, highly vascular, prone to develop deformities, and fractures easily. The disease may involve a single bone (monostotic), but commonly affects multiple bones (polyostotic). The site most frequently affected is the sacrum, followed, in decreasing order, by the spine, femur, skull, sternum, and the pelvis. The growth of bone in the pagetic lesion is not subject to normal controls, does not conform to normal remodeling factors, and may result in invasion of neural foramina or spinal cord compression. Hearing loss is a common complication of this disorder, due either to involvement of the ossicles of the middle ear or to compression of the eighth nerve. Paget's involvement of the facial bones can result in gross facial distortion, and disease of the skull can cause a variety of central nervous system (CNS) lesions including hydrocephalus and pseudobulbar palsy.

The high turnover of bone is responsible for elevation of urinary hydroxyproline excretion (representing collagen breakdown from excessive bone resorption), as well as elevation of serum alkaline phosphatase (representing increased bone formation). The rates of bone resorption and bone formation are generally coupled, and consequently, changes in urinary hydroxyproline and serum alkaline phosphatase are highly correlated. Bone turnover rate may be up to 30 or 40 times normal, imposing a severe metabolic burden on the body, and requiring an increase in cardiac output. High-output congestive heart failure has been reported in patients with extensive disease.

6.3.3. Diagnosis (Table I)

Paget's disease is frequently asymptomatic, but may present with bone pain, increased skin temperature, deformity, fracture, neurologic deficits due to nerve compression or CNS involvement, or congestive heart failure due to high output.

The finding of elevated alkaline phosphatase or the finding of typical lesions on radiographs are the most common confirmatory findings of Paget's disease. The elevation of blood alkaline phosphatase with normal serum calcium and phosphorus, normal liver function, and elevation of urinary hydroxyproline are diagnostic of this disorder. (Hypercalcemia may be seen in patients with extensive Paget's disease who are immobilized, but we have seen a number of cases where Paget's disease and hyperparathyroidism due to a parathyroid adenoma coexisted.)

The radiological picture of cortical thickening, coarse trabeculation, and sclerosis, as well as deformity of the long bones, and the "cotton wool" appearance of the skull are frequently diagnostic. Active (but not "burned-out") pagetic lesions will be found "hot" when a bone scan examination is performed.[126] Occasionally, the radiological picture may mimic metastatic prostatic disease. In such cases, blood acid phosphatase may help in the differential diagnosis.

In less than 1% of patients with Paget's disease, sarcomatous degeneration is seen in a pagetoid lesion.[127] This is heralded by continuous pain and a marked rise in the alkaline phosphatase.

6.3.4. Treatment

As noted above, Paget's disease is frequently asymptomatic and requires no more than careful follow-up. Bone pain, local heat, radiological progression and deformity, fracture, neurologic deficits, congestive heart failure, and planned bone surgery are all indications for medical treatment.

In the geriatric population, one comes across patients who know that they have Paget's disease and who have been told, correctly, some years ago, that this disease has no treatment. The availability of medical therapy should be made known to these patients if they have any of the indications for the therapy previously listed.

It is important to recognize that joints in extremities deformed by Paget's disease are likely to have developed osteoarthritis, and other rheumatologic complications have also been reported.[128] The arthritis may be painful and the patient should be advised that this osteoarthritic symptom will not respond to the Paget's therapy even if the bone pain is relieved. It may be necessary, in such cases, to combine nonsteroidal antiinflammatory medications with the anti-Paget's therapy.

Calcitonin, a hormone elaborated by the medullary cells of the thyroid, has been found useful in the treatment of Paget's disease, although the mechanism is unknown. Salmon calcitonin, an analogue of the human hormone, has been licensed for use in this condition. Fifty Medical Research Council (MRC) units are injected daily subcutaneously. Complete relief of pain is reported by the majority of the patients 2 to 6 weeks after initiation of treatment. Neurological symptoms improve in some patients, although deafness is unaffected. The clinical markers for the disease, serum alkaline phosphatase and urinary hydroxyproline, fall to about 50% of their initial value in the course of treatment.[129] Treatment may be discontinued in 6 to 12 months, and there are reports of prolonged remission after a course of therapy with this agent.[130] Side effects of this therapy include transient nausea and vomiting. Flushing of the hands and face have been observed. The manufacturer (Armour Pharmaceutical Company) recommends skin testing before use.

Diphosphonates are a class of compounds with powerful inhibitory effect on the osteoclastic bone resorption. Etidronate sodium (Didronel®) is a diphosphonate that has been demonstrated to be active against Paget's disease and approved by the FDA for use in this disorder.[131-135] Other diphosphonate compounds that may be more specific and more powerful in their effect on Paget's disease are under investigation.[136] Etidronate sodium is administered orally at a dose of 5 mg/kg 2 hr after breakfast. Like calcitonin, it causes a fall in the biochemical markers of the disease. It is free of side effects when administered at this dose, but the manufacturer (The Proctor and Gamble Company) recommends a limited course of 6 months, following which there may be a period of "remission." The treatment regimen may be repeated if disease activity recurs. Larger doses and more prolonged periods of use may cause the development of symptomatic osteomalacia. Both calcitonin and etidronate sodium can be used concurrently. The combination may be particularly useful in acute neurological complications, such as paraplegia secondary to impingement of the spinal canal by vertebrae involved with Paget's disease.

Another infrequently used method of treatment involves the use of thiazide diuretics and calcium supplementation in order to cause mild elevation of the serum calcium and reduction in serum alkaline phosphatase.[137] Mithramycin, a compound used for the treatment of seminoma, causes damage to osteoblasts and has been used for the treatment of Paget's disease at a dose of 15 to 25 μg/kg.[138] Because of its potential toxicity, this drug has not been widely used in this disorder.

All the therapies outlined above are relatively new, and there is no experience with their effects over periods of decades, neither in terms of the pagetic lesions, nor in terms of the prolonged effects on the patient who is afflicted with this chronic disease.

6.3.5. Summary

Paget's disease is frequently seen in the aging population. In a majority of patients, it is asymptomatic and requires no treatment. In some cases, therapy is indicated and a number of therapeutic approaches is available.

6.4. Age-Related Changes in Thyroid Hormone Economy

6.4.1. Introduction

For years, gerontologists have been intrigued by a possible relationship between senescence and thyroid hormone deficiency. Clinically, it is often difficult even for the most experienced observer to distinguish between hypothyroidism and senescence. Both may be associated with changes in skin, hair, and nails; cardiomegaly; cold tolerance; constipation; and changes in mental status. In addition, thyroid hormone excess may present atypically in the elderly. For these reasons, researchers and clinicians alike have exhaustively studied numerous parameters of thyroid hormone economy and continue to do so. Although a greater understanding of age-related changes has resulted, much confusion still remains.

One of the first observations stimulating additional research was the observed decline in basal metabolic rate (BMR) with increasing age. Until recently, this was thought to be conclusive evidence that aging was associated with some degree of hypothyroidism. A 1977 study by Tzankoff and Norris,[139] however, has provided additional insight into this age-old observation. Studying a population of healthy upper-middle-class volunteers from the Baltimore Longitudinal Aging Study (BLAS), they observed that the decline in BMR with age was due not to age itself, but an age-related decline in lean muscle mass. Data from animal models, however, continue to show an age-related decline in oxygen expenditure even after corrections are made for changes in lean muscle mass.[140] Since the BMR is no longer considered a reliable clinical tool for the assessment of metabolic status, the controversy remains purely academic and of little concern to the practicing clinician. A greater knowledge base, however, may help us gain a better understanding of the aging process.

A comprehensive review of age-related changes in thyroid hormone economy has recently appeared[141] and will not be duplicated in this chapter. Since this review, however, a number of important issues have been raised as well as answered.

6.4.2. Thyroid Function Testing

Perhaps one of the most important questions that arises while caring for the elderly patient is how to interpret thyroid function test results. At present, the determination of serum values of thyroid hormones are universally available and provide the best indicator of thyroid hormone status. Although it is generally agreed that serum levels of 3,5,3'5'-tetra-iodothyronine (T_4, thyroxine) remain constant throughout life in healthy individuals,[142–144] not all studies support this claim.[145,146] More controversial, however, is the effect of age on levels of the more metabolically active thyroid hormone 3,5,3'-tri-iodothyronine (T_3). Much confusion has arisen in the literature due to the difficulty in obtaining healthy subjects in the older age groups. In man, 80% of circulating T_3 comes not from the thyroid gland itself, but from the peripheral conversion of T_4 to T_3. Since illness,[147–151] both acute and chronic, as well as nutritional status[152,153] can alter T_4 to T_3 conversion in the periphery, particular attention must be given to subject selection when studying thyroid hormone economy so that a distinction can clearly be made between those effects that are due to age and those due to illness.

Although some studies report a small decline in serum T_3 values with increasing age,[143,145] others do not.[142] Since the clinician should never diagnose hypothyroidism on the basis of a low serum T_3 value alone, this controversy probably deserves little consideration by the clinician. Some do argue, however, that if serum T_3 declines normally with increasing age, one might diagnose hyperthyroidism due to T_3 toxicosis at a lower level of serum T_3 in an elderly person as compared to a younger individual. In other words, a serum T_3 of 180 mg/dl in an 80-year-old might be considered "high" for that age. As with all clinical practice, a total evaluation of the patient's clinical and laboratory status must be made and if a question still remains, further diagnostic testing pursued.

6.4.3. Effect of Age on Hypothalamic–Pituitary–Thyroid Interrelationships

In the last few years, there has been little new information available concerning this subject. Most studies indicate that serum thyroid-stimulating hormone (TSH) levels are not altered with increasing age.[152,155,156] Some studies,[146,157-158] however, have shown a slight increase in serum TSH with age, yet still within the range of normal for their respective laboratories. This latter finding may reflect an early compensation for a failing thyroid gland in some individuals in an attempt to preserve euthyroidism.[159]

Although there has been a lot written in the past concerning the use of the T_3 suppression test to diagnose an autonomously functioning thyroid gland, it is currently thought that this test has significant risks in elderly subjects and is relatively contraindicated. In addition, thyroid gland autonomy can usually be ascertained by use of the thyrotropin-releasing hormone (TRH) test. The pituitary response to TRH is influenced by circulating levels of thyroid hormone; excess thyroid hormone inhibits and a deficiency of thyroid hormone enhances the pituitary secretion of TSH in response to a TRH challenge. In interpreting TRH test results, it is important that the clinician consider the numerous factors that may influence this test. In addition to a variety of acute and chronic illnesses, psychological depression, steroids, and phenytoin (Dilantin) have been suggested to cause a blunted TSH response. Although still controversial, increasing age may also result in a blunted response.[154,160,160a] This has been described primarily in men over age 50 and seems to be less common in elderly women.[161] In interpreting the TRH test in the elderly, therefore, a rise in the level of serum TSH after the administration of TRH rules out hyperthyroidism. A blunted but not flat response, however, can not be interpreted as indicative of hyperthyroidism. A hyperresponse of serum TSH to TRH administration confirms hypothyroidism; a response less than that cannot, in itself, rule out hypothyroidism in an elderly man due to a possibly blunted TSH response in this age group.

6.5. Hyperthyroidism in the Elderly

6.5.1. Introduction

Thyrotoxicosis is presently being diagnosed more commonly in the elderly. In the 1920s, less than 5% of thyrotoxics were reported being over the age of 65. Present figures place this number closer to 25%. In the elderly, the most common cause of thyrotoxicosis is a toxic nodular goiter. Graves' disease (diffuse toxic goiter) may present at any age, but usually begins in the second, third, or fourth decades of life. In contrast to the female preponderance for thyroid disease in young age groups, elderly men and women appear to be affected about equally with thyroid disorders. The exact prevalence of hyperthyroidism in the elderly is not certain, though a recent study from New Zealand of 559 elderly residing in a variety of domiciles found a prevalence of 0.47%.[162]

6.5.2. Clinical Presentation

The elderly person who becomes thyrotoxic often escapes recognition until late in the course of illness. Approximately 20% of elderly patients with hyperthyroidism fail to have either enlarged or palpable glands. In addition, classical eye findings associated with hyperthyroidism occur less frequently as do other signs of this illness. Often, only one predominant symptom referable to a single organ system is found. The cardiovascular system is the one most frequently involved, presenting with abnormalities in over three-quarters of the cases. Although thyroid hormone excess can lead to cardiovascular compromise despite the absence of preexisting cardiovascular disease, the elderly with a higher prevalence of cardiovascular problems are particularly prone to difficulties.

Palpitations occur in approximately 60%, congestive heart failure in 66%, and angina in 20% of thyrotoxic elderly. Atrial fibrillation is seen in slightly less than half of thyrotoxic elderly patients.

Elderly patients with unexplained atrial fibrillation should have thyroid function screening; approximately 10% will be found to have thyrotoxicosis. The elderly thyrotoxic classically will have atrial fibrillation with a slower apical rate than younger persons and less likelihood of revision back to sinus rhythm despite return to the euthyroid state. It is, therefore, mandatory that the clinician suspect hyperthyroidism in elderly patients who present with new or worsening symptoms of cardiac decompensation, especially when usual therapeutic attempts fail.

Weight loss is a frequent accompaniment occurring in over 50% of elderly thyrotoxics. This latter finding is usually associated with anorexia, in sharp contrast to the increased appetite seen more commonly in younger thyrotoxic individuals. It is presently unknown why age modifies this response; however, recent data from an animal model suggest that thyroid hormone is capable of modifying brain levels of β-endorphin,[163] a response further modified by age.[164] Since CNS β-endorphin has been implicated in satiety and feeding behavior, the association may or may not be causal.

Although diarrhea is less commonly seen in elderly thyrotoxic subjects, preexisting constipation may improve. Almost two-thirds of thyrotoxic elderly complain of heat intolerance. Tremor is often dismissed as due to aging itself.

Although described first in 1931,[165] apathetic hyperthyroidism has received much recent notoriety. Seen almost exclusively in the elderly, this disorder presents with few of the classical features of hyperthyroidism. Patients are characteristically depressed, unanimated, and withdrawn. Often, the clinician diagnoses the patient's condition as being secondary to a psychiatric disorder or malignancy. Classic hallmarks for elderly patients include: (1) a placid, apathetic facies; (2) small goiter; (3) lethargy, depression or indifference; (4) lack of usual ocular signs; (5) substantial muscle weakness or wasting; (6) weight loss; and (7) cardiac dysfunction with or without atrial fibrillation.

The degree to which thyroid function studies are abnormal is quite variable.

Although no specific etiology for this lack of usual symptoms has been found, age-related changes in the autonomic nervous system or tissue resistance to thyroid hormone are likely possibilities, as suggested in animal studies.[166]

Serum T_4 and T_3 resin uptake provides a good assessment of thyroid hormone status. Although age and medications may modify these values, the free T_4 index or free T_4 should not be affected. If these are normal and clinical suspicion of thyrotoxicosis is still high, a serum T_3 by radioimmunoassay may be helpful in diagnosing T_3 toxicosis. A flat response of TSH to TRH administration may also help diagnose hyperthyroidism in borderline cases.

6.5.3. Treatment

Treatment of the thyrotoxic elderly is best done by administering radioactive iodine. There is still controversy over whether a euthyroid state is necessary prior to this treatment. Those who argue in favor of first medically inducing euthyroidism claim that this reduces the chance of a radiation-induced thyroiditis with the potential for an outpouring of thyroid hormone. Others comment that this occurs too rarely to be considered. Some advocate using β-blockers as a fail-safe mechanism, though caution must be advised in those elderly persons with heart disease, diabetes, or pulmonary problems.

6.6. Hypothyroidism

6.6.1. Introduction

Due to many clinical similarities between senescence and the hypothyroid state (i.e., cold intolerance; changes in skin, hair, and nails; cardiomegaly; and constipation), many cases escape detection until late in the course. Estimates of hypothyroidism range from 0.97% to 10%,[162,167-169] depending on the population studied and the interpretation of laboratory tests obtained.

6.6.2. Clinical Presentation

Common causes of hypothyroidism include autoimmune atrophy, Hashimoto's thyroiditis, and iatrogenic causes including past thyroid surgery or radioactive iodine therapy. The thyroid gland itself undergoes numerous micro- and macroscopic changes with increasing age including micro- and macronodule formation, increased fibrosis, and involution. Despite the high number of elderly with this disorder, it is important to remember that clinical manifestations of hypothyroidism are not affected by age, though recognizing these early in the disorder is at times difficult for even the most skilled observer. For these reasons and due to poor medical follow-up for many elderly persons, some geriatricians advocate yearly thyroid function screening. What tests to get still remain controversial, though the serum TSH probably provides the best indicator of thyroid hormone deficiency, either representative of a true hypothyroid state or a failing, but presently compensated, thyroid gland. In a recent report by Sawin et al.,[159] the thyroid status of 344 relatively healthy people over 60 years of age was studied. Twenty-two (5.9%) of those studied had elevated serum TSH levels. Of these, ten subjects had low values of T_4 and free T_4 index, but only one had a low value for serum T_3 or free T_3 index. It was concluded that these subjects were in a compensated euthyroid state despite a failing thyroid gland. Since T_3 is more metabolically active than T_4,[170] the body apparently compensates for a failing thyroid gland by either increasing production of T_3 by the thyroid gland itself or increasing peripheral conversion of T_4 to T_3.

It was also of interest that another 14.4% of the 344 subjects studied by Sawin et al.[159] had what was considered to be a slightly elevated serum TSH value, i.e., $> 5 < 10$ $\mu U/ml$, without changes in either T_4 or free T_4 index. What the eventual outcome will be for these individuals is still uncertain, though most certainly some will eventually go on to frank hypothyroidism without prior intervention.

Studies that diagnose the elderly as hypothyroid purely on the basis of an elevated serum TSH value must be reanalyzed. Apparently, some of these patients have compensated for their failing thyroid gland and remain euthyroid by changes in thyroid hormone production and metabolism. This has also been well illustrated in a study on 27 ambulatory aged patients receiving thyroxine therapy for hypothyroidism.[170b]

Other important considerations in evaluating thyroid status are other clinical diagnoses and the history of drug usage. In a study recently completed by Kaplan et al.,[171] thyroid function tests were analyzed in 98 patients hospitalized for acute medical illnesses. It was concluded that an accurate diagnosis was best made by obtaining a careful history of medication usage and determination of the free T_4 index and TSH levels. Severe illness may result in a transient hypothyroid state due to overwhelming demand and increased thyroid hormone turnover. The diagnosis of hypothyroidism in the aged, therefore, is best made by documenting a low free T_4 index accompanied by an elevation in serum TSH. Although much less common, one must consider hypothyroidism to be due to a pituitary tumor or a pituitary–hypothalamic dysfunction. A low serum TSH in the presence of low free T_4 index should suggest this latter problem, though once again, acute illness among other factors may cloud the diagnosis.

6.6.3. Treatment

Treatment of hypothyroidism in the elderly should be aimed at slowly replacing thyroid hormone. The most commonly used and acceptable preparation for replacement is L-thyroxine. Because of the often coincident findings of coronary insufficiency and arrhythmias, and due to an increased thyroid hormone sensitivity associated with hypothyroidism, the initial dose of thyroid hormone should be either 25 or 50 μg/day orally. Gradual increases in dosage are made only after relatively long intervals of approximately 1 month and close monitoring for potentially harmful side effects is essential. Data now suggest that maintenance levels are less for the elderly as compared to younger populations. Studying 23 elderly (average age: 75.7) and 44 younger ambulatory subjects with primary hypothyroidism, Rosenbaum and Barzel[172] determined that full replacement dosages of L-thyroxine were 118 μg/day versus 158 μg/day, respectively. This confirmed an earlier report by Davis et al.,[173] that increasing age reduced the requirement for thyroid hormone replacement, most likely due to a decreased thyroxine turnover with increasing age.[174]

Although maintenance requirements are physiologically defined by that dose necessary to return the elevated serum TSH to normal, not all elderly subjects can tolerate this amount of thyroid hormone and the increased myocardial oxygen demand that results. It is imperative, therefore, in caring for the elderly hypothyroid person that maximum clinical judgment be used, realizing that even a small amount of thyroid hormone will prevent myxedema coma and that maximum benefit must be weighed against deleterious effects.

Replacement with T_3 should be discouraged due to its short half-life and mode of action described by some as a "burst effect."

6.7. Clinical Aspects of Gonadal and Sexual Function in Elderly Men

6.7.1. Introduction

For centuries, people believed that testicular failure was responsible for the symptoms of old age. For example, in 1889, Brown-Séquard, the renowned French physiologist, prepared a testicular extract and administered it to himself. Although he was convinced that this improved his vigor and capacity for work, his aqueous extract was obviously devoid of any significant quantity of testosterone.[175]

Although we now know that the aging process cannot be attributed to a simple lack of androgens, the development of impotence and/or decreased libido, whether or not due to hormonal changes, are perceived by the general public as definite signs of aging.

6.7.2. Sexual Function in the Elderly

6.7.2.1. The Physiology of the Male Sexual Response

The description of male sexual physiological response as originally described by Masters and Johnson[176] is widely accepted today. According to their observations, regardless of age, sexual response can be divided into four phases: (1) the *excitement* phase, during which in response to various sexual stimuli the heart rate and blood pressure increase; increased blood flow to the pelvis leads to penile erection and some increase in testicular size; other changes include erection of the nipples, flushing of the skin, and increased muscular tension; (2) the *plateau* phase, during which the above state is maintained for variable lengths of time; (3) the *orgasmic* phase, during which muscular tension reaches its peak and contractions of various pelvic muscles occur leading to ejaculation; and (4) the *resolution* phase, during which physiological parameters return gradually to preexcitement levels. This phase includes a *refractory* period, during which new sexual stimuli elicit no response.

6.7.2.2. Effects of Aging on Sexual Activity in Men

The fact that libido and sexual performance decline with age has been widely accepted since, at least, the Golden Era of Athenian culture (more than 24 centuries ago). The Bible does contain, however, several reports of patriarchs who fathered children at a very old age. The first quantitative and scientifically documented data, however, were presented by Kinsey, Pomeroy, and Martin[177] only 35 years ago. According to their data, sexual activity, as determined by the number of ejaculations per week, peaks in the mid- to late-teens and starts declining in the 20s and early 30s, reaching almost zero by the ninth decade of life.

More recently, Martin,[178] who studied the upper-middle-class volunteers in the Baltimore Longitudinal Study of Aging (BLSA), found a steady decrease in frequency of orgasmic events starting in the early 30s. In addition, impotence, relatively rare in the 20s and 30s, increases in later years affecting up to 8% of all men by age 55, 25% by 65, and over 50% by age 75.

6.7.2.3. Alterations in the Physiological Sexual Response with Age

In addition to increased rates of impotence and decreased frequency of orgasmic events, there are other age-related alterations in the physiology of sexual response; knowledge of these can help prevent misunderstanding and, consequently, major psychological problems for many elderly men.

It has been said that "disappointment is discovering for the first time that one cannot do it the second time, and despair discovering for the second time that he cannot do it the first time."[179] Indeed, the earliest age-related change in sexual function is a decline in the capacity for repeated orgasmic events within a short period of time.[177] Multiorgasmic capacity peaks in the early- to mid-teens and declines steadily thereafter. This, according to Masters and Johnson, can be attributed to a prolongation of the refractory period with advancing age[176] with some elderly subjects reporting refractory periods of up to 24 hr or longer. The same authors also reported an age-related increase in stimulation time required for full erection, as well as a prolonged plateau phase and less forceful ejaculation. In addition, vasomotor responses may be attenuated and detumescence more rapid.

Studies of nocturnal penile tumescence (during REM sleep) show a rapid decline in total duration (as percent of total REM sleep time) during the 20s and 30s with a relatively small decline thereafter.[180,181]

Psychological and sociological factors, as well as general health status of both the subject and his spouse, are known to influence sexual performance in the elderly. The role of hormonal changes in sexual function, however, is still unclear.[179,182,183]

6.7.3. The Hypothalamic–Pituitary–Testicular Axis

6.7.3.1. Brief Review of Hormonal Physiology

The testes have a dual function: production of spermatozoa and secretion of sex steroids, mainly testosterone in adult men.[184,185]

While spermatogenesis is under the control of testosterone and the pituitary hormone follicle-stimulating hormone (FSH), testosterone secretion is regulated by another pituitary hormone, luteinizing hormone (LH). LH and FSH are collectively referred to as gonadotropins. Pituitary gonadotropin secretion is under the control of a hypothalamic hormone, known as the luteinizing hormone–releasing hormone (LHRH). LHRH release is regulated by circulating testosterone levels through negative feedback. It now appears that testosterone is first converted to estrogen within the hypothalamus before it exerts its action on the neurons responsible for LHRH secretion.[184,186]

There are indications[184,187] that LHRH secretion and/or action may be modulated, directly or indirectly, by other hormones (estrogens, prolactin, etc.) and neurotransmitters (norepinephrine, dopamine, β-endorphin, enkephalins, hydroxytryptamine).

6.7.3.2. Hormonal Changes in Aging Men

It was previously agreed that (1) although mean levels of circulating serum testosterone decline in men over 50 years of age,[188–192] the variability is such that many aging men retain testosterone levels well within what is considered normal range for young men; (2) the binding of testosterone to plasma testosterone-binding globulin (TeBG) increases with age, resulting in levels of free testosterone lower than would be expected on the basis of total testosterone measurements;[193,195] and (3) the increase in TeBG seems to be related to increased circulating estrogen levels,[196–198] presumably due to increased aromatization of androgen to estrogens.[197]

It has been suggested that decreased testosterone secretion is probably due to testicular failure since (1) gonadotropin levels increase with age,[189,190,196,198] (2) response to exogenous human chorionic gonadotropin (hCG) appears to diminish with age,[196,199,200] and (3) Leydig cell mass may also decline with age.[201,202]

It is apparent, however, that although most studies characterized subjects as not being acutely or chronically ill, the elderly men were recruited from clinic, hospital or nursing home populations.[203] In recent years, data from the study of male volunteers from the BLSA were published.[203,204] Participants in this study are community dwelling, exceptionally well-educated, mostly upper-middle class white men, for whom health history, habits, medications, and a large number of physical and psychological parameters have been recorded longitudinally. From this population, only subjects *without* obesity ($>$ 20% above average body weight), excessive alcohol consumption, chronic illness, other than significant prostatic hypertrophy, and history of prostatectomy or herniorrhaphy with subsequent testicular atrophy, were studied. Subjects taking medications that might interfere with sexual function or hormonal balance were also excluded. Using this population, several hormonal measurements were made both basally and following appropriate hormonal stimulation.[203,204]

As shown in Table III, there was no significant decline in the levels of serum testosterone with advancing age. Similarly, no changes were noted in circulating levels of free testosterone, dihydrotestosterone, estrone, or estradiol.

Afternoon sampling could explain the failure of testosterone to change with age as previously noted, if the only difference between young and old men were an alteration of the circadian rhythm such that older men had a diminished morning secretory peak. If this were so, while men studied in the morning hours would show a difference between young and old, those tested in the afternoon would not. While this was reported in a study of a small number of men,[205] another indicated that testosterone concentrations in morning samples from 180 BLSA men, aged 60 to 80, did not decrease with age; testosterone levels were higher in the morning samples as expected.[180]

Sparrow, Bosse, and Rowe[206] using a population similar to that of the BLSA,

Table III. Effect of Age on Sex Steroid Levels in Serum and on Testosterone Binding to TeBG (Mean $\pm$ SE)[a,b]

Age (yr)	N	T (ng/dl)	FTI (ng/dl)	DHT (ng/dl)	E$_1$ (pg/ml)	E$_2$ (pg/ml)
25–49	24	390 $\pm$ 18	236 $\pm$ 8.6	35.9 $\pm$ 4.3	41.7 $\pm$ 4.1	21.8 $\pm$ 1.6
50–69	23	411 $\pm$ 20	232 $\pm$ 9.7	37.6 $\pm$ 4.5	45.5 $\pm$ 4.4	22.1 $\pm$ 1.6
70–89	22	481 $\pm$ 29[c]	251 $\pm$ 14	49.1 $\pm$ 5.1	41.5 $\pm$ 7.2	22.7 $\pm$ 1.7

[a]Adapted from: Harman, S. M. and Tsitouras, P. D., 1980, Reproductive hormones in aging men. I. Measurement of sex steroids, basal luteinizing hormone, and Leydig cell response to human chorionic gonadotropin, *J. Clin. Endocrinol. Metab.* 51:35–40.
[b](T) Testosterone; (FTI) free testosterone index; (DHT) dihydrotestosterone; (E$_1$) estrone; (E$_2$) estradiol.
[c]$p < 0.05$ compared to group aged 25–49.

the *Boston Normative Study of Aging,* have also reported no change in serum testosterone levels with age as determined by morning sampling.

In summary, it appears that past and present health status may have a major influence on testosterone levels in elderly men. Although it is not unusual to find elderly men with low testosterone levels, it appears that this is not the case for the healthiest segment of the population.

Vermeulen et al.[188] also reported a decrease in the overall rate of metabolism of testosterone with age. Furthermore, dihydrotestosterone (DHT) has been reported to decrease,[207,208] remain unchanged,[203,209] or increase[192] with age. In the study reporting increased DHT levels, it is important to note that the elderly men had significant prostatic hypertrophy. Prostatic tissue contains a 5α-reductase, perhaps explaining the increases observed.

Similarly, investigators are divided as to whether estradiol increases,[191,194,195,196] remains unchanged,[198,203] or declines[199] with age in men. Estrone remains either unchanged[199,203] or increases.[194,196]

6.7.3.3. Pituitary Function in Aging Men

Serum LH and FSH levels show a progressive rise with age (Fig. 1).

This finding is consistent in all studied populations regardless of the presence or absence of decreased testosterone levels in the older men. The increased LH level, despite the maintenance of testosterone levels in the BLSA men, is compatible with a Leydig cell defect that is compensated by enhanced gonadotropic stimulation. An analogous situation has been reported to occur in early thyroid failure ("failing-thyroid syndrome"), where thyroxine levels are maintained within the normal range through increased TSH secretion.[210] The fact that peak testosterone response to hCG is somewhat decreased with age, at least in part, supports this

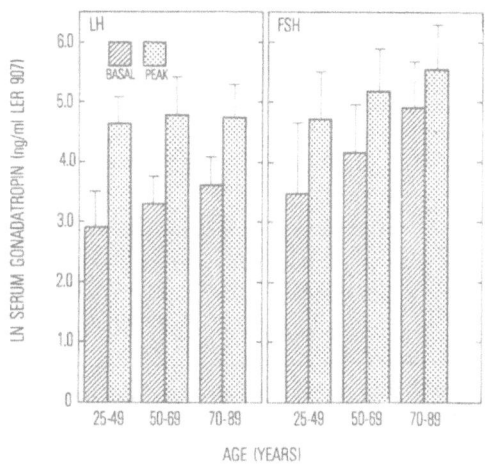

Figure 1. Log-transformed mean basal and peak serum LH and FSH levels obtained for each age group before and after LRH stimulation are shown, with error bars indicating 1 SD. Adapted from: Harman, S. M. and Tsitouras, P. D., 1982, Reproductive hormones in aging men. II. Basal pituitary gonadotropins and gonadotropin responses to luteinizing hormone-releasing hormone, *J. Clin. Endocrinol. Metab.* 54:547–551.

theory.[196,199-201] An alternative explanation for the gonadotropin rise with age invokes a decreasing hypothalamic sensitivity to feedback inhibition by sex steroids with age.[211]

Age-related decreases in gonadotropin responses to LHRH have been reported.[196,200,212,213] In the BLSA study, such a decline in responsiveness was apparent (Fig. 1) only after correcting for increased basal gonadotropin levels.[204,214] This more subtle decrease in LHRH responsivity was most likely due to the excellent health of the men studied. A significant delay in the timing of peak LH response to LHRH was also found in the older men.[204]

6.7.4. Testosterone and Sexual Activity

As mentioned above, there are several reports of decreased sexual activity and decreased serum testosterone in older men; however, the association between these two variables has not been studied in the same population until recently.

The relationship between sexual activity and serum testosterone, as well as the effects of other pathophysiological variables on either of these two parameters, was recently studied in 183 married BLSA volunteers, 60 to 80 years of age.[182] The decline in orgasmic events was found to be rapid and nonlinear. An amount of activity that represents a high level of performance at age 74 might be only low-average performance for a 60-year-old man (Table IV).

Comparison of testosterone levels in the age-adjusted sexual activity groups (tertiles) suggested that older men with high testosterone tended to be more sexually active as compared to men with low testosterone values. Although the difference between the least active men and those with moderate and/or high activity is highly significant ($p < 0.01$), there is a considerable overlap of serum testosterone levels among the groups (Fig. 2). Indeed, the major finding of the study was that only a modest association between testosterone and male sexual vigor was found. A much closer association had been previously assumed. No significant

Table IV. Sexual Activity during the Preceding Year in 183 Married Men

		Sexual activity tertile[a,b]				
Age (years)	n	Least sexual events	n	Medium sexual events	n	Most sexual events
60–64	20	0–21	16	25–30	19	51–136
65–69	13	0–2	16	3–30	16	31–200
70–74	21	0–2	20	3–19	20	20–125
75–79	7	0–3	8	4–27	7	28–76

[a]Adapted from: Tsitouras, P. D., Martin, C., and Harman, S. M., 1982, Relationship of serum testosterone to sexual activity in healthy elderly men, *J. Gerontol.* 37:288–293.
[b]Results are ranges of number of events leading to orgasm that define least, medium, and most active tertiles in each 5-year age range.

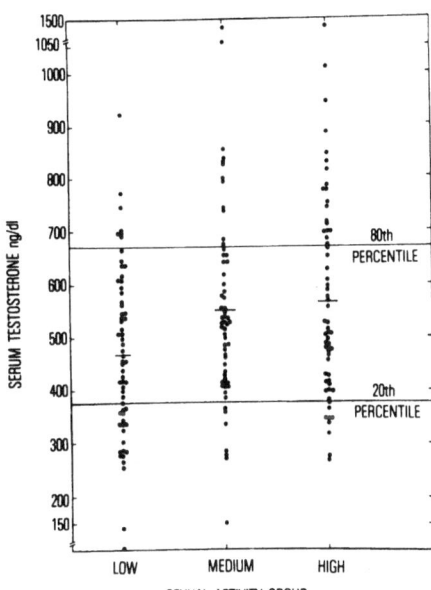

Figure 2. Serum testosterone of individuals in each age-adjusted sexual activity group. Horizontal lines in each group indicate the means. Adapted from: Tsitouras, P. D., Martin, C. E., and Harman, S. M., 1982, Relationship of serum testosterone to sexual activity in healthy elderly men, *J. Gerontol.* 37(3):288–293.

relationship was found between coronary heart disease, muscle mass, or smoking and either serum testosterone or sexual activity. Although a negative association ($r = -0.263$, $p < 0.001$) between percent of body weight estimated to be fat and serum testosterone was reported, obesity was found to have no influence on sexual activity. Consumption of ethanol in moderately heavy amounts (4 to 8 oz/day), although too small to influence overall testosterone levels, was nonetheless associated with decreased sexual activity. Heavier ethanol consumption leads to a decline in both parameters.[215,216]

Such data confirm a modest association between sexual activity and serum testosterone, but do *not* justify the belief that decreased serum testosterone *causes* diminished sexual activity in older men. In fact, only a small fraction of the older men with low sexual activity had abnormally low serum testosterone levels. It is also possible that the level of sexual activity was responsible for the maintenance of higher testosterone levels in some men, rather than the opposite. Recent evidence, indeed, suggests such a relationship in lower primates.[217]

In summary, the level of testosterone appears to be only one of several factors that may contribute to a decline in sexual activity with age. For example, Martin[218] reported, in the same BLSA men, that frequency of sexual activity in the first year or two of marriage and the general level of activity between 20 and 39 years of age highly correlated with sexual frequency in later life. However, age per se appears to be the most important determinant of sexual activity so far identified. These data suggest that other, as yet undefined, age-related factors must have a strong influence on sexual activity.

6.7.5. Other Causes of Impotence in the Elderly

There are numerous causes of impotence to be considered in elderly men. Although psychological factors, including the health of the patient and his spouse,[219] are probably responsible for many of these cases, such diagnosis should not be made before other "organic" causes of impotence have been excluded. Nocturnal penile tumescence studies can usually help differentiate between "organic" and "psychological" impotence.

The most common "organic cause" of impotence results from drug usage. The list of drugs proven or suspected to cause impotence is long and includes several commonly used agents (Table V), both prescribed and over-the-counter.

Several other diseases associated with the development of impotence in elderly men are summarized in Table VI.

Table V. Commonly Used Drugs Associated with the Development of Impotence

(1) Antihypertensive agents	Reserpine
	Methyldopa
	Clonidine
	β-adrenergic blockers[a]
	Prazosin
	Guanethidine
	Bethanidine
(2) Psychotropic agents	Tricyclic antidepressants
	Phenothiazines
	Butyrophenones
	Barbiturates
	Benzodiazepines
	Lithium carbonate[a]
	Phenytoin
	Carbamazepine
	Narcotic analgesics
	Cannabis[a]
	Alcohol
(3) Other	Atropine, benzatropine
	Disopyramide
	Phenoxybenzamine
	Clofibrate
	Metoclopramide
	Cimetidine[a]
	Serotonin antagonists[a]
	Estrogens
	Cyproterone
	Spironolactone
	Adrenal steroids[a]
	Liquorice

[a]Suspected but not adequately proven association.

Table VI.   Diseases Associated with Impotence and / or Reduced Libido

(1) Endocrine	Hypothyroidism
	Hyperthyroidism
	Increased endogenous estrogens (usually tumors)
	Addison's disease
	Pituitary adenomas (mostly the ones producing prolactin or growth hormone)
	Hypogonadism
(2) Metabolic	Diabetes mellitus
	Haemochromatosis
(3) Neurological	Organic brain lesions (commonly: temporal lobe)
	Spinal cord (injury, multiple sclerosis, tabes dorsalis, spina bifida)
	Pelvic nerve lesions
	Limbic system lesions
(4) Vascular	Sickle cell anemia
	Leriche syndrome
(5) Genital	Peyronie's disease
	Phimosis
(6) Surgical	Lumbar sympathetectomy (usually impaired ejaculation only)
	Radical prostatectomy
	Castration
(7) Hepatic	Cirrhosis
(8) Chronic illness	Renal failure
	Malignant neoplasms
	Chronic infections
	Other

6.7.6. Evaluating Impotence

It is essential that all elderly men experiencing difficulty in sexual performance, and who are concerned enough to seek the physician's attention, undergo thorough diagnostic evaluation. Symptoms must not be attributed to the process of aging and/or treatments initiated prior to a thorough investigation.

Based on available information, a flow-chart is presented as one approach to the evaluation of the impotent elderly patient (Fig. 3).

6.7.7. Conclusions

The available literature confirms the common popular belief that aging is accompanied by decreased sexual activity and/or potency. Serum testosterone levels in the elderly are variable; in the extremely healthy, no decline is noted in serum testosterone, although LH and FSH levels may be elevated.

Although a modest association between testosterone levels and sexual vigor

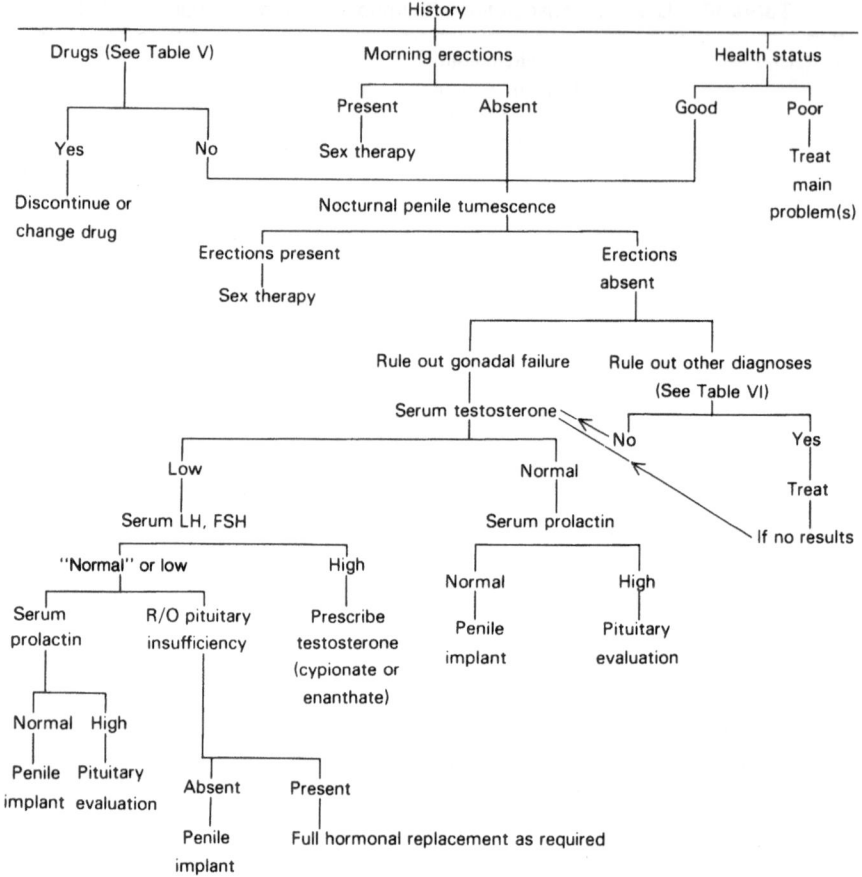

Figure 3. Evaluation of male impotence—a flowsheet.

exists, a cause-and-effect relationship has not been proven. Other factors, including previous life patterns, health status, and other psychological parameters may play an important role as well. Various diseases, including endocrine and neurological, can cause impotence. In addition, a vast array of drugs can adversely affect potency and/or levels of sexual activity in elderly men.

The effectiveness of testosterone "replacement" therapy for the treatment of impotence in the elderly has not yet been proven, although studies on a small number of subjects report short-term effectiveness.[198,220,221] The use of testosterone in the elderly should, at present, be restricted to the overtly hypogonadal, as long-term risks of testosterone therapy are yet unknown. Every effort should be made to diagnose other potentially reversible, causes of impotence.

6.8. Menopause

6.8.1. Introduction

Menopause connotes the termination of menstrual bleeding resulting from a sharp and dramatic decline of the ovarian secretion of estrogens and progesterone; this most likely is the result of primary ovarian failure.

Although the term *menopause* refers to a woman's last physiologic menstrual event, the term *climacteric* defines the rather long perimenopausal period of transition from a reproductive to a nonreproductive phase of life, usually covering many years before and after the last menstrual event.[222,223] Unfortunately, these two terms are still being used interchangeably in the medical literature.

Menopause is an inevitable result of aging. As a result of increasing life span, more than 40 million women in the U.S. are more than 50 years old with an average life expectancy of 28 to 30 years. The average age of menopause in North America is presently 51 years.[224-227] As a result of demographic changes, clinical problems related to the menopause have become more prevalent. Despite the fact that 4 out of 5 postmenopausal women have some symptoms of estrogen deficiency, it is estimated only 10 to 20% of them will seek medical attention.

The vast majority of these elderly women, as well as younger ones with surgically induced menopause (oophorectomy) can benefit from estrogen therapy. The hormonal management of the peri- and postmenopausal period, however, remains one of the most controversial issues in modern medicine.

In this section, we shall review the endocrine alterations of the peri- and postmenopausal period, the clinical consequences of menopause, the evidence of a relationship between clinical events and hormonal changes, and, finally, the benefits and risks of hormonal replacement. The clinician must personally evaluate the information presented and make his/her own decision on whether, when, and how to use hormonal replacement therapy in the management of these patients.

6.8.2. Hormonal Changes in the Peri- and Postmenopausal Period

Changes in hormonal secretion can be observed years before the last menstrual period. Rising gonadotropins, primarily FSH, can be observed as early as 10 years before menopause. Although FSH elevations can be observed in the majority of premenopausal women over 45 years of age, LH elevations are not usually seen despite a moderate reduction in estradiol levels throughout the cycle.[225,228,229] Mean levels of progesterone remain unchanged with age, despite a greater variability of values as compared to young women (18 to 20 years old).

In postmenopausal women, FSH levels are almost always elevated, although LH elevations are less pronounced or even absent in a significant fraction of peri- or early postmenopausal women. Such a disproportionate increase of FSH versus LH is seen in both normal (age-related) and oophorectomy-induced menopause.

Furthermore, despite the fact that women in their late 30s and early 40s experience decreasing frequency of ovulation and fertility, significant changes in the frequency and length of menstruation do not become common until women are in their mid- to late 40s. The explanation of these discrepancies is not known. Possibilities include (1) inability of existing radioimmunoassays to detect small changes in estrogen and progesterone secretion, (2) progressive loss of a substance, perhaps analogous to inhibin, which modulates FSH secretion, and (3) an age-related decrease in hypothalamic–pituitary sensitivity to feedback inhibition. This latter theory is supported by recent reports indicating that higher doses of estrogens and testosterone are needed to suppress LH levels in aging men,[230] and that, in postmenopausal women, even "high" doses of conjugated estrogens fail to suppress FSH and LH to levels found in the premenopausal period.[231]

Since the metabolic clearance rates of both LH and FSH are not significantly reduced in postmenopausal women, increased pituitary production of gonadotropins appears responsible for the increased circulating levels.

Pulsatile gonadotropin release in postmenopausal women occurs at 1- to 2-hr intervals; the pulses are larger than those observed in young cycling women. Hyperresponsiveness of the pituitary to gonadotropin-releasing hormone (Gn-RH or LH-RH) and increased pituitary content in postmenopausal women were recently reported.[232] Such changes are similar to those found in other failing endocrine organs (i.e., primary thyroid failure) and provide additional support for a primary ovarian failure in the aged woman.[233]

6.8.3. Sex Steroids

The universal loss of estrogen production in aging women should be contrasted to the unpredictable and less pronounced decrease of testosterone in the aging man.[188,234] Estradiol, the principal premenopausal estrogen, declines approximately 85% postmenopausally; estrone by about 70%. Similar reductions of serum estrogen levels are observed following oophorectomy in premenopausal women.[235–238] Oophorectomy in postmenopausal women causes little, if any, change in serum estradiol, estrone, and androstenedione. This suggests that the small amounts of estradiol, estrone, and androstenedione circulating in postmenopausal women are, for the most part, produced by extraovarian sites: estradiol from peripheral conversion of estrone and testosterone, and estrone from androstenedione which is primarily secreted from the adrenals. A small amount of androstenedione may still be produced in the ovaries (as indicated by a fourfold higher concentration in the ovarian vein as compared to the serum level). Postmenopausally, ovarian vein testosterone concentration is 10 to 20 times higher than circulating levels. Since oophorectomy induces a 60 to 70% decline in serum testosterone, it is certain that the postmenopausal ovary is still secreting testosterone in these women.[222,236]

The rate of extragonadal conversion of androstenedione and estradiol to estrone increases with advancing age.[239] It is not clear, however, whether this is a direct effect of aging or is due to an age-related increase in fat tissue, the major site for conversion of estradiol to estrone.[227,240]

Despite popular belief, the normal adrenal gland does not secrete significant amounts of estrogens.[222]

6.9. Clinical Problems of the Climacteric

6.9.1. Introduction

The endocrinologic changes described above coincide with the development of certain clinical phenomena. Some are directly attributable to estrogen deficiency, i.e., atrophic vulvitis and vaginitis; some are related with but not necessarily the result of estrogen withdrawal, i.e., hot flushes and osteoporosis; and some, although chronologically related to menopause, may or may not be caused by estrogen deficiency, i.e., insomnia, depression, anxiety. A causal relationship between psychological phenomena and lack of estrogen secretion is difficult to assess; in fact, evidence suggests that estrogen therapy may have no effect on psychological well-being.[227,241]

6.9.2. Vasomotor Symptoms

Perhaps the most dramatic symptoms brought to the attention of the physician by the menopausal woman include hot flushes and night sweats. Hot flushes are often described as a sensation of heat associated with perspiration, usually involving the upper half of the body (chest, face, head). Their etiology still remains a mystery. Although, in the past, they were attributed to estrogen deficiency, recent reports indicate that environmental factors may play a role in their pathogenesis.[222,227,242] More than half of all postmenopausal women will develop these symptoms; their frequency and severity, however, is quite variable. Despite the common belief that they disappear within 1 to 2 years, a recent study indicates that approximately half of oophorectomized women who developed early symptoms were still symptomatic 8 years afterwards.[227,243]

Until recently, some argued that increased gonadotropin levels, rather than decreased estrogens, were responsible for the development of vasomotor symptomatology. Recent findings have put this theory to rest. Approximately half of the women undergoing normal menopause and almost one-third of oophorectomized women never develop flushes despite the fact that they exhibit similar gonadotropin elevations. Estrogen doses adequate for treatment of hot flushes are too low to fully suppress gonadotropin secretion;[231] hot flushes can develop despite total hypophysectomy.[244] In addition, although the flush is associated with a synchronized pulse of LH release,[244,245] acute estrogen administration in doses adequate to suppress LH release fails to promptly inhibit the hot flushes.[222]

Recent studies using recordings of finger skin temperatures (an objective measurable criterion of the occurrence of hot flushes) have yielded interesting results. Meldrum et al.[244] reported that hot flushes were associated with a significant increase (35%) in serum LH levels within 5 to 10 min of the onset of finger temperature elevation. Other hormonal responses included a 56% rise of dihydroepiandrosterone, an 18% rise in androstenedione, and a 45% rise in cortisol. A smaller increase in progesterone was also reported. FSH, estrone, and estradiol did not change. Similarly, Casper, Yen, and Wilkes[246] reported that hot flushes were associated with a pulsatile pituitary release of LH. Although a small but significant parallel rise in serum FSH was also found, no change in the levels of serum prolactin, dopamine, epinephrine, or norepinephrine was observed. These findings suggest a link between central (CNS) neuroendocrine mechanisms responsible for the initiation of episodic LHRH release and those determining the onset of flush episodes. It does not, however, indicate direct hormonal cause for the initiation of these symptoms.[246]

The most effective treatment for flushes is the administration of estrogens. Doses of up to 0.625 mg of conjugated estrogens (or equivalent) are effective in the vast majority of patients. Only a few patients will require higher dosages (1.25 mg). Estrogens should probably be continued at this level for a few months; a *gradual* decrease in the dosage with eventual withdrawal can be achieved in most women over a 1-year period usually with minimal symptom recurrence.

In cases where estrogens are contraindicated or the patient does not wish to use them, progestogens can be tried although they are less effective in most cases.[227,247] Finally, clonidine at doses of 25 to 75 mg twice daily can offer symptomatic relief without serious side effects in the majority of these women.[248] It should be noted, however, that estrogen treatment is more effective than either alternative.

6.9.3. Osteoporosis

A detailed discussion of this subject is found earlier in this chapter. In summary, estrogen depletion either due to oophorectomy or aging may lead to accelerated bone loss which can be prevented by *long-term* estrogen therapy.[79,107,249–252]

6.9.4. Atrophy of the Genitalia

Vaginal atrophy is a consequence of the decline in estrogen levels and occurs almost universally following menopause. Although dyspareunia may result, this appears to be less prevalent in women who have regular sexual activity following menopause.[253]

Estrogen administration is highly effective in reversing atrophic changes of the genitalia and, subsequently, controlling dyspareunia.[221,254] Intravaginal estrogen administration has been advocated by some in the hope of avoiding systemic side effects. Although effective, estrogens given intravaginally are absorbed well[254–257] with circulating levels almost as high as with oral administration. Therefore, intravaginal estrogen administration appears to be no safer than oral estrogen usage.

6.9.5. Cardiovascular Disease

The role of estrogens in the pathogenesis or prevention of atherosclerotic diseases in postmenopausal women remains unclear. Although epidemiologic evidence suggest a sharp increase in the incidence of myocardial infarction in women after age 40,[258] a cause-and-effect relationship between decreased estrogen levels and increased incidence of myocardial infarction has not been well established.

Estrogens are capable of reducing low-density lipoproteins and increasing high-density lipoprotein cholesterol.[259] Such changes should, in theory, lead to decreased atherogenesis. Experimental evidence to date, however, does not support this theoretical proposition. Most reports[260,261] show no effect of estrogen administration on the prevalence of coronary artery disease in postmenopausal women, although one report claimed some benefit,[262] while another suggested the opposite.[263] Furthermore, estrogen given to men to prevent recurrent myocardial infarction actually leads to an increased recurrence rate.[264]

Tikkanen et al.[265] reported that a 12-month trial of estradiol in postmenopausal women reduced low-density lipoprotein cholesterol by 22% while increasing high-density lipoprotein cholesterol by 21%. No significant effect on total lipoproteins was found despite a 67% increase in high-density lipoprotein triglycerides.

Varma[266] reported that piperazine estrone sulfate had no effect on serum cholesterol or triglyceride levels after 12 months of treatment. Largelius et al.,[267] however, using similar doses of the same drug had discrepant data. Although triglycerides showed no change even after a 12-month interval, an 8% reduction in total serum cholesterol concentration and a 12% increase in high-density lipoprotein cholesterol was reported.

The addition of certain progestogens to the therapeutic regimen (for prevention of endometrial carcinoma; see below) complicates the metabolic picture even more. Silfverstolpe et al.[268] studied what effect progestogens alone had on various lipid parameters. In summary, although all progestogens tested had no effect on very-low-density lipoproteins, the use of "anabolic"-type progestogens (norethisterone acetate, Norgestrel®) resulted in decreased serum cholesterol and phospholipids while medroxyprogesterone acetate had no effect. Norethisterone acetate decreased total high-density lipoproteins as well as total cholesterol and triglyceride levels. The other two progestogens tested (Norgestrel and medroxyprogesterone acetate) exhibited no significant influence on serum levels. Norethisterone acetate was also associated with decreased glucose tolerance; during medroxyprogesterone acetate administration, *both* fasting and postglucose challenge blood glucose values increased.

The effects of combined estrogen and progestogen administration are even more complicated,[269-272] depending not only on the type of progestogen used but also on other parameters, possibly including dose of estrogen and duration of progestogen administration.

With most authorities at present tilting towards cyclic estrogen, with or without progestogen regimens, any effort to predict their effects on cardiovascular disease appears futile.

It is important to remember that, unlike the oral contraceptive literature, no significant increase in thromboembolic episodes has been reported in postmenopausal women treated with estrogens.

6.10. Estrogen Use in Postmenopausal Women

6.10.1. Benefits and Risks

The benefits for estrogen therapy can be classified in two categories. The proven benefits are (1) control of vasomotor symptoms, (2) prevention of osteoporosis, and (3) treatment of atrophic vaginitis. The questionable benefits are (1) prevention of atherosclerosis, and (2) treatment of postmenopausal depression, anxiety, etc.

Similarly the risks can be divided into: (1) undocumented risks, i.e., breast cancer, cardiovascular diseases, hypercoagulability, and obesity,[273,274] and (2) reasonably well-documented risks, i.e., endometrial carcinoma.[275-278]

The issue of increased incidence of endometrial carcinoma in postmenopausal estrogen users deserves a closer review.

Studies performed in experimental animals[279-281] 40 to 50 years ago provided good evidence for a carcinogenic potential for estrogens. The coexistence of high rates of endometrial cancer and higher-than-average estrogen levels in obese women and those with polycystic ovaries was described more than 20 years ago. Based on such evidence, Ziel and Finkle[275] and Smith and co-workers[276] designed studies to prove an association between the use of estrogens and endometrial carcinoma in postmenopausal women. The publication of their results in 1975 started one of the longest-lasting and most bitterly debated medical controversies of recent times.

In late 1975, Smith et al.[276] in Seattle and Ziel and Finkle[275] in Los Angeles reported a 7.5-fold increased risk of endometrial carcinoma in postmenopausal estrogen users. A few months later, the FDA responded by issuing a warning recommending low-dose, cyclic use of estrogens. The next year a report from Mack[282] in southern California indicated an 8-fold increase in risk, and Weiss,

Szekely, and Austin[278] using tumor registries, discovered a 10% increase in endometrial cancer incidence within a period of 5 years. More support came in 1977 from McDonald et al.[277] New reports were forthcoming from around the globe, e.g., Czechoslovakia, Finland, etc.[283]

As more studies were reported, this association became less clear.[284,285] Since 1975, an enormous amount of data has amassed on this subject, some of questionable quality. Trying to evaluate all the evidence is an impossible task, although the overall findings can probably be summarized in the following way:

(1) There appears to be an increased incidence of endometrial cancer among estrogen users.

(2) Relative risk appears to be higher in the U.S. than in most Western European countries.[283]

(3) The *overall* incidence of endometrial cancer is between 10 and 20 cases per 100,000 women of any age, per year.

(4) Whereas the incidence for women over 50 is approximately 40 per 100,000 in England, in the U.S. 80 to 200 new cases per 100,000 were reported in 1975.[283]

(5) The death rate from endometrial cancer is approximately 100 to 200 per million women over 55.

(6) The relative risk of developing of endometrial carcinoma appears to be proportional to the total duration and dosage of estrogen used.[286]

(7) Cyclical low-dose estrogen therapy is associated with a much smaller incidence of endometrial cancer.[287]

(8) Cyclical low-dose estrogen *plus* progestogen (for the last 7 to 10 days of each cycle) is *not* associated with a significant increase in the risk of developing endometrial cancer.[287–291]

(9) Cytological examination of small samples of the endometrium by suction biopsy may not be adequate for the diagnosis of early-stage endometrial cancers.[292]

(10) Any periodic episodes of uterine bleeding in postmenopausal estrogen users requires prompt attention.[292]

(11) Obese women have a higher risk for endometrial carcinona.

6.10.2. Conclusions

Based on the available evidence, it appears that estrogen use in postmenopausal women has significant beneficial effects as well as potential risks. More detailed information regarding the actual benefit:risk ratio is not yet available.

It is advised that any recommendation concerning estrogen usage by postmenopausal women follow the guidelines of the 1979 NIH Consensus Development Conference on Estrogen Use in Postmenopausal Women, which states that: "... the patient should be given as much information as possible about the evidence for the effectiveness of estrogens in treating specific menopausal conditions and the risks that their use may entail."[293,294]

When agreed upon by both clinician and patient, ideally a cyclic low-dose estrogen regimen combined with 7 to 10 days of progestogen should be started.

If "menstrual type" bleeding is not acceptable to the patient, a low-dose estrogen regimen alone should be used.

Any episode of uterine bleeding should be *promptly* investigated.

It should be noted that there are no *proven risks* associated with estrogen use following hysterectomy.

References

1. Barzel, U. S. (ed.), 1970, *Osteoporosis,* Grune and Stratton, New York.
2. Barzel, U. S. (ed.), 1979, *Osteoporosis II,* Grune and Stratton, New York.
3. DeLuca, H. F., Frost, H. M., Jee, W. S., Johnston, C. C., Jr., and Parfitt, A. M. (eds.), 1980, *Osteoporosis: Recent Advances in Pathogenesis and Treatment,* University Park Press, Baltimore.
4. Raisz, L. G., 1977, Bone metabolism and calcium regulation, in: *Metabolic Bone Disease,* Volume 1 (L. V. Avioli and S. M. Krane, eds.), Academic Press, New York, pp. 1–48.
5. Avioli, L. V. and Raisz, L. G., 1980, Bone metabolism and disease, in: *Metabolic Control and Disease,* 8th ed. (P. K. Bondy and L. E. Rosenberg, eds.), W. B. Saunders, Philadelphia, pp. 1709–1814.
6. Parfitt, A. M., 1979, Quantum concept of bone remodeling and turnover: Implications for the pathogenesis of osteoporosis, *Calcif. Tissue Int.* 28:1–5.
7. Meunier, P. J., Courpron, P., Edouard, C., Alexandre, C., Bressot, C., Lips, P., and Boyce, B. F., 1979, Bone histomorphometry in osteoporotic states, in: *Osteoporosis II* (U. S. Barzel, ed.), Grune and Stratton, New York, pp. 27–48.
8. Teitelbaum, S. L., Rosenberg, E. M., Richardson, C. A., and Avioli, L. V., 1976, Histological studies of bone from normocalcemic postmenopausal osteoporotic patients with increased circulating parathyroid, *J. Clin. Endocrinol. Metab.* 42:537–543.
9. Gallagher, J. C., Riggs, B. L., Jerpbak, M., and Arnaud, C. D., 1980, The effect of age on serum immunoreactive parathyroid hormone in normal and osteoporotic women, *J. Lab. Clin. Med.* 95:373.
10. Avioli, L. V., McDonald, J. E., and Lee, S. W., 1965, The influence of age on the intestinal absorption of ^{47}Ca in women and its relation to ^{47}Ca absorption in postmenopausal osteoporosis, *J. Clin. Invest.* 44:1960–1967.
11. Alevizaki, C. C., Ikkos, D. C., and Singuelakis, P., 1973, Progressive decrease of true intestinal calcium absorption with age in normal man, *J. Nucl. Med.* 14:760–762.
12. Bullamore, J. R., Wilkinson, R., Gallagher, J. C., Nordin, B. E. C., and Marshall, D. H., 1970, Effects of age on calcium absorption, *Lancet* ii:535–537.
13. Gallagher, J. C., Riggs, B. L., Eisman, J., Hamstra, A., Arnaud, S. B., and

DeLuca, H. F., 1979, Intestinal calcium absorption and serum vitamin D metabolites in normal subjects and osteoporotic patients, *J. Clin. Invest.* 64:729–736.

14. Matkovic, V., Kostial, K., Siminovic, I., Brodarec, A., and Buzina, R., 1977, Influence of calcium intake, age and sex on bone, *Calcif. Tissue Res.* 22(Suppl):393–396.

15. Nordin, B. E. C., 1961, The pathogenesis of osteoporosis, *Lancet* i:1011–1014.

16. Smith, R. W., Jr. and Frame, B., 1965, Concurrent axial and appendicular osteoporosis: Its relation to calcium consumption, *N. Engl. J. Med.* 273:73–78.

17. Nordin, B. E. C., 1962, Calcium balance and calcium requirement in spinal osteoporosis, *Am. J. Clin. Nutr.* 10:384–390.

18. Heaney, R. P., Recker, R. R., and Saville, P. D., 1977, Calcium balance and calcium requirements in middle-aged women, *Am. J. Clin. Nutr.* 30:1603–1611.

19. Recker. R. R., Saville, P. D., and Heaney, R. P., 1977, Effect of estrogens and calcium carbonate on bone loss in postmenopausal women, *Ann. Intern. Med.* 87:649–655.

20. Horsman, A., Gallagher, J. C., Simpson, M., and Nordin, B. E. C., 1977, Prospective trial of oestrogen and calcium in postmenopausal women, *Br. Med. J.* 2:789–792.

21. Nordin, B. E. C., Horsman, A., Marshall, D. H., Simpson, M., and Waterhouse, G. M., 1979, Calcium requirements and calcium therapy, *Clin. Orthop.* 10:216–239.

22. Nordin, B. E. C., Horsman, A., Crilly, R. G., Marshall, D. H., and Simpson, M., 1980, Treatment of spinal osteoporosis in postmenopausal women, *Br. Med. J.* 280:4451–4454.

23. Barzel, U. S., 1970, The role of bone in acid base metabolism, in: *Osteoporosis* (U. S. Barzel, ed.), Grune and Stratton, New York, pp. 199–206.

24. Barzel, U. S. and Jowsey, J., 1969, The effects of chronic acid and alkali administration on bone turnover in adult rats, *Clin. Sci.* 36:517–524.

25. Barzel, U. S., 1975, Acid induced osteoporosis: An experimental model of human osteoporosis, in: *Calcified Tissues 1975* (Nielsen, S. P. and Hjørting-Hansen, E., eds.) FADL's FORLAG, Copenhagen, pp. 417–422.

26. Johnson, N. E., Alcantara, E. N., and Linkswiler, H. M., 1970, Effect of level of protein intake on urinary and fecal calcium and calcium retention of young adult males, *J. Nutr.* 100:1425–1430.

27. Anand, C. R. and Linkswiler, M. D., 1974, Effect of protein intake on calcium balance of young men given 500 mg calcium daily, *J. Nutr.* 104:695–700.

28. Walker, R. M. and Linkswiler, H. M., 1972, Calcium retention in the adult human male as affected by protein intake, *J. Nutr.* 102:1297–1302.

29. Margen, S., Chu, J. Y., Kaufman, N. A., and Calloway, O. H., 1974, Studies in calcium metabolism. I. The calciuretic effect of dietary protein, *Am. J. Clin. Nutr.* 27:584–589.

30. Chu, J. Y., Margen, S., and Costa, F. M., 1975, Studies in calcium metabolism. II. Effects of low calcium and variable protein intake on human calcium metabolism, *Am. J. Clin. Nutr.* 28:1028–1035.

31. Spencer, H., Kramer, L., and Osis, D., 1978, Effect of a high protein (meat) intake on calcium metabolism in man, *Am. J. Clin. Nutr.* 31:2167–2180.

32. Spencer, H., Kramer, L., Osis, D., and Norris, C., 1978, Effect of phosphorus on the absorption of calcium and on the calcium balance in man, *J. Nutr.* 108:447–457.

33. Heaney, R. P., 1981, Nutritional, hormonal, and mechanical factors in age-related bone loss, International Symposium on Osteoporosis, Jerusalem, Israel, May 31–June 4, 1981, in press.

34. Nordin, B. E. C., Horsman, A., Brook, R., and Williams, D. A., 1976, The relationship between oestrogen status and bone loss in postmenopausal women, *Clin. Endocrinol.* 5(Suppl.):S353–S361.

35. Cohn, S. H., Vaswani, A., Zanzi, I., and Ellis, K. J., 1976, Effect of aging on bone mass in adult women, *Am. J. Physiol.* 230:143–148.

36. Smith, D. M., Khairi, M. R. A., Norton, J., and Johnston, C. C., Jr., 1976, Age and activity effects on rate of bone mineral loss, *J. Clin. Invest.* 68:716–721.

37. Lindsay, R., Aitken, J. M., Anderson, J. B., Hart, D. N., MacDonald, E. B., and Clark, A. C., 1976, Long-term prevention of postmenopausal osteoporosis by estrogen, *Lancet* i:1038–1041.

38. Horsman, A., Gallagher, J. C., Simpson, M., and Nordin, B. E. C., 1977, Prospective trial of oestrogen and calcium in postmenopausal women, *Br. Med. J.* 2:789–792.

39. Lindsay, R., MacLean, A., Kraszewsky, A., Hart, D. M., Clark, A. C., and Garwood, J., 1978, Bone response to termination of oestrogen treatment, *Lancet* i:1325–1327.

40. Horsman, A., Nordin, B. E. C., and Crilly, R. G., 1979, Effect on bone of withdrawal of oestrogen therapy, *Lancet* ii:33.

41. Frumar, A. M., Meldrum, D. R., Geola, F., Shamonki, I. M., Tataryn, I. V., Deftos, L. J., and Judd, H. L., 1980, Relationship of fasting urinary calcium to circulating estrogen and body weight in postmenopausal women, *J. Clin. Endocrinol. Metabol.* 50:70.

42. Caputo, C. B., Meadows, D., and Raisz, L. G., 1976, Failure of estrogens and androgens to inhibit bone resorption in tissue culture, *Endocrinology* 98:1065–1068.

43. van Paassen, H. C., Poortman, J., Borgart-Creutzburg, I. H. C., Thijsson, J. H., and Duursma, S. A., 1978, Oestrogen binding proteins in bone cell cytosol, *Calcif. Tissue Res.* 25:249–254.

44. Chen, T. L. and Feldman, D., 1978, Distinction between alpha-fetoprotein and intracellular estrogen receptors: Evidence against the presence of estradiol receptors in rat bone, *Endocrinology* 102:236–244.

45. Schweikert, H. U., Rulf, W., Niederle, N., Schaefer, H. E., and Kruck, E., 1979, Dihydrotestosterone formation in normal and osteoporotic human bone, in: *Osteoporosis II* (U. S. Barzel, ed.), Grune and Stratton, New York, p. 247.

46. Heaney, R. P., Recker, R. R., and Saville, P. D., 1978, Menopausal changes in calcium balance performance, *J. Lab. Clin. Med.* 92:953–963.

47. Gallagher, J. C., Riggs, B. L., Hamstra, A., and DeLuca, H. F., 1978, Effect of estrogen therapy on calcium absorption and vitamin D metabolism in postmenopausal osteoporosis, *Clin. Res.* 26:415a.

48. Spencer, H., Kramer, L., Gatza, C. A., and Lender, M., 1979, Calcium loss, calcium absorption, and calcium requirement in osteoporosis, in: *Osteoporosis II* (U. S. Barzel, ed.), Grune and Stratton, New York, pp. 65–89.

49. Dalen, N. and Lamke, B., 1976, Bone mineral losses in alcoholics, *Acta Orthop. Scand.* 197:353.

50. Baran, D. T., Teitelbaum, S. L., Bergfeld, M. A., Hamilton, J. B., Hahn, A. J., Hahn, T. J., and Avioli, L. V., 1980, Effect of alcohol ingestion on bone and mineral metabolism in rats, *Am. J. Physiol.* 238:E507–E510.

51. Dalen, N., Hallberg, D., and Lamke, B., 1975, Bone mass in obese subjects, *Acta Med. Scand.* 197:353.

52. Daniell, H. W., 1976, Osteoporosis of the slender smoker—Vertebral compression fractures and loss of metacarpal cortex in relation to postmenopausal cigarette smoking and lack of obesity, *Arch. Intern. Med.* 136:298–304.

53. Lindquist, O. and Bengtsson, C., 1979, The effect of smoking on menopausal age, *Maturitas* 1:171–173.

54. Lindquist, O., Bengtsson, C., Hansson, T., and Roos, B., 1979, Age at menopause and its relation to osteoporosis, *Maturitas* 1:175–181.

55. Heaney, R. P. and Recker, R. R., 1982, Effects of nitrogen, phosphorus, and caffeine on calcium balance in women, *J. Lab. Clin. Med.* 99:46–55.

56. Minaire, P., Meunier, P., Edouard, C., Berhard, J., and Courpron, P., 1975, Osteomorphometric and biochemical data on osteoporosis resulting from immobilization, *Rev. Rheum.* 42:479–488.

57. Uhthoff, H. K. and Jaworski, Z. F. G., 1978, Bone loss in response to long-term immobilisation, *J. Bone Joint Surg.* 60B:420–429.

58. Avioli, L. V., 1978, What to do with "postmenopausal osteoporosis?" *Am. J. Med.* 65:881–884.

59. Habener, J. F. and Mahaffey, J. E., 1978, Osteomalacia and disorders of vitamin D metabolism, *Ann. Rev. Med.* 29:327–342.

60. Mundy, G. R., Cove, D. H., and Fisken, R., 1980, Primary hyperparathyroidism: Changes in the pattern of clinical presentation, *Lancet* i:1317.

61. Heath, H., III, Hodgson, S. F., and Kennedy, M. A., 1980, Primary hyperparathyroidism: Incidence, morbidity, and potential economic impact in a community, *N. Engl. J. Med.* 302:189–193.

62. Aloia, J. F., Petrak, Z., Ellis, K., and Cohn, S. H., 1976, Body composition and skeletal metabolism following pituitary irradiation in acromegaly, *Am. J. Med.* 61:59–63.

63. Avioli, L., Jost, R. G., Cryer, P., Slatopolsky, E., Teitelbaum, S. T., Coxe, W., and Whyte, M., 1980, Vertebral compression fractures with accelerated bone turnover in a patient with Cushing's disease. *Am. J. Med.* 68:932.

64. Mundy, G. R., Shapiro, J. L., Bandelin, J. G., Canalis, G. M., and Raisz, L. G., 1976, Direct stimulation of bone resorption by thyroid hormones. *J. Clin. Invest.* 58:529–534.

65. Condon, J. R., Dent, C. E., Nassim, J. R., Hilb, A., and Stainthorpe, E. M., 1978, Possible prevention and treatment of steroid-induced osteoporosis, *Postgrad. Med. J.* 54:249–253.

66. Hahn, T. J., Halstead, L. R., Teitelbaum, S. L., and Hahn, B. H., Altered mineral metabolism in glucocorticoid-induced osteopenia: Effect of 25-hydroxyvitamin D administration, *J. Clin. Invest.* 64:655–665.

67. Avioli, L. V., 1975, Heparin-induced osteopenia: An appraisal, *Adv. Exp. Med. Biol.* 52:375.

68. Wise, P. H. and Hall, A. J., 1980, Heparin-induced osteopenia in pregnancy, *Br. Med. J.* 281:110–111.

69. Long, R. G., 1980, Hepatic osteodystrophy: Outlook good but some problems unsolved, *Gastroenterology* 78:644–647.

70. Aloia, J. F., Cohn, S. H., Ostuni, J. A., Cane, R., and Ellis, K., 1978, Prevention of involutional bone loss by exercise, *Ann. Intern. Med.* 89:356–358.

71. Huddleston, A. L., Rockwell, D., Kulund, D. N., and Harrison, R. B., 1980, Bone mass in lifetime tennis athletes, *JAMA* 244:1107–1109.

72. Aloia, J. F., Cohn, S. H., Babu, T., Abesamis, C., Kalici, N., and Ellis, K., 1978, Skeletal mass and body composition in marathon runners, *Metabolism* 27:1793–1796.

73. Smith, D. M., Nance, W. E., Kang, K. W., Christian, J. C., and Johnston, C. C., Jr., 1973, Genetic factors in determining bone mass, *J. Clin. Invest.* 52:2800–2808.

74. Cohn, S. H., Abesamis, C., Yasumura, S., Aloia, J. F., Zanzi, I., and Ellis, K. J., 1977, Comparative skeletal mass and radial bone mineral content in black and white women, *Metabolism* 26:171–178.

75. Lindsay, R., Hart, D. M., Purdie, D., Ferguson, M. M., Clark, A. C., and Kraszewsky, A., 1978, Comparative effects of oestrogen and a progestogen on bone loss in postmenopausal women, *Clin. Sci. Mol. Med.* 54:193–195.

76. Lindsay, R., Hart, D. M., Maclean, A., Garwood, J., Clark, A. C., and Kraszewski, A., 1979, Bone loss during oestriol therapy in postmenopausal women, *Maturitas* 1:279–285.

77. Dequeker, J., De Muylder, E., and Ferin, J., 1977, The effect of long-term lynestrenol treatment on bone mass in cycling women, *Contraception* 15:717–723.

78. Hutchinson, I. A., Polansky, S. M., and Feinstein, A. R., 1979, Postmenopausal oestrogens protect against fractures of hip and distal radius: A case-control study, *Lancet* ii:705.

79. Nachtigall, L. E., Nachtigall, R. H., Nachtigall, R. D., and Beckman, E. M., 1979, Estrogen replacement therapy. I: A 10-year prospective study in the relationship to osteoporosis, *Obstet. Gynecol.* 53:277–281.

80. Chestnut, C. H., III, Nelp, W. B., Baylink, D. J., and Denney, J. D., 1977, Effect of methandrostenolone on postmenopausal bone wasting as assessed by changes in total bone mineral mass, *Metabolism* 26:267–277.

81. Lindsay, R., Hart, D. M., and Kraszewski, A., 1980, Prospective double-blind trial of synthetic steroid (Org OD 14) for preventing postmenopausal osteoporosis, *Br. Med. J.* 280:1207–1209.

82. Bloch-Michel, H., Milhaud, G., and Cortris, G., 1970, Prolonged treatment of osteoporosis with thyrocalcitonin. Report of 7 cases, *Rev. Rheum.* 37:629.

83. Aloia, J. F., Zanzi, I., Ellis, K., and Cohn, S. H., 1977, Combination therapy for osteoporosis, *Metabolism* 26:787–792.

84. Jowsey, J., Riggs, B. L., Kelly, P. H., and Hoffman, D. L., 1978, Calcium and salmon calcitonin in treatment of osteoporosis, *J. Clin. Endocrinol. Metab.* 47:633–639.
85. Wallach, S., Cohn, S. H., Atkins, H. L., Ellis, K. J., Kohberger, R., Aloia, J. F., and Zanzi, I., 1977, Effect of salmon calcitonin on skeletal mass in osteoporosis, *Curr. Ther. Res.* 22:556–572.
86. Rasmussen, H., Bordier, P., Marie, P., Auquier, L., Eisinger, J. B., Kuntz, O., Caulin, F., Argemi, B., Gueris, S., and Julien, A., 1980, Effect of combined therapy with phosphate and calcitonin on bone volume in osteoporosis, *Metab. Bone Dis. Rel. Res.* 2:107–111.
87. Reeve, J., Hesp, R., Williams, D., Hulme, P., Klenerman, L., Zanelli, J. M., Darby, A. J., Tregear, G. W., and Parsons, J. A., 1976, Anabolic effect of low doses of a fragment of human parathyroid hormone on the skeleton in postmenopausal osteoporosis, *Lancet* i:1035–1038.
88. Riggs, B. L., Jowsey, J., Kelly, P. J., Hoffman, D. L., and Arnaud, G. D., 1976, Effects of oral therapy with calcium and vitamin D in primary osteoporosis, *J. Clin. Endocrinol. Metab.* 42:1139–1144.
89. Lawoyin, S., Zerwekh, J. E., Glass, K., and Pak, C. Y. C., 1980, Ability of 25-hydroxyvitamin D_3 therapy to augment serum 1,25- and 24,25-dihydroxyvitamin D in postmenopausal osteoporosis, *J. Clin. Endocrinol. Metab.* 60:595–596.
90. Cohen, H. N., Farrah, D., Fogelman, I., Goll, C. C., Beastall, G. H., McIntosh, W. B., Fletcher, M., and Boyle, I. T., 1980, A low dose regime of 1-alpha-hydroxyvitamin D_3 in the management of senile osteoporosis: A pilot study, *Clin. Endocrinol.* 12:537–542.
91. Hoikka, V., Alhava, E. M., Aro, A., Karjalai, P., and Rehnberg, V., 1980, Treatment of osteoporosis with 1-alpha-hydroxycholecalciferol and calcium, *Acta Med. Scand.* 207:221–224.
92. Wandless, I., Jarvis, S., Evans, J. G., Aird, E. G. A., and Stevens, J., 1980, Vitamin D_3 in osteoporosis, *Br. Med. J.* 280:1320.
93. Heaney, R. P. and Saville, P. D., 1976, Etidronate disodium in post-menopausal osteoporosis, *Clin. Pharmacol. Ther.* 20:593–604.
94. Jowsey, J., Riggs, B. L., Kelly, P. J., and Hoffman, D. L., 1972, Effect of combined therapy with sodium fluoride, vitamin D and calcium in osteoporosis, *Am. J. Med.* 53:43–49.
95. Compston, J. E., Chadha, S., and Merrett, A. L., 1980, Osteomalacia developing during treatment of osteoporosis with sodium fluoride and vitamin D, *Br. Med. J.* 281:910–911.
96. Riggs, B. L., Hodgson, S. F., Hoffman, D. L., Kelly, P. J., Johnson, K. A., and Taves, D., 1980, Treatment of primary osteoporosis with fluoride and calcium, *JAMA* 243:446–449.
97. Reutter, F. W. and Olaf, A. J., 1978, Bone biopsy findings and clinical observations in long-term treatment of osteoporosis with sodium fluoride and vitamin D_3, in: *Fluoride and Bone* (B. Courvoisier, A. Donath, and C. A. Baud, eds.) Hans Huker, Berne.
98. Dequeker, J., 1976, Quantitative radiology: Radiogrammetry of cortical bone, *Br. J. Radiol.* 49:912–920.

99. Dunn, W. L., Wahner, H. W., and Riggs, B. L., 1980, Measurement of bone mineral content in human vertebrae and hip by dual photon absorptiometry, *Radiology* 136:485–487.

100. Jensen, P. S., Orphanoudakis, S. C., Rauschkolb, E. N., Baron, R., Lang, R., and Rassmusen, H., Assessment of bone mass in the radius by computed tomography, *Am. J. Roentgenol.* 134:285–292.

101. Boyce, B. F., Dourpron, P., and Meunier, P. J., 1978, Amount of bone in osteoporosis and physiological senile osteopenia. Comparison of two histomorphometric parameters, *Metab. Bone Dis. Rel. Res.* 1:35–38.

102. Lauffenburger, T., Olah, A. J., Dambacher, M. A., Guncaga, J., Leutner, C., and Haas, H. G., 1977, Bone remodeling and calcium metabolism: A correlated histomorphometric, calcium kinetic, and biochemical study in patients with osteoporosis and Paget's disease, *Metabolism* 26:589–606.

103. Manzke, E., Chestnut. C. H., III, Wergedal, J. E., Baylink, D. J., and Nelp, W. B., 1975, Relationship between local and total bone mass in osteoporosis, *Metabolism* 24:605–615.

104. Cohn, S. H., Vaswani, A., Zanzi, I., Aloia, J. F., Roginsky, M. S., and Ellis, K. J., 1976, Changes in body chemical composition with age measured by total-body neutron activation, *Metabolism* 25:85–96.

105. Harrison, J. E., McNeill, K. G., Hitchman, A. J., and Britt, B. A., 1979, Bone mineral measurements of the central skeleton by in vivo neutron activation analysis for routine investigation of osteopenia, *Invest. Radiol.* 14:27–34.

106. Aloia, J. F., Cohn, S. H., Ross, P., Vaswani, A., Abesamis, C., Ellis, K., and Zanzi, I., 1978, Skeletal mass in post-menopausal women, *Am. J. Physiol.* 235:E82–E87.

107. Riggs, B. L., Seeman, E., Hodgson, S. F., Taves, D. R., and O'Fallon, W. M., 1982, Effect of the fluoride/calcium regimen on vertebral fracture occurrence in postmenopausal osteoporosis, *N. Engl. J. Med.* 306:446–450.

108. Habener, J. F. and Mahaffey, J. E., 1978, Osteomalacia and disorders of vitamin-D metabolism, *Ann. Rev. Med.* 29:327.

109. Dent, C. E. and Stamp, T. C. B., 1977, Vitamin D, rickets, and osteomalacia, in: *Metabolic Bone Disease* (L. V. Avioli and S. M. Krane, eds.), Academic Press, New York.

110. Frame, B. and Parfitt, A. M., 1978, Osteomalacia: Current concepts, *Ann. Intern. Med.* 89:966–982.

111. Jowsey, J., 1977, *Metabolic Diseases of Bone,* W. B. Saunders, Philadelphia.

112. Mallette, L. E., Patten, B. M., and Engel, W. K., 1975, Neuromuscular disease in secondary hyperparathyroidism, *Ann. Intern. Med.* 82:474–483.

113. Schott, G. D. and Wills, M. R., 1976, Muscle weakness in osteomalacia, *Lancet* i:626–629.

114. Sokoloff, L., 1978, Occult osteomalacia in American (USA) patients with fracture of the hip, *Am. J. Surg. Pathol.* 2:21–30.

115. Adams, J. S., Clemen, T. L., Parrish, J. A., and Holick, M. F., 1982, Vitamin-D synthesis and metabolism after ultraviolet irradiation of normal and vitamin-D-deficient subjects, *N. Engl. J. Med.* 306:722–725.

116. Hahn, T. J. and Avioli, L. V., 1975, Anticonvulsant osteomalacia, *Arch. Intern. Med.* 135:997–1000.

117. Thompson, W. G. and Thompson, G. R., 1969, Effect of cholestyramine on the absorption of vitamin D₃ and calcium, *Gut* 10:717–722.

118. Kantrowitz, F. G., Byrne, M. H., and Krane, S. M., 1975, Clinical and biochemical effects of the diphosphonate in Paget's disease of bone, *Arthritis Rheum.* 18:407.

119. Long, R. G., Skinner, R. K., Wills, M. R., and Sherlock, S., 1976, Serum 25-hydroxyvitamin D in untreated parenchymal and cholestatic liver disease, *Lancet* ii:650–652.

120. Marx, S. J., Spiegel, A. M., Brown, E. M., Gardner, D. G., Downs, R. W., Attie, M., Hamstra, A. J., and DeLuca, H. F., 1978, Familial syndrome of decrease in sensitivity to 1,25-dihydroxyvitamin D, *J. Clin. Endocrinol. Metab.* 47:1303–1310.

121. Rasmussen, H. and Anast, C., 1978, Familial hypophosphatemic (vitamin D-resistant) rickets and vitamin D-dependent rickets, in: *Metabolic Basis of Inherited Disease,* 4th ed. (J. B. Stanbury and J. B. Wyngaarden, eds.), McGraw-Hill, New York, p. 1537.

122. Drezner, M. K. and Feinglos, M. N., 1977, Osteomalacia due to 1-alpha,25-dihydroxycholecalciferol deficiency. Association with a giant cell tumor of bone, *J. Clin. Invest.* 60:1046.

123. Singer, F. R., 1977, *Paget's Disease of Bone,* Plenum Press, New York.

124. Rebel, A., Basle, M., Poupcard, A., Kouyoumdkoam, S., Filmon, R., and Lepatelour, A., 1980, Viral antigens in osteoclasts from Paget's disease of bone, *Lancet* ii:344–346.

125. Mills, B. G. and Singer, F. R., 1976, Nuclear inclusions in Paget's disease of bone, *Science* 194:201–202.

126. Miller, S. W., Castronovo, F. P., Prendergrass, H. P., and Potsaid, M. S., 1974, Technetium 99M labeled diphosphonate bone scanning in Paget's disease, *Am. J. Roentgenol.* 121:177–183.

127. Ross, F. G. M., Middlemiss, J. H., and Fitton, J. M., 1973, Paget's sarcoma in bone—a radiological study, in: *Bone—Certain Aspects of Neoplasia* (C. H. G. Price and F. G. M. Ross, eds.), Buttersworths, London.

128. Franck, W. A., Bress, N. M., Singer, F. R., and Krane, S. M., 1974, Rheumatic manifestations of Paget's disease of bone, *Am. J. Med.* 56:592–603.

129. DeRose, J., Singer, F. R., Avramides, A., Flores, A., Dziadiw, R., Baker, R. K., and Wallach, S., 1974, Response of Paget's disease to porcine and salmon calcitonins, *Am. J. Med.* 56:858–866.

130. Avramides, A., Flores, A., DeRose, J., and Wallach, S., 1976, Paget's disease of the bone: Observations after cessation of long-term synthetic salmon calcitonin treatment, *J. Clin. Endocrinol. Metab.* 42:459–463.

131. Kantrowitz, F. G., Byrne, M. H., and Krane, S. M., 1975, Clinical and metabolic effect of diphosphonate EHDP in Paget's disease of bone, *Clin. Res.* 23:445A.

132. Canfield, R., Rosner, W., Skinner, J., McWhorter, J., Resnick, L., Feldman, F., Kammerman, S., Ryan, K., Kunigonis, M., and Bohne, W., 1977, Diphosphonate therapy of Paget's disease of bone, *J. Clin. Endocrinol. Metab.* 44:96–106.

133. Khairi, M. R. A., Altman, R. D., DeRose, G. P., Zimmerman, J., Schenk, R. K., and Johnston, C. C., Jr., 1977, Sodium etidronate in the treatment of Paget's disease of bone: A study of long term results, *Ann. Intern. Med.* 87:656–663.

134. Johnston, C. C., Jr., Khairi, M. R. A., and Meunier, P. J., 1980, Use of etidronate (EHDP) in Paget's disease of bone, *Arthritis Rheum.* 23:1172–1176.

135. Siris, E. S., Canfield, R. E., Jacobs, T. P., and Baquiran, D. C., 1980, Long-term therapy of Paget's disease of bone with EHDP, *Arthritis Rheum.* 23:1177–1184.

136. Delmas, P. D., Chapuy, M. C., Vignon, E., Charhon, S., Briancon, D., Alexandre, C., Eduard, C., and Meunier, P. J., 1982, Long term effects of dichloromethylene diphosphonate in Paget's disease of bone, *J. Clin. Endocrinol. Metab.* 54:837–844.

137. Evans, R. A., 1977, A cheap oral therapy for Paget's disease of bone, *Aust. N.Z. J. Med.* 7:259–261.

138. Russell, A. S., Chalmers, I. M., Percy, J. S., and Lentle, B. C., 1979, Long term effectiveness of low dose mithramycin for Paget's disease of bone, *Arthritis Rheum.* 22:215–218.

139. Tzankoff, S. P. and Norris, A. H., 1977, Effect of muscle mass decrease in age-related BMR changes, *J. Appl. Physiol.* 43:1001–1006.

140. Denckla, W. D., 1974, Role of the pituitary and thyroid glands on the decline of minimal O_2 consumption with age, *J. Clin. Invest.* 53:572–581.

141. Ingbar, S., 1978, The influence of aging on human thyroid economy, in: *Geriatric Endocrinology* (R. B. Greenblatt, eds.), Raven Press, New York.

142. Braverman, L., Dawber, N., and Ingbar, S., 1966, Observations concerning the binding of thyroid hormone in the sera of normal subjects of varying ages, *J. Clin. Invest.* 45:1273–1279.

143. Hesch, R. D., Gatz, J., and Pope, J., 1976, Total and free triiodothyronine and thyroid-binding globulin concentration in elderly human persons, *Eur. J. Clin. Invest.* 6:139–145.

144. Davis, P. and Davis, F., 1974, Hyperthyroidism in patients over the age of 60 years, *Medicine,* 53:161–181.

145. Hermann, J., Rusche, H. J., Kroll, H. J., Hilger, P., and Kruskemper, H. L., 1974, Free triiodothyronine (T_3) and thyroxine (T_4) serum levels in old age, *Horm. Metab. Res.* 6:239–240.

146. Wenzel, K. W. and Horn, W. R., June 1975, Triiodothyronine (T_3) and thyroxine (T_4) kinetics in aged men. Program, 7th International Thyroid Conference, Boston, *Excerpta Medica,* ICS #361, Abstract No. 154.

147. Chopra, I. J. and Smith, S. R., 1975, Circulating thyroid hormones and thyrotropin in adult patients with protein-caloric malnutrition, *J. Clin. Endocrinol. Metab.* 40:221–227.

148. Mashang, T., Jr., Parks, J. S., Baker, L., Vaidya, V., Utiger, R. D., Bongiovanni, A. M., and Snyder, P. J., 1975, Low serum triiodothyronine in patients with anorexia nervosa, *J. Clin. Endocrinol. Metab.* 40:470–473.

149. Chopra, I. J., Chopra, U., Smith, S. R., Reza, M., and Solomon, D., 1975, Reciprocal changes in serum concentrations of 3,3′,5′-triiodothyronine (reverse T_3) and 3,3′,5-triiodothyronine (T_3) in systemic illnesses, *J. Clin. Endocrinol. Metab.* 41:1043–1049.

150. Bermudez, F., Surks, M. I., and Oppenheimer, J. H., 1975, High incidence of decreased serum triiodothyronine concentration in patients with nonthyroidal disease, *J. Clin. Endocrinol. Metab.* 41:27–40.

151. Burrows, A. W., Cooper, E., Shakespear, R. A., Aickin, C. M., Hesch, R. D., and

Burke, C. W., 1977, Low serum T_3 levels in the elderly sick: Protein binding, thyroid and pituitary responsiveness and reverse T_3 concentrations, *Clin. Endocrinol.* 7:289-292.

152. Vagenakis, A. G., Burger, A., Portnay, G. I., Rudolph, M., O'Brien, J. T., Azizi, F., Arky, R. A., Nicod, P., Ingbar, S. H., and Braverman, L. E., 1975, Diversion of peripheral thyroxine metabolism from activating to inactivating pathways during complete fasting, *J. Clin. Endocrinol. Metab.* 41:191-194.

153. Balsam, A. and Ingbar, S. H., 1978, The influence of fasting, diabetes, and several pharmacological agents in the pathways of thyroxine metabolism in rat liver, *J. Clin. Invest.* 63:415-424.

154. Snyder, P. and Utiger, R., 1972, Response to TRH in normal man. *J. Clin. Endocrinol. Metab.* 34:380-385.

155. Azizi, F., Vagenakis, G. I., Portnay, B., Rapoport, B., Ingbar, S. H., and Braverman, L. E., 1975, Pituitary-thyroid responsiveness to intramuscular thyrotropin-releasing hormone based on analyses of serum thyroxine, triiodothyronine and thyrotropin concentrations, *N. Engl. J. Med.* 292:273-276.

156. Cuttelod, S., Lemarchand-Beraud, T., Magnenat, P., Perret, C., Poli, S., and Venotti, A., 1974, Effect of age and role of kidneys and liver on thyrotropin turnover in man, *Metabolism* 23:101-113.

157. Lemarchand-Beraud, T. H. and Vanotti, A., 1969, Relationships between blood thyrotropin levels, protein bound iodine and free thyroxine concentration in man under normal physiological conditions, *Acta Endocrinol.* 60:315-317.

158. Ohara, H., Kobayaski, T., Shiraishi, M., and Wada, T., 1974, Thyroid function of the aged as viewed from the pituitary-thyroid system. *Endocrinol. Jpn.* 21:377-381.

159. Sawin, C. T., Chopra, D., Azizi, F., Mannix, J. E., and Bacharach, P., 1979, The aging thyroid: Increased prevalence of elevated serum thyrotropin levels in the elderly, *J. Am. Med. Soc.* 242:247-250.

160. Snyder, P. J. and Utiger, R. D., 1972, Thyrotropin response to thyrotropin releasing hormone in normal females over forty, *J. Clin. Endocrinol. Metab.* 34:1096-1101.

160a. Ordene, K. W., Pan, C., Barzel, U. S., and Surks, M. F., 1982, Abnormal TSH regulation in aging patients, *Clin. Res.* 30:553A (Abstract).

161. Wenzel, K. W., Meinhold, H., Herpich, M., Adlkofer, F., and Schleusener, H., 1974, TRH-Stimulationstest mit alters-und geschlechsabhangigem TSH-Antieg bein Normalpersonen, *Klin. Wochenschr.* 52:721-724.

162. Campbell, A. J., Reinken, J., and Allan, B. C., 1981, Thyroid disease in the elderly community, *Age Ageing* 10:47-52.

163. Gambert, S. R., Garthwaite, T. L., Pontzer, C. H., and Hagen, T. C., 1980, Age-related changes in central nervous system beta-endorphin and ACTH, *Neuroendocrinology* 31:252-255.

164. Gambert, S. R., 1981, Interaction of age and thyroid hormone status on beta-endorphin content in rat corpus striatum and hypothalamus, *Neuroendocrinology* 32:114-117.

165. Lahey, F. H., 1931, Non-activated (apathetic) type of hyperthyroidism, *N. Engl. J. Med.* 204:747-748.

166. Gambert, S. R., Ingbar, S. H., and Hagen, T. C., 1980, Interaction of age and

thyroid hormone status on Na^+-K^+ ATPase in rat renal cortex and liver, *Endocrinology* 108:27–30.

167. Jeffreys, P., 1972, The prevalence of thyroid disease in patients admitted to a geriatric department, *Age Ageing* 1:33–37.

168. Bahemuka, M. and Hodkinson, H., 1957, Screening for hypothyroidism in elderly patients, *Br. Med. J.* 2:601–605.

169. Ahconheim, J. and Libow, L., 1981, High occurrence rate of hypothyroidism in a frail elderly population. *Proceedings of the 34th Annual Meeting of the Gerontological Society of America,* Toronto, Canada, Abstract No. 162.

170. Ingbar, S. H. and Braverman, L. E., 1975, Active form of the thyroid hormone, *Ann. Rev. Med.* 26:443–447.

170a. Rosenbaum, R. L. and Barzel, U. S., 1981, Clinical hyperthyroidism in the elderly, *J. Am. Geriatr. Soc.* 29:221–223.

171. Kaplan, M. M., Larsen, P. R., Crantz, F. R., Dzau, V. J., and Rossing, T. H., 1982, Prevalence of abnormal thyroid function test results in patients with acute medical illnesses, *Am. J. Med.* 72:9–16.

172. Rosenbaum, R. L. and Barzel, U. S., 1982, Levothyroxine replacement dose for primary hypothyroidism decreases with age, *Ann. Int. Med.* 96:53–55.

173. Davis, E. B., Lamantia, R. S., Sapulding, S. W., and Davis, P. J., 1980, Conventional therapy overtreats elderly hypothyroid patients. *Proceedings of the 62nd Annual Meeting of the Endocrine Society,* Annaheim, California, Abstract No. 33.

174. Gregerman, R. I., Gaffney, G. W., and Shock, N. W., 1962, Thyroxine turnover in euthyroid man with special reference to changes with age, *J. Clin. Invest.* 41:2065–2074.

175. Murad, F. and Haynes, R. C., Jr., 1980, Androgens and anabolic steroids, in: *The Pharmacological Basis of Therapeutics* (A. Goodman Gilman, L. S. Goodman, and A. Gilman, eds.), MacMillan Publishing Co., New York, p. 1448.

176. Masters, W. H. and Johnson, V. E., 1966, *Human Sexual Response,* Little, Brown and Co., Boston, pp. 248–270.

177. Kinsey, A. C., Pomeroy, W. B., and Martin, C. E., 1948, *Sexual Behavior in the Human Male,* W. B. Saunders, Philadelphia.

178. Martin, C. E., 1977, Sexual activity in the aging male, in: *Handbook of Sexology* (J. Money and H. Mousafh, eds.), Elsevier, Amsterdam, pp. 813–824.

179. Harman, S. M., 1978, Clinical aspects of aging of the male reproductive system, in: *The Aging Reproductive System, Aging,* Volume 4 (E. L. Schneider, ed.), Raven Press, New York, pp. 29–58.

180. Karacan, I., Williams, R. L., Thronby, J. I., and Salis, P. J., 1975, Sleep related penile tumescence as a function of age, *Am. J. Psychiatry,* 132:932–937.

181. Johnson, J., 1975, Impotence, *Br. J. Psychiatry* 9:206–211.

182. Tsitouras, P. D., Martin, C. E., and Harman, S. M., 1982, Relationship of serum testosterone to sexual activity in healthy elderly men, *J. Gerontol.* 37(3):288–293.

183. Gregerman, R. I. and Bierman, E. L., 1981, Aging and hormones, in: *Textbook of Endocrinology* (R. H. Williams, ed.), W. B. Saunders, Philadelphia, pp. 1192–1212.

184. Bardin, C. W. and Paulsen, C. A., 1981, The testes, in: *Textbook of Endocrinology* (R. H. Williams, ed.), W. B. Saunders, Philadelphia, pp. 293–354.

185. Eik-Nes, K. B., 1975, Biosynthesis and secretion of testicular steroids, in: *Handbook of Physiology*, Section 7: Endocrinology, Volume V: Male reproductive system (D. W. Hamilton and R. O. Greep, eds.), Williams and Wilkins, Baltimore, pp. 95–116.

186. Kastin, A. J. and Schally, A. V., 1972, Release of LH and FSH after administration of synthetic LHRH, *J. Clin. Endocrinol. Metab.* 34:753–757.

187. Reichlin, S., 1981, Neuroendocrinology, in: *Textbook of Endocrinology* (R. H. Williams, ed.), W. B. Saunders, Philadelphia, pp. 588–644.

188. Vermeulen, A., Rubens, R., and Verdonck, L., 1972, Testosterone secretion and metabolism in male senescence, *J. Clin. Endocrinol. Metab.* 34:730–735.

189. Stearns, E. L., MacDonald, J. A., Kaufman, B. J., Lucman, T. S., Winter, J. S., and Faiman, C., 1974, Declining testicular function with age, hormonal and clinical correlates, *Am. J. Med.* 57(5):761–766.

190. Baker, H. W. G., Brenner, W. J., Burger, H. G., DeKretser, D. M., Dulmans, A., Eddie, L. W., Hudson, B., Keogh, E. J., Lee, V. W. K., and Rennie, G. C., 1976, Testicular control of follicle stimulating hormone secretion, *Recent Prog. Horm. Res.* 32:429–476.

191. Pirke, K. M. and Doerr, P., 1973, Age related changes and interrelationships between plasma testosterone, estradiol, and testosterone binding globulin in normal adult males, *Acta Endocrinol.* 74:729–800.

192. Horton, R., Hsieh, P., Barberia, J., Pages, L., and Cosgrove, M., 1975, Altered blood androgens in elderly men with prostate hyperplasia, *J. Clin. Endocrinol. Metab.* 41(4):793–796.

193. Vermeulen, A. and Verdonck, L., 1972, Some studies on the biological significance of free testosterone, *J. Steroid. Biochem.* 3:421–426.

194. Kley, H. K., Nieschlag, E., Bidlingmaier, F., and Krüskemper, H. L., 1974, Possible age-dependent influence of estrogens on the binding of testosterone in plasma of adult men, *Horm. Metab. Res.* 6:213–216.

195. Pirke, K. M. and Doerr, P., 1975, Age related changes in free plasma testosterone, dihydrotestosterone, and estradiol, *Acta. Endocrinol.* 80 (1):171–178.

196. Rubens, R. M., Dhout, M., and Vermeulen, A., 1974, Further studies on Leydig cell function in old age, *J. Clin. Endocrinol. Metab.* 39:40–45.

197. Hemsell, D. L., Grodin, J. M., Brenner, P. F., Siiteri, P. K., and McDonald, P. C., 1974, Plasma precursors of estrogen. II: Correlation of the extent of conversion of plasma androstenedione to estrone with age, *J. Clin. Endocrinol. Metab.* 38:476–479.

198. Greenblatt, R. B., Oettinger, M., and Bohler, C. S. S., 1976, Estrogen-androgen levels in aging men and women, therapeutic considerations, *J. Am. Geriatr. Soc.* 24:173–178.

199. Longcope, C., 1973, The effect of human chorionic gonadotrophin on plasma steroid levels in young and old men, *Steroids* 21:583–592.

200. Mazzi, C., Riva, L. R., and Bernasconi, D., 1974, Gonadotrophins and plasma testosterone in senescence, in: *The Endocrine Function of the Human Testis*, Volume 2 (V. H. T. James, M. Serio, and L. Martin, eds.), Academic Press, New York, pp. 51–62.

201. Tillenger, L. G., Birke, G., Franksson, C., and Plantin, L. O., 1955, The steroid

production of the testicles and the relation to the number and morphology of Leydig cells, *Acta Endocrinol.* 19:340–348.

202. Kaler, L. W. and Neaves, W. B., 1978, Attrition of the human Leydig cell population with advancing age, *Anat. Rec.* 192(4):513–518.

203. Harman, S. M. and Tsitouras, P. D., 1980, Reproductive hormones in aging men. I. Measurement of sex steroids, basal luteinizing hormone, and Leydig cell response to human chorionic gonadotropin, *J. Clin. Endocrinol. Metab.* 51:35–40.

204. Harman, S. M. and Tsitouras, P. D., 1982, Reproductive hormones in aging men. II. Basal pituitary gonadotropins and gonadotropin responses to luteinizing hormone-releasing hormone, *J. Clin. Endocrinol. Metab.* 54:547–551.

205. Brenner, W. J. and Prinz, P. N., 1981, The diurnal rhythm in testosterone levels is lost with aging in normal men, *63rd Annual Meeting of the Endocrine Society*, Abstract No. 480, Cincinnati, Ohio, Endocrine Society.

206. Sparrow, D., Bosse, R., and Rowe, J. W., 1980, The influence of age, alcohol consumption and body build on gonadal function in men, *J. Clin. Endocrinol. Metab.* 51:508–512.

207. Pazzagli, M., Forti, G., Capellini, A., and Serio, M., 1975, Radioimmunoassay of plasma dihydrotestosterone in normal and hypogonadal men, *Clin. Endocrinol.* 4:513–520.

208. Giusti, G., Gonelli, P., Borreli, D., Fiorelli, G., Forti, G., Pazzagli, M., and Serio, M., 1975, Age-related secretion of androstenedione, testosterone, and dihydrotestosterone by the human testis, *Exp. Gerontol.* 10(5):241–245.

209. Pirke, K. M. and Doerr, P., 1975, Plasma dihydrotestosterone in normal adult males and its relation to testosterone, *Acta Endocrinol.* 79:357–365.

210. Sawin, C. T., Chopra, D., Azizi, F., Mannix, J. E., and Bacharach, P., 1979, The aging thyroid. Increased prevalence of elevated serum thyrotropin levels in the elderly, *JAMA* 242(3):247–250.

211. Muta, K., Kato, K., Akamine, Y., and Ibayishi, H., 1981, Age related changes in the feedback regulation of gonadotropin secretion by sex steroids in men, *Acta Endocrinol.* 96:154–162.

212. Snyder, P. J., Reitano, J. F., and Utiger, R. D., 1975, Serum LH and FSH responses to synthetic gonadotrophin releasing hormone in normal men, *J. Clin. Endocrinol. Metab.* 41(5):938–945.

213. Hang, E. A., Aakvaag, A., Sand, T., and Torjesen, P. A., 1974, The gonadotrophin response to synthetic GnRH in males in relation to age, dose, and basal serum levels of estradiol-17-β and gonadotrophins, *Acta Endocrinol.* 77(4):625–635.

214. Harman, S. M., Tsitouras, P. D., Costa, P. T., Loriaux, D. L., and Sherins, R. J., 1982, Evaluation of pituitary gonadotropic function in men: Value of luteinizing hormone-releasing hormone response versus basal luteinizing hormone level for discrimination of diagnosis, *J. Clin. Endocrinol. Metab.* 54:196–200.

215. Gordon, G. G., Altman, K., Southern, A. L., Rubin, E., and Lieber, C. S., 1976, Effects of alcohol on sex-hormone metabolism in normal men, *N. Engl. J. Med.* 295:793–797.

216. Turner, T. B., Mezey, E., and Kimball, A. W., 1977, Measurement of alcohol-related effects in man: Chronic effects in relation to level of alcohol consumption, *Johns Hopkins Med. J.* 141:235–248.

217. Michael, R. P. and Zympe, D., 1978, Potency in male rhesus monkeys: Effect of continuously receptive females, *Science* 200:451–453.
218. Martin, C. E., 1981, Factors affecting sexual functioning in 60 to 79 year old married males, *Arch. Sex. Behav.* 5:399–420.
219. Kent, J. Z. and Acone, A. B., 1966, Plasma androgens and aging, in: *Androgens in Normal and Pathological Conditions* (A. Vermeulen and D. Exley, eds.), Excerpta Medica Foundation ICS #101, Amsterdam, pp. 31–40.
220. Wesson, M. B., 1964, The value of testosterone in men past middle age, *J. Am. Geriatr. Soc.* 12:1149–1153.
221. Reiter, T., 1963, Testosterone implantation: A clinical study of 240 implantations in aging males, *J. Am. Geriatr. Soc.* 11:540–550.
222. Vaughn, T. C. and Hammond, C. B., 1981, Estrogen replacement therapy, *Clin. Obstet. Gynecol.* 24(1):253–283.
223. Notelovitz, M., 1978, Gynecologic problems of menopausal women. I. Changes in genital tissue, *Geriatrics* 33(8):24–30.
224. Quigley, M. M. and Hammond, C. B., 1979, Estrogen-replacement therapy: Help or hazard? *N. Engl. J. Med.* 301:646–648.
225. Jaffe, R. B., 1978, The menopause and perimenopausal period, in: *Reproductive Endocrinology: Physiology, Pathophysiology, and Clinical Management* (S. S. C. Yen and R. B. Jaffe, eds.), W. B. Saunders, Philadelphia, pp. 261–270.
226. Jaszmann, L. J. B., 1976, Epidemiology of the climacteric syndrome, in: *The Management of the Menopause and Post-Menopausal Years* (S. Campbell, ed.), University Park Press, Baltimore, pp. 11–23.
227. Gregerman, R. I. and Bierman, E. L., 1981, Aging and hormones, in: *Textbook of Endocrinology* (R. H. Williams, ed.), W. B. Saunders, Philadelphia, pp. 1192–1209.
228. Sherman, B. M. and Korenman, S. G., 1975, Hormonal characteristics of the human menstrual cycle throughout reproductive life, *J. Clin. Invest.* 55:699–706.
229. Sherman, B. M., West, J. H., and Korenman, S. J., 1976, The menopausal transition: Analysis of LH, FSH, estradiol, and progesterone concentrations during menstrual cycles of older women, *J. Clin. Endocrinol. Metab.* 42:629–636.
230. Muta, K., Kato, K., Akamine, Y., and Ibayishi, H., 1981, Age related changes in the feedback regulation of gonadotropin secretion by sex steroids in men, *Acta Endocrinol.* 96:154–162.
231. Geola, F. L., Frimar, A. M., Tataryn, I. V., Lu, K. H., Hershman, J. M., Eggena, P., Sambhi, M. P., and Judd, H. L., 1980, Biological effects of various doses of equine conjugated estrogens in postmenopausal women, *J. Clin. Endocrinol. Metab.* 51:620–625.
232. Yen, S. S. C., Tsai, C. C., Naftolin, F., Vandenburg, G., and Ajabor, L., 1972, Pulsatile patterns of gonadotropin release in subjects with and without ovarian function, *J. Clin. Endocrinol. Metab.* 34:671–675.
233. Silver, T. M. and Yen, S. S. C., 1973, Augmented gonadotropin response to synthetic LRF in hypogonadal state, *J. Clin. Endocrinol. Metab.* 37:491–494.
234. Harman, S. M. and Tsitouras, P. D., 1980, Reproductive hormones in aging men. I. Measurement of sex steroids, basal LH and Leydig cell response to hCG, *J. Clin. Endocrinol. Metab.* 51:35–40.

235. Hutton, J. D., Jacobs, H. S., and James, V. H. T., 1979, Steroid endocrinology after the menopause: A review, *J. R. Soc. Med.* 72(11):835–841.
236. Judd, H. L., 1976, Hormonal dynamics associated with the menopause, *Clin. Obstet. Gynecol.* 19:775–788.
237. Judd, H. L., 1980, Reproductive hormone metabolism in postmenopausal women, in: *Menopause, Comprehensive Management* (B. A. Eskin, ed.), Masson Publishing Co., New York, pp. 55–71.
238. Aksel, S., Schomberg, D. W., Tyrey, L., and Hammond, C. B., 1976, Vasomotor symptoms, serum estrogens and gonadotropin levels in surgical menopause, *Am. J. Obstet. Gynecol.* 126:165–169.
239. Grodin, J. M., Siiteri, P. K., and MacDonald, B. C., 1973, Source of estrogen production in postmenopausal women, *J. Clin. Endocrinol. Metab.* 36:207–214.
240. Elahi, D., Muler, D., Tzankoff, S., Andres, R., and Tobin, J. D., 1978, Effect of age and obesity on fasting levels of glucose, insulin, glucagon, and GH, *The Gerontologist* 18(part 2):68 (Abstract).
241. Thompson, J. and Oswald, I., 1977, Effect of estrogen on the sleep, mood and anxiety of menopausal women, *Br. Med. J.* 2:1317–1319.
242. Yen, S. S. C., 1977, The biology of menopause, *J. Reprod. Med.* 18:287–296.
243. Aitken, J. M., Davidson, A., and England, P., 1974, The relationship between menopausal vasomotor symptoms and gonadotropin excretion in urine after oophorectomy, *J. Obstet. Gynaecol. Br. Commonw.* 81:150–154.
244. Meldrum, D. R., Erlik, Y., Lu, J. K. H., and Judd, H. L., 1981, Objectively recorded hot flushes in patients with pituitary insufficiency, *J. Clin. Endocrinol. Metab.* 52:684–689.
245. Meldrum, D. R., Tataryn, I. V., Frumar, A. M., Erlik, Y., Lu, K. H., and Judd, H., 1980, Gonadotropins, estrogens and adrenal steroids during the menopausal hot flash, *J. Clin. Endocrinol. Metab.* 50:685–689.
246. Casper, R. F., Yen, S. S. C., and Wilkes, M. M., 1979, Menopausal flushes: A neuroendocrine link with pulsatile luteinizing hormone secretion, *Science* 205:823–825.
247. Albrecht, B. H., Schiff, I., Tulchinsky, D., and Ryan, K. J., 1981, Objective evidence that placebo and oral medroxyprogesterone acetate therapy diminish menopausal vasomotor flashes, *Am. J. Obstet. Gynecol.* 139:631–635.
248. Clayden, J. R., Bell, J. W., and Pollard, P., 1974, Menopausal flushing: Double-blind trial of a nonhormonal medication, *Br. Med. J.* 1(9 March):409–412.
249. Worley, R. J., 1981, Age, estrogen and bone density, *Clin. Obstet. Gynecol.* 24(1):203–218.
250. Johnson, R. E. and Specht, E. E., 1981, The risk of hip fracture in postmenopausal females with and without estrogen drug exposure, *Am. J. Pub. Health* 71:138–144.
251. Christiansen, C., Christensen, M. S., and Transbol, I., 1981, Bone mass in postmenopausal women after withdrawal of estrogen-gestagen replacement therapy, *Lancet* i:459–461.
252. Nordin, B. E. C., Horsman, A., Crilly, R. J., Marshall, D. H., and Simpson, M., 1980, Treatment of spinal osteoporosis in postmenopausal women, *Br. Med. J.* 280(6212):451–455.

253. Masters, W. H. and Johnson, V. E., 1970, *Human Sexual Inadequacy,* Little, Brown and Co., Boston.
254. Maoz, B. and Durst, N., 1980, The effects of estrogen therapy on the sex life of postmenopausal women, *Maturitas* 2:327–336.
255. Deutsch, S., Ossowski, R., and Benjamin, I., 1981, Comparison between degree of systemic absorption of vaginally and orally administered estrogens at different dose levels in postmenopausal women, *Am. J. Obstet. Gynecol.* 139:967–968.
256. Schiff, I., Tulchinsky, D., Ryan, K. J., Kadner, S., and Levitz, M., 1980, Plasma estriol and its conjugates following oral and vaginal adminstration of estriol to postmenopausal women: Correlations with gonadotropin levels, *Am. J. Obstet. Gynecol.* 138:1137–1141.
257. Keller, T. J., Riedmann, R., and Fischer, M., 1980, Ostron-Ostradiol-und Ostriolgehart nach intravaginaler Applikation von Ostriol in der Postmenopause, *Gynaek. Rundsch.* 20(Suppl 1):77–79.
258. Oliver, M. F., 1976, The menopause and coronary heart disease, in: *The Management of the Menopause and Postmenopausal Years* (S. Campbell, ed.), University Park Press, Baltimore.
259. Ryan, K. J., 1976, Estrogen and atherosclerosis, *Clin. Obstet. Gynecol.* 19:805–815.
260. Nachtigall, L. E., Nachtigall, R. H., Nachtigall, R. D., and Beckman, E. M., 1979, Estrogen replacement therapy. II. A prospective study in the relationship to carcinoma, cardiovascular and metabolic problems, *Obstet. Gynecol.* 54:74–79.
261. Pfeffer, R. I., Whipple, G. H., Kurosaki, T. T., and Chapman, J. M., 1978, Coronary risk and estrogen use in postmenopausal women, *Am. J. Epidemiol.* 107:479–487.
262. Hammond, C. B., Jelovsek, F. R., Lee, K. L., Greasman, W. T., and Parker, R. T., 1979, Effects of long-term estrogen replacement therapy: I. Metabolic effects, *Am. J. Obstet. Gynecol.* 133:525–536.
263. Cordon, T., Kannel, W. B., Hjortland, M. C., and McNamara, P. M., 1978, Menopause and coronary heart disease. The Framingham Study, *Ann. Intern. Med.* 89:157–161.
264. The Coronary Drug Research Group, 1973, The coronary drug project, *JAMA* 226(6):652–657.
265. Tikkanen, M. J., Kuusi, T., Vartiainen, E., and Nikkila, E. A., 1979, Treatment of post-menopausal hypercholesterolemia with estradiol, *Acta Obstet. Gynecol. Scand.,* 88(Suppl.):83–88.
266. Varma, T. R., 1980, Effect of estrogen on fasting serum cholesterol and triglyceride levels in post-menopausal women, *Int. J. Gynaecol. Obstet.* 17:551–555.
267. Largelius, A., Johnson, P., Lunell, N.-O., and Samsioe, G., 1981, Treatment with oral estrone sulfate in the female climacteric. I. Influence on lipids, *Acta Obstet. Gynecol. Scand.* 60:27–31.
268. Silfverstolpe, G., Gustafson, A., Samsioe, G., and Svanborg, A., 1979, Lipid metabolic studies in oophorectomized women, *Acta Obstet. Gynaecol. Scand.* 88(Suppl.):89–95.
269. Krauss, R. M., Lindgren, F. T., Wingerd, J., Bradley, D. D., and Ramcharan, S., 1979, Effects of estrogens and progestins on high density lipoproteins, *Lipids* 14:114–118.

270. Lillienberg, L., Adlercreutz, H., and Svanborg, A., 1979, Effect of a sequential estrogen-progestin therapy on the plasma level of estrogens and lipids on post-menopausal women, *Acta Endocrinol.* 92:319–329.

271. Paterson, M. E. L., Sturdee, D. W., Moore, B., and Whitehead, T. P., 1980, The effect of various regimens of hormone therapy on serum cholesterol and triglyceride concentration in post-menopausal women, *Br. J. Obstet. Gynecol.* 87:552–560.

272. Hirvonen, E., Malkomen, M., and Manninen, D., 1981, Effects of different progestogens on lipoproteins during post-menopausal replacement therapy, *N. Engl. J. Med.* 304:560–563.

273. Bland, K. I., Buchanan, J. B., Weisberg, B. F., Hagan, T., and Grey, L. A., 1980, The effects of exogenous estrogen replacement therapy of the breast: Breast cancer risk and mammographic parenchymal patterns, *Cancer* 45:3027–3033.

274. Gambrell, R. D., Massey, F. M., Castaneda, T. A., and Boddie, A., 1980, Estrogen therapy and breast cancer in postmenopausal women, *J. Am. Geriatr. Soc.* 28:251–257.

275. Ziel, H. K. and Finkle, W. D., 1975, Increased risk of endometrial carcinoma among users of conjugated estrogens, *N. Engl. J. Med.* 293:1167–1170.

276. Smith, D. C., Prentice, R., Thompson, D. J., and Hermann, W. L., 1975, Association of exogenous estrogen and endometrial carcinoma, *N. Engl. J. Med.* 293:1164–1166.

277. McDonald, T. W., Annegers, J. F., O'Fallon, W. M., Dockerty, M. B., Malkasian, G. D., and Kurlan, L. T., 1977, Exogenous estrogen and endometrial carcinoma. Case-control and incidence study, *Am. J. Obstet. Gynecol.* 127:572–580.

278. Weiss, N. S., Szekely, D. R., and Austin, D. F., 1976, Increasing incidence of endometrial cancer in the United States, *N. Engl. J. Med.* 294:1259–1262.

279. Gardner, W. V., 1944, Tumors in experimental animals receiving steroid hormones, *Surgery* 6:8–32.

280. Perry, I. H. and Ginzton, L. L., 1937, Development of tumors in female mice treated with 1,2,5,6-dibenzanthracene and theelin, *Am. J. Cancer* 29:680–704.

281. Cook, J. W. and Dodds, E. C., 1933, Sex hormones and cancer producing compounds, *Nature* (London) 131:205–206.

282. Mack, T. M., 1978, Exogenous estrogens and endometrial carcinoma: Studies, Criticisms and Current Status, in: *International Symposium on Endometrial Cancer* (M. G. Brush, R. J. King, and R. Taylor, eds.), Bailliere Tindall, London, pp. 17–28.

283. Klopper, A., 1980, The risk of endometrial carcinoma from estrogen therapy of the menopause, *Acta Endocrinol.* 233 (Suppl.):29–35.

284. Salini, T., 1980, Endometrial carcinoma risk factors with special reference to the use of estrogens, *Acta Endocrinol.* 233(Suppl.):37–43.

285. Volker, W., Kannengiesser, U., Majewski, A., and Vasterling, H. W., 1978, Ostrogentherapie und Endometriumkarzinom, *Geburtschilfe Frauenheilkd.* 38:735–743.

286. Hulka, B. S., Kaufman, D. G., Fowler, W. C., Grimson, R. C., and Greenberg, B. G., 1980, Predominance of early endometrial cancers after long-term estrogen use, *JAMA* 244:2419–2422.

287. Paterson, M. E. L., Wade-Evans, T., Sturdee, D. W., Thom, M. H., and Studd,

J. W. W., 1980, Endometrial disease after treatment with estrogens and progestogens in the climacteric, *Br. Med. J.* 1(March):822–824.

288. King, R. J. B., Whitehead, M. I., Campbell, S., and Minardi, J., 1979, Effect of estrogen and progestin treatments on endometria from post-menopausal women, *Cancer Res.* 39:1094–1101.

289. Gambrell, R. D., Massey, F. M., and Castameda, T. A., 1979, Reduced incidence of endometrial cancer among postmenopausal women treated with progestogens, *J. Am. Geriatr. Soc.* 27:389–394.

290. Thom, M. H., White, P. J., Williams, R. M., Sturdee, D. W., Paterson, M. E. L., Wade-Evans, T., and Studd, J. W. W., 1979, Prevention and treatment of endometrial disease in climacteric women receiving estrogen therapy, *Lancet* ii:455–457.

291. Aiman, J., 1981, Age, estrogen, and the endometrium, *Clin. Obstet. Gynecol.* 24:193–202.

292. Studd, J. W. W., Thom, M., Dische, F., Driver, M., Wade-Evans, T., and Williams, D., 1979, Value of cytology for detecting endometrial abnormalities in climacteric women receiving hormone replacement therapy, *Br. Med. J.* 280(6167):846–848.

293. Estrogen use and postmenopausal women, 1979, *Ann. Intern. Med.* 91:921–922.

294. Estrogen use and postmenopausal women, 1979, National Institutes of Health Consensus Development Conference, Vol. 2, No. 8, NIH, Bethesda, MD.

Neuropsychiatric Problems in the Elderly

Gabe J. Maletta

7.1. Introduction

The fact that persons 65 years and older (the "elderly") comprise the most rapidly growing portion of the U.S. population is now well known. The number has increased steadily in the twentieth century, and is now approximately 24 million (11% of the population); and by 2035, 20% of the population of the U.S. has been estimated to be over 65, or approximately 56 million people.[1]

The elderly are at considerable risk for a varied multitude of physical and psychiatric problems. Although they represent 11% of the population, they account for more than 14% of the outpatient visits to health care facilities. Also, they are admitted to general hospitals at a rate of more than double that of younger patients, and remain in the hospital longer. Elderly persons occupy 85% of the 1.2 million nursing home and extended-care facility beds in the U.S.[2]

Psychiatric diseases among the elderly are more prevalent than in their younger counterparts,[3] even accounting for the observation that there is a societal reluctance to identify disorders in the elderly as psychiatric, and to tolerate deviant behavior in this group for longer periods of time.[4] Because of this situation, it is difficult to accurately assess the true prevalence of psychiatric disorders in this

GABE J. MALETTA • Geriatric Research, Education, and Clinical Center, Minneapolis Veterans Administration Medical Center, Minneapolis, Minnesota 55417.

population. The numbers range from 20 to 45% in the 95% of elderly individuals residing in the community, and is much higher, approaching 90%, in nursing home residents.[5,6]

To enlarge on the difficulty of accurately assessing the prevalence of psychiatric disorders in the elderly, the concepts of "neuropsychiatric" versus "psychiatric" must be considered.

It is common practice to categorize disturbed behavior into "organic" or "functional" groups, implying that the etiology of the former is strictly biologic and the behavior of the latter group is due to environmental rather than biologic causes. This rather artificial separation is particularly prevalent in elderly patients, with the added confusion of considering most patients in this age group that exhibit disturbed behavior as "senile."[7] This label suggests another vague category, somehow neither totally "organic" nor totally "functional"; the only thing clear about this nosology is that it tends to be totally confusing.

Individuals with disturbed CNS function have only a limited number of ways to express this dysfunction, regardless of whether the etiology is "functional" or "organic" (the "final common pathway"). Thus, similar problems with attention, perception, memory, orientation, or thinking; speech dysfunction; and emotional lability may be seen in an elderly patient with a dementing illness, as well as in a patient suffering from a psychotic depression or schizophrenia. The concept that a patient with a "functional" psychosis will have a concomitant clear sensorium is much more valid in younger patients than in older ones. Conversely, patients with dementing illnesses frequently exhibit thought disorders in the form of delusions, and a loss of reality-testing in the form of hallucinations or illusions along with their sensorium deficits. Moreover, the relationship between environmental stresses and strains (primarily involving uncontrolled and inexorable losses) and the physiological response of a compromised older host are much more complex than with younger individuals, making separation into effective diagnostic categories much more difficult (Fig. 1).[9] This is an excellent example of the biopsychosocial model of Engel.[8] Besides physiologic changes in various systems with

Table I. Physiological Stresses for the Elderly

Multiple chronic diseases
Insidious degenerative processes
Increased risk of injury
Impaired metabolism
Impaired neuromuscular/musculoskeletal/integrative systems
Hemeostatic imbalances
Nutritional deficiencies
Decreased sensory activity
Gastrointestinal/genitourinary disorders
Cardiovascular–renal disorders

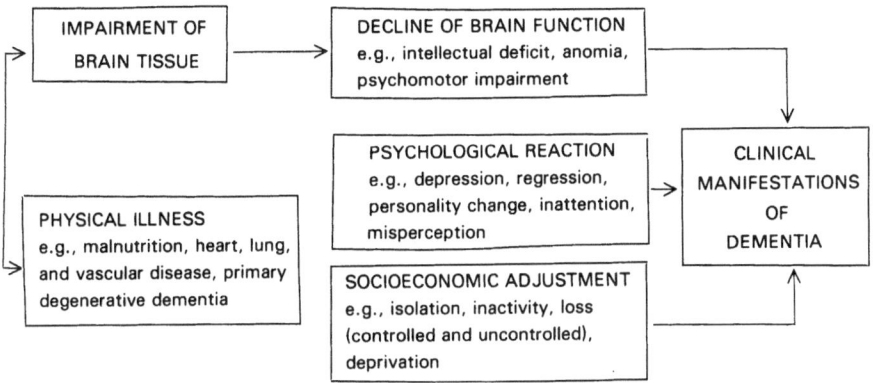

Figure 1. Multidimentional view of dementia.

aging that affect the CNS, both directly and indirectly (Table I), there are morphologic changes in the CNS at the system, organ, tissue, cellular, and subcellular levels with aging that are directly associated with functional changes in cognition and behavior.[10,11] For a more comprehensive treatment of this subject, the reader is directed elsewhere.[12]

In keeping faith with the concept of neuropsychiatric problems in the elderly, this chapter is divided into the following sections: psychiatric problems, drugs of abuse, and organic mental disorders, as well as Parkinson's and other relevant neurologic diseases in the elderly.

Although, with the exception of the organic mental disorders, treatment will not be addressed in this discussion, it is clear that in medicine, the correct diagnosis is crucial for two reasons, i.e., a guide to appropriate treatment, as well as provision of a prognosis. Therefore, not only should one appreciate the complexity of diagnosing disturbed behavior, but also there is a need for the correct diagnosis to ensure proper treatment and the best possible prognosis for both the elderly patient and his family.[13]

7.2. Psychiatric Problems

The term *psychiatric* here refers not to the broad dysfunction, which encompasses drugs of abuse and the organic mental disorders, but rather to a more narrow dysfunction which includes the so-called functional brain disorders.[14] Therefore, this section will discuss psychogenic thought and affective disorders, neuroses, and special problems of the elderly, including stress, the relationship between functional disorders and physical illness, and suicide.[3,5,15]

7.2.1. Thought Disorders

Thought disorders secondary to affective and organic mental disorders will be discussed in the appropriate sections.

7.2.1.1. Schizophrenia

Schizophrenia is primarily a chronic disorder in the elderly and is probably better defined as a syndrome rather than a disease. Psychotic thought disorders are now considered to be common problems in the aged population. However, some confusion exists in terms of time of onset.

It is generally accepted that most older schizophrenics developed the problem in their early years and carried it with them into old age, with few having the initial onset of illness late in life. Usually the onset is seen in the late teens or young adult period, so that a 65-year-old may have a 40- to 50-year history of illness, the so-called chronic schizophrenic so frequently seen in the back wards of some state mental hospitals. Most of these patients were admitted long before the introduction in the mid-1950s of effective psychotropic drug treatment for their disorder. There are unique groups of elderly patients who are considered by some to be psychotic or schizophrenic (unfortunately, these two words are frequently and inappropriately used synonymously). One group of these elderly patients present with a seemingly first-time, acute onset of a schizophreniform illness and no evidence of dementia. Another is a group of patients with a long-standing dementia who may have little or no observable thought disorder or hallucinations, but do have enough disorientation and general intellectual impairment to cause considerable distress to themselves or those around them.

As in early life, although usually not as fulminant, schizophrenias in the elderly are characterized by disturbances in thinking (delusional), mood (blunted or inappropriate), and behavior (grossly disorganized). Loss of reality testing, such as hallucinations (usually auditory) or illusions, may also be present. These observations fit into the DMS-III *symptomatic* criteria for schizophrenia.[16] The other two criteria necessary for diagnosis of schizophrenia are *impairment* (deterioration from a previous level of functioning in work, social functioning, etc.) and *duration* (continuous signs of the illness for at least 6 months). Similar signs lasting a shorter time, between 2 weeks and 6 months, are designated as *schizophreniform*, rather than schizophrenic.[17]

7.2.1.2. Late-Occurring Paranoid States

Although paranoid thinking may be a part of the symptom complex seen in schizophrenia, it is listed separately because late-occurring paranoid conditions in an elderly patient frequently represent a first-time presentation of mental illness.[18] This phenomenon has been given a specific name, i.e., paraphrenia. Symptoms of this psychotic illness, generally characterized by well-circumscribed delusions and/or hallucinations of a grandiose or persecutory type, may not occur until age 60 or later.[19] It is thought by some[20] that this late onset of paranoid symptomatology may represent an unconscious "face-saving" device by the elderly patient against the gradual loss of self-mastery and control that is being experienced, and the fear and helplessness implicit with it.

Another theoretical explanation for the increase in paranoia in the elderly is as follows:

(1) Aging is associated with a variety of changes involving uncontrolled loss (psychosocial as well as physical) including job, friends, loved ones, income, physical strength, perceptual ability, hearing, memory, even hair.

(2) What characterizes many of these losses is that they are not under the control of the individual. He or she progressively *loses control* over the environment. This inability to maintain control is a key issue in many of the problems associated with elderly individuals.

(3) This progression of losses leads to a search for some explanation.

(4) Using the primitive defense of projection, the etiology of one's problems could well reside in some outside person or force; consequently, there is a valid reason to be on guard and suspicious of others.

One can arbitrarily distinguish among four increasing degrees of intensity of paranoid ideation in the elderly: (1) suspiciousness, (2) transitional paranoid reaction, (3) paraphrenia (late-onset paranoia without other evidence of schizophrenic illness), (4) paranoia associated with schizophrenia.[20]

It is important to point out that paranoid symptoms in the elderly frequently have a basis in reality, and may require a thorough examination of the psychosocial and family situation, rather than medications. Also, one should always think of the normal sensory decline (primarily decreased audition of high-frequency tones and a decrease in visual acuity and color perception) when examining an old patient with a late onset of "paranoia." Sensory decline is an important area in the elderly that is all too frequently overlooked during the mental status examination.

7.2.1.3. Thought Disorders Secondary to an Organic Mental Disorder

Organic mental disorders (OMD) are the major cause of psychiatric illness in the elderly population.

Beside the obvious cognitive deficits in the areas of orientation, attention, perception, and memory, elderly patients with OMD frequently exhibit disorders of thought. These may range from a very circumscribed delusional system to a more wide-ranging disorder of thought and reality testing which mimics a schizophrenic illness. The difference between these patients and patients with functional ("nonorganic") psychosis is the clear sensorium associated with the thinking disorder seen in those patients with functional problems. Thought disorders may be seen in elderly patients with a variety of acute (delirium) or chronic (dementia) organic mental disorders.[21]

7.2.2. Affective Disorders

When discussing affective disorders in the elderly, one usually means depression, although mania must also be included.[22] Affective disorders may be acute or chronic, and may present with or without psychotic features, i.e., disorders of thought.[23]

7.2.2.1. Depression

If there is a predominant psychologic disturbance in the elderly, it is depression.[25] Depression can be viewed as a syndrome interrelating psychic, somatic, and behavioral symptoms and signs, lasting at least 2 weeks.

Prominent psychic signs and symptoms include a persistent dysphoric mood (sad, "depressed," "blue"), irritability, anhedonia (inability to experience pleasure), guilt feelings, difficulty in concentration, pessimism, loss of interest, somatic concerns or delusions, helplessness, hopelessness, and suicidal thoughts.

Some common somatic manifestations include: anorexia, insomnia (or hypersomnia), fatigue, reduced sex drive, headache, amenorrhea where applicable, and constipation.

Behavioral signs are exemplified by: poor grooming, withdrawal, crying, motor retardation (or agitation), self-reproach, and suicide attempts.

These features may include a thinking disorder (e.g., delusions) and/or loss or impairment of reality testing, i.e., hallucinations, illusions, or even a depressive stupor. The psychotic features may be either mood-congruent (i.e., the content of the disordered thinking is consistent with depressive themes of inadequacy, guilt, deserved punishment, death, etc.); or they may be mood-incongruent (i.e., persecution, grandiosity, thought-insertion, thought-broadcasting, control, etc.). The significance or importance of the mood congruency or incongruency of psychotic features in affective disorders is currently controversial.

Depression in senescence is commonly overlooked, because it does not always follow the same pattern or have the same symptoms and signs as in the younger age group. The onset is likely to be more gradual and is likely to be primarily somatic in its manifestation, thereby being easily confused with the physical illnesses that are so common in the older patient. The usual affective symptoms and signs of depression such as sadness, crying spells, guilt, and self-deprecation may be absent, and instead an atypical clinical picture may be seen.

Depressed elderly patients may demonstrate a considerable impairment of memory, attention, concentration, and comprehension, along with psychomotor retardation and loss of initiative. These dysfunctional cognitive signs may be so prominent as to easily confuse a depression with a dementing illness. Depression in the elderly is often referred to as "atypical" or "masked."

It is essential that this differential diagnosis be made, because frequently an elderly patient who is depressed receives a diagnosis of dementia and is then treated by staff accordingly. This treatment unfortunately may result in the elderly patient beginning to conform to the situational ambience of his environment, with demented activity and behavior eventually following. Depression in the elderly is an eminently treatable problem.[25] Late-onset depressives, in comparison with early-onset patients, seem to have had better premorbid emotional, social, and psychosexual adjustment. The majority of severe late-onset depressive attacks appear after the age of 60, in both men and women. It appears that the onset may follow the occurrence of some traumatic event, which also differs from younger depressed patients, where specific precipitants are usually not evident.

These precipitating events can be classified as the occurrence, in a depression-prone individual, of multiple losses, either experienced or feared. These losses include: health, bereavement over death of spouse, relatives, and friends, loss of the work role because of retirement, loss of financial security, moving away of children, loss of status, loss of familiar physical surroundings, and an underlying fear of the inexorably approaching end of life.

7.2.2.2. Mania

Although manias are far less frequent in late life than are depressions, they do occur. Frequently, these episodes are part of a bipolar disorder, which may have been overlooked in the elderly patient. It usually follows a depressive reaction, and the manic symptoms, e.g., pressured speech, flight of ideas, etc., may be mistaken for aggressiveness or overactivity and the diagnosis overlooked. Hostile and/or paranoid behaviors of delusional proportion may also be present in these elderly patients, which may further complicate the diagnosis of mania.

7.2.3. Neurotic Disorders

In keeping with the DSM-III definition, neurotic disorders is here used as a descriptive term, rather than implying an etiologic concept. Although some authors suggest that neurotic disorders seem to improve with aging, their prevalence is pronounced in the elderly. Neuroses are much more frequent in the aged than are psychoses. However, since they manifest neither gross personality disorganization nor gross distortion of external reality, much less attention is paid to them than to the more visible psychoses. For purposes of familiarity, neurotic disorders in the elderly are classified here according to their predominating symptoms and signs.

7.2.3.1. Anxiety Neurosis

Anxiety is defined as an apprehension that stems from the anticipation of danger, the source of which is largely unknown. This disorder is characterized by increased muscle tension, gastrointestinal and urinary system disturbances, head-aches, irritability, disturbances in regular heart rhythm, excessive perspiration, and even a vague sense of impending doom.

Since all too often, real-life situations that are anxiety-provoking occur quite frequently in the older patient, it is not unusual that in this age group anxiety states are common.[26]

7.2.3.2. Compulsive Neurosis

These kinds of disorders that occur in the elderly are similar to those which occur earlier in life. Orderliness, perfectionism, attention to minute details, self-doubt, and feelings of inadequacy are some common signs of the compulsive person. Repeated acts of a penitential nature occasionally appear in elderly patients, and may be an attempt at protection against particular guilt-arousing fantasies.

7.2.3.3. Hysterical Neurosis

Signs of these disorders, especially the conversion type, i.e., loss of function of a particular body part, are uncommon in the elderly. However, what is frequently seen in older patients is a preoccupation and possible exaggeration of the severity of minor physical symptoms and complaints.

7.2.3.4. Chronic Fatigue

This disorder is also known as neuroasthenia, and is characterized by complaints of chronic weakness, fatigue, and exhaustion. It is obviously difficult to highlight this particular problem in older patients because of their propensity to tire quickly and recover more slowly from a stressor than younger individuals. One theory for the increase in emotional fatigability in the aged is that as gratifying experiences decrease with advanced age, so does an individual's interest, and therefore he is apt to tire more quickly.

It should be stressed that a regimen of satisfying accomplishments is more in order for an older patient with this problem than the often-heard suggestion to "take a long vacation and get away from it all." "Rests" of this type may actually exacerbate the lethargy and emotional fatigue.

7.2.3.5. Hypochondriasis

The prevalence of this disorder in the elderly population is extremely high. Hypochondriasis, or the inordinate preoccupation with one's body functions, is an especially common disorder in the aged.[7]

The symptoms seem to be focused mostly on various aspects of the gastrointestinal system, although no system is excluded from involvement. It has been suggested that this preoccupation among the elderly with feeding, digestion, and evacuation is involved psychodynamically with the unconscious expression of dependency needs, i.e., the desire to be taken care of, as when one was an infant.

7.2.4. Special Problems

7.2.4.1. Sleep Disturbances

It is generally thought that older individuals need somewhat less sleep than they did in their earlier years. Periods of sleep may be shorter and less sound, i.e., less stage 4 sleep, and complaints about lack of sleep are so common and intense among elderly individuals, that they often approach the level of a neurotic disorder. It is better to categorize those appropriate complaints as sleep disturbances, rather than sleeplessness. These disturbances may be due to more frequent nocturia than when younger, with a subsequent inability to fall back to sleep quickly. Also, many uninvolved, inactive older persons take several naps during a typical day, thereby obviating the ability, or the need, to achieve an uninterrupted full night's sleep.

7.2.4.2. Stress

Aged persons are susceptible to many stresses and strains that significantly influence not only physical and mental parameters, but also the capacity for social self-maintenance and self-sufficiency.

The stresses include physiologic stress related to decreased functional capacity, as well as acute and chronic illness, and psychologic stresses involved with feelings of dependence, isolation, loneliness, and intra- and interpersonal and intrafamily conflicts. Also, socioeconomic stresses occur, primarily related to losses related to retirement, widowhood, loss of family and friends, and loss of occupational status, and adequate economic support.[28] Some of the stress factors common to the elderly patient are illustrated in Tables I–IV.

The summated detrimental effects of this multitude of stresses over a long period of time are crucial regarding the outcome of illness in the elderly, and in fact may be as important as the specific effects of a particular mental or physical disorder.[9]

Table II. Economic Stresses for the Elderly

Compulsory retirement
Reduced income/inflation
Substandard housing
Increased expenses for medical care/food/rent
Inadequate retirement benefits/insurance/Social Security

Table III. Psychological
Stresses for the Elderly

Situational reactions
Psychiatric crises
Dementias
Neurotic episodes

7.2.4.3. Relationship between Functional Disorder and Physical Illness

The intertwining of physical illness and mental status must be strongly emphasized. Physical health may be more relevant to psychiatric impairment than any other factor studied, both in hospitalized and community-resident elderly patients. There is a general decrease in physical capacity with time as one ages, usually heralded by a lessening of strength, vigor, and coordination. There is also an increase in the likelihood of developing a chronic disabling disease, e.g., cardiovascular, renal, or pulmonary, as well as osteo- or rheumatoid arthritis. Older individuals are increasingly more vulnerable to serious illnesses related to infection, malnutrition, accidents, and drug and alcohol abuse. All of these may be associated with evidence of mental and/or emotional problems.

A decrease in sensory acuity occurs with aging. Visual defects or blindness occur in 4% of individuals in their 60s, and in 15% of those in their 80s. Hearing defects occur in 5% of those in their 60s, and in 25% of those in their 80s. Functional changes are known to occur at the level of sensory receptors, with an increase in the threshold level of stimulation necessary for activation. Also, functional changes occur in the afferent pathway to the brain with aging, as evidenced by a small decrease in nerve condition velocity.

Changes in the nervous system at the sensory receptor and the afferent pathway account for only about 4% of the decrease in function noted in the aging nervous system. Most of the functional changes occur within the brain itself with possible alterations occurring in resting membrane potential threshold, neuroglial regulation, synaptic receptor number and sensitivity, change in excitation inhibition ratios, or focal changes in blood–brain barrier.

In an aged individual, changes become evident in all sensory modalities, including vision, audition, olfaction, taste, touch, vibration, and pain. In terms of vision, there is a decrease in visual acuity, as well as a decrease in the ability to discriminate among colors (especially blue and green), leading to problems with

Table IV. Sociocultural Stresses for the Elderly

Diminished social role	Societal rejection/social desolation
Loss of authority	Withdrawal/isolation
Dependence on others	Denial of aging
Deflated ego	Mortality anticipation
Communication breakdown	

proper depth perception. Specific auditory problems of the aged, e.g., presbycusis, are manifested by a decreased acuity for high-frequency sounds, as well as a decrease in the ability to discriminate among sounds.

Decreases in visual and particularly auditory sensation with aging are significant, since these changes tend to amplify the feelings of loneliness and isolation, which may already be prevalent in many elderly people due to psychologic factors. In fact, this situation of isolation, coupled with a borderline sensorium, and under conditions of severe stress, may frequently lead to an abrupt onset situation of delirium in an elderly individual, known colloquially as "sundowning." The name is derived from the frequent observation in hospitals that many elderly patients whose mental functioning is borderline during the day, frequently decompensate totally at night, when their already compromised sensory input is even more severely curtailed.

Inadequate nutrition is a significant problem in the elderly. Problems in this area are due to a variety of reasons, including lack of understanding of good nutrition, lack of money, and sometimes an inability to get out and shop. Also, feelings of loneliness, apathy, and depression contribute to the lack of interest in eating and the unwillingness to try to achieve a good diet.

7.2.4.4. Suicide

Suicide occurs with fairly high frequency among the elderly, predominantly among white men. In fact, the highest rates for suicide in the entire population are for white male divorced individuals over 65. The high rate is thought to be directly related to ill health and depressive reactions, with the correlation depending, in part, on the fear of chronic disability and dependence that characterize many elderly. Suicide among the elderly is a serious problem, which in many cases is not really appreciated, either by professionals or the lay public. The seriousness of this danger is underscored by the fact that successful suicide attempts are more common than unsuccessful ones in old age. Also, the methods most frequently used for suicide, especially among aged men, i.e., shooting, hanging, and drowning, indicate the severity of the suicide intent.

There is some indication that suicide in the older age group in recent years may be decreasing, for reasons that are not at all clear; but suicide still represents a serious problem in the elderly population.

7.3. Drugs of Abuse

7.3.1. Introduction

Chemical dependence is arbitrarily defined as use of a drug for a minimum duration of 1 month, with social complications evolving from this use, and the exhibition of either a psychological dependence or pathological use pattern. Further, there is evidence with usage of a buildup of tolerance, or the onset of untoward signs and symptoms following withdrawal.

Another view is simply to classify it as "an inappropriate need for drugs."

Chemical dependency is a common problem in the elderly but is frequently overlooked for a variety of reasons, both personal and societal. These include the fact that the elderly are usually not arrested or prosecuted by society for minor crimes, and therefore never come to the attention of society; many are retired, and therefore do not come to the attention of employers, and elderly abusers frequently deny that a problem exists or are isolated and hidden by their families. This makes a valid determination of numbers of elderly abusers extremely difficult.

7.3.2. Comparison of Drugs of Abuse—Young versus Aged

It is interesting to compare the types of drugs used by young and old individuals. For example, in the younger abuser, loosely defined as 10 to 20 years old, the three major classes of drugs utilized are narcotics, nonnarcotics (barbiturates, stimulants, hallucinogens, and marijuana), and alcohol. The older abuser also utilizes narcotics and alcohol, but except for similar barbiturate abuse, has a very different list of nonnarcotics. This includes antianxiety and hypnotic agents, analgesics (including aspirin and acetaminophen), antihistamines, anticholinergics, and laxatives. Also, unlike his younger counterpart, who prefers heroin, the older narcotic abuser utilizes primarily Dilaudid®, possibly because it can be taken by mouth, has a better dose standardization, and is easier to obtain from legitimate and conventional sources.

7.3.3. The Elderly Abuser

In elderly narcotic and alcohol abusers, there seems to be a subgrouping into two distinct categories, one being the younger abuser who simply survived into the elderly population, while another group is composed of those who began de novo at an advanced age, frequently in their late 50s or 60s. These groups have been referred to as "early-onset" and "late-onset" drug abusers.

This phenomenon is particularly interesting in those older alcohol users, and is useful in clarifying and distinguishing between the elderly alcoholic who has been drinking for many years and the individual who drinks heavily for the first time in old age.

The most distinctive feature of the early-onset group is the exhibition of a social isolation and an almost total lack of interpersonal relationships. These drinkers are stereotyped as the "wino" or "skid-row bum."[29,30]

It is noteworthy that this early-onset group of alcoholics, mostly men, have few mementos of their past, e.g., photographs, address books. They generally have no contact with family or friends, and do not know the whereabouts of spouse and children or even if grandchildren exist. They may not even own the clothes they are wearing and may have received them from Salvation Army or police benevolence.

Following their discharge from the hospital, where they're usually admitted for malnourishment, exacerbation of chronic problems like peptic ulcers, chronic obstructive lung disease, and frequently with varying degrees of cognitive impairment, they almost never return for any follow-up clinic appointments. Members of this early-onset group could be considered as the dregs of society and should, by all rights, be the saddest of individuals. Paradoxically, there are frequent reports of clear-cut remnants of a social charm in many of these men. They are definitely societal survivors, which must require distinctive social skills. Therefore, psychopathology must be considered an important aspect of the early-onset drinker.

In contrast, those in the late-onset group are represented by both sexes, in a larger group than the early-onset one, and frequently were referred to as "social drinkers" earlier in life; or they may even have abstained totally from alcohol. If there were earlier periods of drinking, they were usually in response to some societal stress, and these episodes were never considered to be problematic.

Alcohol became a serious problem with them late in life, perhaps as an attempt at coping with disappointments associated with their aging. It's important to stress that life circumstances for many older individuals are often quite different from those of their younger counterparts, and may be due to society's still extant, frequently calloused, handling of the elderly, including poverty and rejection.

Rather than exhibiting the psychopathology of the early-onset drinkers, it is more appropriate to consider a psychosocial causation, perhaps complicated by chronic disease, with the late-onset drinkers. They may be responding to the "reactive" factors described by Rosin and Glatt.[31]

Instead of exuding remnants of social charm, members of the late-onset drinking group are frequently depressed and even suicidal on admission to hospital, and may present as hostile and withdrawn. These are individuals who, earlier in life, had many social and occupational affiliations and corresponding stresses and strains. They are also most likely to live with their families throughout much of their lives.

Late-onset patients usually do much better with treatment than the early-onset group, and their prognosis is somewhat better. Psychotherapy, antidepressant, or antianxiety pharmacotherapy, and Alcoholics Anonymous (AA) may be helpful. AA provides a new social support system where the individual can be subjected to an expanded and higher order philosophy, and where serving as a sponsor to others is beneficial toward providing a sense of purpose, dignity, and increased self-esteem.

A more comprehensive treatment of alcohol abuse in the elderly may be found elsewhere.[32]

The elderly nonnarcotic abusers can be divided into those individuals who actively seek to abuse drugs and those who inadvertently misuse drugs.

Those who seek out drugs to abuse receive them from a variety of sources including the doctor (or doctors), friends, relatives, drugstore over-the-counter (OTC) preparations, as well as street "drug pushers." There is much evidence to show that the abuse of sedatives, analgesics, and other prescription items increases markedly with age in both men and women, primarily due to the increase in medication usage in elderly individuals.[12]

Also, usage of antihistamines and anticholinergics, found in many OTC cold remedies and antianxiety preparations, markedly increases with aging. These drugs are notorious causes of delirium in elderly individuals.

The inadvertent drug abuser may be defined as an individual who, for whatever reason, does not take medications appropriately and ends up encountering an adverse drug reaction.

Some common reasons for this situation include: dementia, leading to confusion regarding use of prescribed drugs; inability to read the label or hear directions because of decreased sensory acuity with aging; confusing directions on the label; lack of education concerning potential adverse drug—food or drug—drug interactions; and sharing medications (often updated) with friends and family. Another significant reason is physician ignorance of the pharmacologic uniqueness of elderly patients.

7.3.4. Thought on Causation of Alcohol Abuse in the Elderly

No one cause for alcoholism in the elderly is known to exist at present. There are a number of hypotheses that attempt to relate the unique psychosocial problems of the elderly with the specific problem of alcohol abuse. In fact, it has been suggested that alcohol abuse in the elderly is not so much a medical or genetic as it is a social problem. Some of the common hypotheses involve feelings of uselessness and rejection; the transition from independence to dependence; poverty; reaction to low societal status and alienation.

A particularly interesting theory is the sense of loss of life-structure and subsequent feelings of loneliness and self-worthlessness that may follow the leaving home of grown children. These feelings may then lead the individual into the development of alcohol abuse in attempt to "drown" one's increasing perceived life problems.

However, despite these many problems, a large majority of older people who experience some or all of these stresses never develop into alcohol abusers. Therefore, although there is a clear association between biopsychosocial hardships and growing old, and an association between growing old and abusing drugs, there are no good data directly linking these two observations. Moreover, there are few data that compare the characteristics of those older problem drinkers with those older individuals who drink socially, or not at all.

Also, and very crucial, there are no studies comparing older to younger individuals in terms of reasons for drinking. It would be very helpful to look at some of the maladaptive behavior patterns in individual problem drinkers that may have led to that situation. For example, the well-known problems of dependency and denial seen in many abusers might be considered, as well as viewing these people in relation to psychic developmental problems and at their ability to manage feelings and impairments.

It may be that these particular maladaptive behavior patterns play a significant role in whether an individual, predisposed genetically or medically by an inadequate "threshold," becomes an alcohol abuser, either early- or late-onset.

These comments are relevant to elderly abusers of drugs other than alcohol and are important relationships to consider and study.

7.4. Organic Mental Disorders

7.4.1. Introduction

The term *organic mental disorders* was specifically used in the title in order to reinforce the clarity of definition in this complex area now offered by DSM-III. The focus is on the dementing illnesses and their differential diagnosis, with a particular emphasis on the elderly patient.

It is well known that there are many synonyms utilized by both professionals and lay people when discussing the definitive diagnosis for global cognitive and behavioral deterioration. These include *senility, organic brain syndrome, chronic brain syndrome, cerebral arteriosclerosis, and old brain syndrome.* Clearly all these words, including the word *dementia,* are buzz words, i.e., they are without real substance in meaning. DMS-III makes for communication regarding the organic mental disorders in a more valid, effective, reliable, and reproducible manner. The diagnostic entities are clearly defined, and inclusion as well as exclusion criteria are provided for precision of diagnosis. An essential feature of the Organic Mental Disorders section of DSM-III is the presence of the concept of either transient (reversible) or permanent (irreversible) brain dysfunction, attributable to specific organic (pathophysiologic) factors judged as *necessary* for the dysfunction.

To ensure clarity, two concepts must be reviewed, i.e., organic brain syndrome and organic mental disorders. Organic brain syndrome is defined in DSM-III as a constellation of psychological or behavioral signs and symptoms *without reference to etiology* (for example, delirium or dementia).[16]

This concept of organic brain syndrome must be differentiated from the earlier version of the term OBS, which was an all-inclusive, nonsubstantive diagnosis, and is synonymous with the other nondiagnoses previously mentioned. Following this logic, DSM-III next defines the concept of organic mental disorder as "a *particular organic brain syndrome* in which the etiology is known or presumed (for example, multi-infarct dementia or ethanol withdrawal delirium)."[16]

Another way of stating it is that the organic brain syndromes are clusters of signs and symptoms which are the clinical manifestations of the organic mental disorders. Therefore, using these definitions, dementia, as a general concept, falls into the category of an organic brain syndrome, and dementias with specific or known etiologies fall into the category of organic mental disorders.

There are three classes of organic mental disorders, i.e., age-related; substance-induced, and special. The first two are etiologically defined by the diagnoses themselves, whereas the third (or special) is composed of the aforementioned nondefined organic brain syndromes which need further information regarding etiology before the diagnosis can be completed.

Regarding age-related organic mental disorders, there are two types; one is the so-called primary degenerative dementia (PDD, which is synonymous with Alzheimer's disease or senile dementia Alzheimer's type, depending on age of onset); and multi-infarct dementia (MID).

This brief overview of the DSM-III concept of organic mental disorders is important and necessary in terms of pointing out and understanding where the concept of dementia fits, especially in the elderly. Dementia is defined as a clinical symptom complex in a patient marked by gradual deterioration of intellectual and emotional function with no loss of consciousness. This deterioration is due to chronic progressive degeneration of brain tissue, and may be progressive, static, or remitting. There are several key words in this definition, i.e., clinical symptom complex, gradual, no loss of consciousness, progressive, and degeneration. DMS-III adds to this definition specifics regarding the deteriorating cognitive and behavioral criteria, including: memory, abstract thinking, judgment, impulse control, and personality change. It also adds that dementia should "interfere with social and occupational functioning." These parameters can be enlarged to also include problems with perception, attention, orientation, lability of affect, speech (e.g., anomias, paranomias, and paraphasias). It should be noted that memory loss in this context is not to be confused in the elderly patient with the concept of "benign senescent forgetfulness."[33]

There are three major points that must be considered concerning dementia: (1) All unusual behavior in the elderly is not necessarily dementia; therefore, the differential diagnosis is very important, and it follows that the subsequent treatment modes will substantially differ. (2) If the unusual behavior is dementia, it can be due to a wide variety of organic causes, both intracranial and extracranial. (3) Following the biopsychosocial model in medicine of Engel, dementia must be considered as a multifaceted problem, not just a medical one, but also one which involves physiologic, socioeconomic, and psychologic parameters.

Organic mental disorders are known to be the most prevalent psychiatric disorders of later life. Because the number of people over 65 is becoming ever greater, the necessity of appropriate differential diagnosis of disturbed behavior in the elderly becomes clear and significant. It is also of interest that by the year 1990, 2 of 3 men over age 60 in the U.S. will be veterans, and, by the year 2000, there will be approximately 9 million veterans over the age of 65 in the United

States (there are approximately 3 million at present).[34] Even though the incidence of dementia does increase with aging, it is a myth that dementia will strike everyone at the age of 65. That is to say, dementia is not a normal physiologic consequence of getting older; it is considered a disease process, i.e., pathologic, in those patients who have become demented. Only 5% of persons over 65 have signs of severe dementia.[35] When combined severe and mild signs are reviewed, the number of patients involved only increases to approximately 10 to 18%.[36] By age 80, those with signs of severe dementia increase to approximately 20 to 25%. Although the percentage was thought to increase markedly over age 85, there is some evidence that this may in fact not be the case; however, these are not clear data at present.

It is well known that the elderly have problems maintaining homeostasis in the face of either an internal or external stress, perhaps due to the concept of "decreased cerebral reserve." When one considers the physiology of the brain as an organ (i.e., even though it only is 2% of the body weight, but, at any given time, uses 65% of the glucose in the circulation and 20% of the oxygen), it is easy to understand why a small deficit in either of these nutrients for whatever reason, even for a short time, may lead to severe dysfunction in the elderly.

7.4.2. Causes of Dementia

There are many causes of dementia, but in terms of the elderly population, by far the two major causes of dementia are PDD (Alzheimer's disease) and MID. These two entities make up approximately 75 to 80% of all the reported cases of dementia in the elderly. The remainder of the major causes are listed in Table V.

As far as PDD and MID are concerned, PDD makes up approximately 50%

Table V. Major Causes of Dementia

Alzheimer's disease	Nutritional dementias
Multi-infarct dementia (lacunar infarcts)	Folate deficiency(?)
Space-occupying brain lesions	Niacin deficiency (pellagra)
Chronic subdural	Pyridoxine deficiency
Chronic abscess	Thiamine deficiency (amnestic syndrome)
Frontal meningioma or a metastatic lesion	Alcoholic dementia
Myxedema (hypothyroidism) or other *chronic*	Chronic normal pressure hydrocephalus
endocrine causes	Dementia pugilistica
Pernicious anemia (vitamin B_{12} deficiency)	Neurosyphilis
Chronic arsenic, mercury, or lead intoxication	Other infectious agents (viral, tuberculous,
Chronic hepatic, renal, or other metabolic	cryptococcal)
deficiency	Specific neurologic syndromes (including
Carbon monoxide poisoning	Wilson's, Parkinson's, Creutzfeldt–Jakob,
Dialysis dementia	Huntington's, progressive supranuclear
	palsy (?), cerebellar degeneration, and
	multiple sclerosis)

10 to 20% and those with combined PPD and MID make up about 10%. PDD (Alzheimer's disease) is an enormous topic in itself, and will be discussed later. When MID is compared with PDD, it appears to be more common in men than women. MID refers to the cognitive loss resulting from multiple occlusions of small cerebral arteries. It has a more rapid onset than PDD, and there is a so-called stuttering progression (rather than inexorable), and sometimes focal neurologic signs are seen along with the cognitive deficit, including numbness, tingling, weakness, slurred speech, and even seizures. Frequently, there is also a history of high blood pressure, and sometimes hyperlipidemia. Pseudobulbar palsy with emotional lability is common, as is dysarthria and dysphasia. Also, patients exhibit abrupt ischemic episodes which frequently lead to weakness, slowness, hyperreflexia, and sometimes even a positive extensor plantar reflex. The primary vascular lesions causing MID are usually found in extracranial arteries or in the heart, rather than being primarily due to the cerebral arteries themselves. The Hachinski Index has been helpful in attempting to differentiate MID from PDD in elderly patients.[37]

CT scan may be useful in the diagnosis if one or more small areas of lucency can be seen, but lacunar infarcts are often too small for CT resolution. Focal or asymmetrical areas of slowing on the EEG help differentiate MID from PDD.

Nutritional dementias are a good example of the biopsychosocial concept of dementia. Nutritional dementia is a multifaceted problem. There are many factors involved, including malnutrition due to financial problems, physical problems of aging (dentures, GI upset, physically unable to shop), sensory problems (a decrease in olfaction and gustatory abilities), and psychologic factors (loneliness, unattractive or unpalatable food, depression, etc.).

7.4.3. Dementia as a Biopsychosocial Problem

Dementia in an elderly patient must be considered a multifaceted problem, with psychologic, social, economic, and physiologic factors being important contributors, along with the strictly biomedical problems involved.

Therefore, besides physical illness, one must take into account factors such as isolation, a sense of uncontrolled loss, financial problems, depression, sensory deficiencies, etc., when attempting to fully understand the clinical manifestations of dementia. The interrelationship among these various contributing factors is expressed in Fig. 1.

Another important related issue is the stress transmitted to the patient with dementia by the family trying somehow to effectively cope at home with the ever-increasing problems seen during the gradual deterioration over time. This increase in stress fuels a vicious cycle, clearly contributing to an increase in signs and symptoms of the disease, thereby making the stress worse. Significantly, there is also an increasing stress on the family unit regarding their attempts at dealing with feelings of anger, guilt, and the clear-cut ambivalence they feel toward their loved one, which only increases the longer the deteriorating patient remains at home. The clinician can be of immense service to the family by empathic counseling around the issue of appropriate time and optimum location for placement.

7.4.4. Differential Diagnosis

The diagnosis of dementia is based primarily on clinical observation, which makes it easy to confuse with other syndromes with similar signs and symptoms. Although dementia is sometimes underdiagnosed, it is most frequently overdiagnosed in the elderly patient. This occurs even in patients exhibiting severe neuroses, affective disorders, or paranoid psychoses, despite a clear sensorium; these misdiagnoses usually happen simply because the patient exhibiting the disturbed cognitive behavior is elderly.

There is a final common pathway of signs of cognitive dysfunction as discussed in the definition of dementia, common not only to dementia, but to other clinical syndromes in the elderly, including delirium and depression. Therefore, it is crucial to look at causes of unusual or even bizarre behavior in patients of this age group in an organized manner in order to make the appropriate diagnosis. Only in this way can effective treatment course be planned.

Delirium is one of the clinical syndromes in the elderly that can mimic dementia. One definition of delirium (also known as acute confusional state) is a fluctuating disorder of attention and wakefulness, with associated dysfunction of perception, memory, orientation, thinking, and judgment.

There may also be a frequent lability of affect, psychomotor disturbances, and a loss of reality testing (manifested by hallucinations and/or illusions). Delirium is rapid in onset and reversible in character, and is caused by an acute disruption of brain metabolism. In patients with delirium, the level of consciousness varies over time, and the hallucinations seen are commonly visual, but may also be auditory. Fear, anger, depression, sensory misperceptions, and fearfulness (greater at night due to a decrease in sensory input, i.e., "sundowning") are also seen in delirium, and this syndrome rarely lasts more than 1 month. At the outset, the only clinical difference observed between dementia and delirium in a patient may be the fluctuating level of consciousness in delirium, leading to a disordered attention span, the most prominent feature. This difference would be difficult to differentiate if the elderly patient was seen only for a brief time and there was no history known either of onset of the problem or of premorbid functioning. If the patient is seen for a long enough period, or a good history is obtained from a reliable informant, the differentiation of delirium from dementia is rather straightforward. However, if the aged patient is seen in a one-shot, brief situation, as frequently occurs in an emergency room, there may be some early difficulty in deciding on the correct diagnosis.

There are many known causes of delirium, and evidence suggests approxi-

Table VI. Major Causes of Delirium

Drug toxicity (prescribed, street, over-the-counter)
    Psychotropics (especially anticholinergics), bromide, and anti-parkinsonians, including L-dopa
    Digitalis, diuretics, antihypertensives, corticosteroids, disulfiram.
Central nervous system
    Head trauma
    Subarachnoid or epidural hemorrhage
    Intracranial mass lesion
    Transient ischemic attack (TIA)
    Meningitis (acute and chronic)
    Emboli leading to minor stroke (CVA)
    Seizure (ictal or postictal)
    Lupus vasculitis
Systemic
    Infections, systemic or CNS (with or without fever)
    Dehydration and electrolyte imbalance
    Burns, multiple trauma
    Acute hepatic failure or insufficiency
    Acute renal failure or insufficiency (uremia)
    Acute porphyria
Miscellaneous
    Fecal impaction in the elderly
    Urinary bladder distension in the elderly
    Withdrawal from addiction to alcohol, sedatives, hypnotics
    Postoperative state (particularly cardiac and eye surgery)
    Intensive care unit syndrome
    Extreme isolation or fatigue
    Hypothermia
    Postpartum state
Cardiovascular pulmonary
    Anemia (dietary or GI bleed)
    "Silent" myocardial infarction in the elderly
    "Silent" pneumonia in the elderly
    Onset of arrhythmia
    Congestive cardiac failure
    Pulmonary insufficiency
Metabolic and endocrine
    Diabetes mellitus
    Hypoglycemia (also nonketotic hyperglycemia)
    Hyperglucocorticoidism (also hypoglucocorticoidism)
    Hypothyroidism (also hyperthyroidism)
    Hypercalcemia
    Lipoprotein disturbances

mately 1 in 10 elderly patients diagnosed as demented may in fact be delirious instead. By far, the primary cause of delirium in the elderly is drug toxicity. This includes not only prescribed drugs, but OTC as well as street drugs, social drugs and drugs shared by family and friends. The drug itself may cause the delirium, or side effects of a drug (especially anticholinergic ones), an excess dose, a "normal" dose given to a frail aged patient, and/or drug–drug or drug–system interactions all may contribute toward causing a delirious elderly patient (see Table VI).

Other causes of delirium may involve the central nervous system, the cardiovascular–pulmonary–renal system, metabolic and endocrine, systemic and miscellaneous causes. In a frail elderly patient, such straightforward phenomena as fecal impaction or urinary bladder distention, as well as extreme isolation, fatigue, or intensive care unit syndrome, may be enough to precipitate a delirium.

Depression in an elderly patient is easy to confuse with dementia. This is because of the frequent atypical signs and symptoms of depression seen in the elderly that were discussed previously. These include psychomotor retardation and/or a decrease in attention, perception, concentration, and memory, which can easily be misdiagnosed as delirium or dementia. *Pseudodementia* is a term utilized by some to refer solely to patients with depression who present with signs and symptoms of dementia. However, the word as first employed[38] and subsequently used[39] refers to any patient who appears demented, but may have a variety of psychiatric diagnoses, including mania, schizophrenia, hysteria, and character disorders. Part of this confusion in terms may be because, among older individuals, pseudodementia occurs most often in the context of depression.[40]

Besides causing delirium, drugs can also cause depression in an elderly patient. There are several drugs which fall into this category including: methyldopa (Aldomet®), reserpine, clonidine, propranolol, bromides, alcohol, barbiturates, benzodiazepines, digitalis, glucocorticoids, and occasionally some of the antipsychotics (particularly depot Prolixin®).

Evidence suggests that anywhere from 9 to 25% of the elderly patients diagnosed as demented are, in fact, depressed.[41] There is some suggestion that depression may be more commonly seen in those elderly patients with MID rather than PDD, but this has yet to be substantiated.

It is important and should be stressed under the topic of differential diagnosis that, rather than a single cause of disturbed behavior in an elderly patient, a combination of etiologies is usually seen, e.g., a dementia plus a depression, and even on occasion a dementia plus a depression with an overlaying delirium.

7.4.5. Specifics Regarding Diagnosis of Dementia

It is obvious that an accurate diagnosis is crucial, not only among the various dementias, but also among dementia, delirium, and depression, in order to effect appropriate treatment. Following a comprehensive history, the most orderly way to begin this process is to attempt to differentiate the depressed group from the dementia versus delirium group; this may be done, or at least initiated, at the bedside. There are many paradigms for carrying out this initial separation; one of the most effective, since it includes neurologic (frontal release signs) as well as psychiatric parameters, is the screening battery for diffuse cortical dysfunction described by Jenkyn et al.[42] If the patients falls into the dementia/delirium group following the initial differentiation, the well-known basic battery of tests (UA, CBC, SMA-12, and for folate, B_{12}, thyroid, drugs, heavy metals, and other possible influencing factors) plus a well-standardized mental status examination,[43] and neuropsychological testing are indicated. The premorbid capacity of the patient is, of course, of the utmost importance in differentiating delirium from dementia. An EEG and CT scan should be included in the workup. An abnormal CT scan is not pathognomonic for dementia, since much overlap is seen between the normal and demented elderly patient, but the data may be helpful regarding the final diagnostic decision.

7.4.6. Alzheimer's Disease

7.4.6.1. Epidemiology

A major impediment to progress in identifying etiological and risk factors in Alzheimer's disease is the lack of adequate epidemiological information.[44] At present, only prevalence data on Alzheimer's in persons over 65 in Western Europe and two U.S. communities are available.[45,46] These data suggest that the prevalence of Alzheimer's disease in the U.S. in patients over 65 years of age is approximately 3% or approximately 750,000 people; this is about 50% of all causes of dementia in this age cohort. These numbers are for people over 65 who are not presently living in institutions. The prevalence of Alzheimer's disease for those patients in institutions is thought to be much higher, on the order of approximately 30%. Dementia in patients in nursing homes and institutions accounts for about 60% of the residents (with the aforementioned 30% of them probably having Alzheimer's disease).

It is reported that Alzheimer's disease occurs more frequently in women than in men, but these data are difficult to quantify since there are more females than males in the population being studied in general.[47] There does not seem to be any relationship between the incidence of Alzheimer's disease and premorbid intelligence. It is well known that patients with Alzheimer's disease do have significantly shorter life expectancies than those age-matched individuals without the disease, although it is not clear why this occurs. Without question, those with Alzheimer's disease are less able to handle their activities of daily living and are therefore more prone to life-shortening infections, nutritional deficiencies, and other hazards, but it is not clear whether this is the only factor involved. Descriptive epidemiology could provide essential data needed on age-specific incidences and prevalence in Caucasian populations as well as comparisons with black and Spanish-speaking populations and other cross-cultural studies. This kind of research has yet to be done. Some questions that might be answered would be whether the incidence of Alzheimer's rises smoothly with age, as might be expected if a single group of etiological factors were involved, or whether there is a biomodal distribution of age incidence (as suspected by some clinicians), which would suggest differing etiologic factors. Also, documentation of the suggested decline reported by some researchers in incidence of Alzheimer's after age 90 would be useful in the search for etiology.

A specific cross-sectional case-control approach for the study of epidemiology of Alzheimer's would be particularly useful for the short-term investigation of possible etiological hypotheses and the study of familial relationships in an attempt to try to validate genetic hypotheses. The occurrence of Alzheimer's disease in "punch drunk" boxers (dementia puglistica) has been well documented. Do other forms of head injury predispose to Alzheimer's? What is the role of alcoholism, dietary deficiencies, specific nutrient cachexias? These questions could be addressed using a case–control study format. Recent evidence suggested a direct relationship between the increased age of parents and the incidence of Alzheimer's disease in their children.[48] Subsequent studies to replicate this finding have not supported any association (L. Heston, personal communication; J. Mortimer, personal communication).

7.4.6.2. Etiological/Risk Factors

7.4.6.2a. Genetic Hypotheses. There is now well-established evidence that the rate of occurrence of Alzheimer's disease [as well as senile dementia of the Alzheimer's type (SDAT)] has increased in near relatives of patients.[49] Earlier studies suggested a simple Mendelian dominant relationship in SDAT, with age-associated incomplete penetrance,[50] but this hypothesis is now not accepted by most geneticists, except as applicable to a small group of patients with clear-cut familial pre-senile Alzheimer's disease. Indeed, for SDAT, there does not appear to be sufficient evidence to support a genetic inheritance—autosomal dominant or multi-factorial (polygenic) (J. Mortimer, personal communication). If, as believed by many investigators, this disease occurs as a result of the interaction of environmental and genetic factors,[53] then the understanding of such genetic factors would help identify the population at risk and would greatly assist in determining the important environmental factors in this population at risk.

Thus, genetic studies designed to identify these modes of inheritance are clearly needed.[54] For example, genetic studies should be undertaken, especially concerning chromosome number 21, since this chromosome is related to Down's syndrome with its well-known frequent development into Alzheimer's disease. It is felt that, in those patients with Down's syndrome (trisomy 21), the incidence of development into Alzheimer's is well over 95%.[53] There has also been a recent correlation seen between Alzheimer's disease and Down's syndrome within families, as well as a relationship within families of Alzheimer's and certain myeloproliferative disorders, for example, leukemia.[54] Chromosome 16 should also be explored, since this is the site of the gene related to haptoglobin expression and there seems to be a particular relationship between Alzheimer's disease and one of the haptoglobins. It would also be worthwhile to study a genetically determined susceptability to aluminum.

Familial Alzheimer's disease must be explored in many respects, including ascertaining the pattern of Mendelian dominance, and the relationship between familial Alzheimer's disease and other dementing illnesses, for example, Creutz-feldt–Jakob disease.

7.4.6.2b. Neurotransmitters. The study of CNS distribution of neurotransmitters has grown to primary importance in view of the recent demonstration that a deficiency of the cortical cholinergic system exists in certain brain areas of patients with Alzheimer's disease.[55,56]

It is known that the density (or number) of receptors specific to acetylcholine decreases in certain brain areas of patients with Alzheimer's. It is important to broaden the study of the anatomy of the transmitter systems in primates and humans, so that correlations between symptomatology and changes in neurotransmitters may be made. Not only is acetylcholine thought to be important but also GABA and glutamate (glutamic acid) are of great potential importance because of their putative neurotransmitter function.[57] Circadian alterations in transmitter concentrations should be analyzed, and the knowledge of concentrations of these transmitter substances in tissues and fluids other than brain in patients would be helpful regarding possible diagnosis and ultimate treatment.[58] Determinations must be made concerning the stability of transmitter-related enzymes in post-mortem tissue so that the data gleaned from autopsy material may be validated.

7.4.6.2c. Aluminum. A several-fold increase in aluminum levels in patients with Alzheimer's disease has been established.[59] It is not known whether the aluminum is a primary contributing factor or whether it accumulates as a secondary phenomenon.[60] There are no data available regarding the epidemiology of aluminum intoxication in those high risk areas such as factory workers and miners. Also the cytotoxicity of aluminum has not been established in reference to human tissue, or even in animal cells in vivo or in vitro.

7.4.6.2d. Latent Viruses. Virus infection as a cause of senile dementia of the Alzheimer's type has been suggested on the basis of two kinds of evidence. First, tissue from two cases out of six familial Alzheimer's disease are said to have been transmitted to primates where they were expressed as spongy encephalopathy rather than a specific lesion of Alzheimer's disease.[61] This work must be verified, amplified, and extended obviously to nonprimates. Since sheep are so susceptable to another spongy encephalopathy (scrapie), this species might be tried as a recipient of Alzheimer's tissue.[62] It is well known that Creutzfeldt–Jakob disease has been transmitted to several small laboratory animals, and it is tempting to think that Alzheimer's disease might also be the result of an infectious process.[63] Second, certain strains of the virus that causes scrapie infected into strains of recipient mice have resulted in lesions strongly reminiscent of the human senile plaque seen in the brains of patients with Alzheimer's disease. This research certainly needs to be amplified. There seems to be a particular propensity of certain viruses to replicate in association with neurofibers, especially the neurotubule. Can certain virus infections alter the neurofibers to cause the characteristic interneuronal tangles (neurofibrillary tangles) found so prominently in Alzheimer's disease?

7.4.6.2e. Structural Proteins. Abnormalities in structural proteins are clearly important in Alzheimer's disease. The presence in the cerebral cortex of neurofibrillary tangles containing abnormal paired helical filaments is a constant feature of this disorder. Biochemical studies of normal neurofibers are progressing, but those of abnormal neurofibers are in their infancy. The relationship between the structural proteins on the one hand, and metals, viruses, ischemia, and other factors on the other hand, is worth investigating.

7.4.6.2f. Immunologic Factors. The immunologic aspects of the cerebral dysfunction in Alzheimer's disease are only minimally understood.[64] So far, there has been a demonstration of a so-called antibrain antibody, the nature of which is not known at all, nor whether or not it is psychotoxic. Some evidence has been presented concerning altered serum concentration of immunoglobulins correlated with diminished cerebral function. The effect of antibodies to specific neurocomplement might well be of considerable importance in regard to the formation of structural or functional lesions in the brain. Amyloid is a prominent component of the brains of patients with Alzheimer's disease, and its chemical nature, origin, and significance, if any, must be studied further.

In regard to abnormal immune function, it would be interesting to know the fate of those children who, many years ago, may have been thymectomized for a variety of reasons, since the function of the thymus gland in immune activities in human is now well established.

7.4.6.3. Pathological Correlations

The brains of patients with Alzheimer's present a general shrunken appearance with changes especially pronounced in the frontal and temporal lobes. There is symmetric enlargement of the lateral and sometimes the third ventricles. The initial pathologic studies done by Alzheimer also described occipital degeneration.[65,66] Microscopically, there is a widespread loss of neurons, especially prominent in the frontal and temporal lobes of the cerebral cortex. Loss also is often present in the basal ganglia with secondary neuroglial proliferation. Characteristic senile plaques are seen throughout the cortex. They are amorphous, granular, amyloidlike material scattered throughout the cerebral cortex, most easily seen with silver staining.[67] Their significance at the present time is unknown. Also seen are characteristic neurofibrillary tangles, which are thick fiberlike strands of silver-staining material often in the form of loops, coils, or tangled masses seen within the neuronal cytoplasm. Their significance is also unknown.

Much of the recent progress and understanding in Alzheimer's disease (and senile dementia–Alzheimer's type) has depended upon quantitative correlations of clinical and pathological findings.[68] Quantitative morphometric studies of the anatomic distribution of specific Alzheimer's lesions, like the neurofibrillary tangles and senile plaques must be correlated with behavior and cognitive changes as well as with cerebral blood flow, EEG changes, and CT changes.[69,70,71] Morphometric and morphologic studies that need to be encouraged include further analysis of cell numbers and types of animal and tissue volumes in various parts of human brains and in relevant animal models.

Along with the cerebral cortex, this should include deeper structures such as hypothalamus and white matter.[72] The pathology of small vessels, i.e., arterioles, capillaries, and venules must be studied further as to the altered structure of their walls and of their innervention.[73] Also, the blood–brain barrier might be altered in age and/or in Alzheimer's disease, and the nature and significance of such alterations must be studied.

The findings of age-specific differences in distributions of tangles and plaques in Alzheimer's patients must be expanded, and the question of whether these are associated with any clinical differences during life among patients must be determined. It is well known that anywhere from 10 to 20% of the patients with Alzheimer's disease have coexisting infarcts. Does this add to or hasten the dementia by perhaps reducing the metabolic reserve of the brain? It must be determined whether, in fact, the degree of dementia in these "mixed" patients is a function of the amount of brain tissue destroyed, or the distribution of the Alzheimer's-type lesions.

Another area suggested for specific study involves those instances where there is pathologic evidence of Alzheimer's disease in terms of large numbers of plaques and neurofibrillary tangles where that patient in life had relatively intact psychological status, i.e., where the disease perhaps was subclinical. The questions that need to be explored are the distribution of these lesions and whether some other factors exist in that brain that can explain the fact that some patients have less psychological impairment in the presence of what appears to be a very widespread instance of this disorder when viewed pathologically.

It is important to remember that the diagnosis of Alzheimer's disease is both a clinical and a pathological one. Although a high degree of diagnostic accuracy can be achieved by history, examination, and concurrence of psychometric, EEG, CT, and cerebrospinal fluid (CSF) findings, as well as exclusion of other causes of dementia, both an improvement in the overall diagnostic accuracy and the identification of very early stages of even persons at risk could be achieved if a clinical method for identifying the presence of tangles and plaques, or perhaps even a biochemical change, could be found.

Other pathological changes in Alzheimer's are the loss of dendritic spines as well as the loss of neurones in the hippocampus and the cortex. Also, granulovacuolar lesions are noted in the extracellular space.[74]

7.4.6.4. Pick's Disease—The Clinical/Pathological Comparison with Alzheimer's

Pick's disease is thought to be an autosomal dominant trait with a high degree of penetrance, but this is not clear. There seems to be a symmetrical degeneration of the frontal lobes as well as the tips of the temporal lobes and perhaps even some posterior parietal involvement. Pick's may be thought of as a "diffuse frontal lobe disease." For example, there are problems with language much more than with Alzheimer's disease. Echolalia, euphoria, and a lack of anxiety ("la belle indiffér-ence") may be seen in Pick's disease.

Even though in theory this is true, there is no way of differentiating between the two in life ("Pick's versus Alzheimer's") because they are both clinically similar. It is of no practical importance to differentiate between the two.

It is thought that Pick's occurs more in females than in males, and that this disease rarely occurs over the age of 65. It usually is seen before the age of 60 and is in that sense a true "presenile" dementia. Pathologically, one sees the same severe atrophy in the cerebral cortex as with Alzheimer's, but as stated before, it is located in the anterior frontal lobe and tips of the temporal lobes. There may even be a specific line of demarcation between the atrophied portions and the rest of the brain, which appears grossly normal. There is also atrophy of subcortical structures in Pick's, including the caudate nucleus, the putamen, thalamus, and substantia nigra, as well as in the descending frontopintine fiber system. Extensive destruction of white matter is also seen in the affected areas of cortex.

There are no neurofibrillary tangles seen in Pick's disease and the density of senile plaques is not much greater than that seen in normal patients. There are also so-called "Pick cells" seen, which are swollen, ballooned-out neurons in the atrophic regions. Also, deeply silver staining, spherical, intracytoplasmic significance of these cells is unclear. It should be noted that the Pick cells are usually seen only in the first three layers of the cerebral cortex.

Pick's is much rarer than Alzheimer's, although specific numbers are not presently available.

7.4.6.5. Treatment

It is inappropriate to separate dementias into treatable versus nontreatable types. When one says "nontreatable," that usually refers to a progressive, presently noncurable type of dementia like PDD or MID. Further, even though some dementias are not curable in the strict sense, they are certainly arrestable in terms of their progression and in that sense are, in fact, treatable. Some dementias are even remitting following effective treatment. Even those dementias which are nontreatable to cure can be treated by psychotherapeutic and/or pharmacotherapeutic modes involving patients and/or family. Most causes of delirium, some dementias, and depression will usually have clear-cut treatment paradigms and are therefore straightforward to treat once the specific diagnosis has been elucidated. Combination diagnoses are more difficult to treat. One interesting example is the use of electroconvulsive therapy in a patient with combined depression and dementia. This treatment has usually been contraindicated because, although possibly effecting a positive treatment result for the depression, it is thought that the signs of dementia will worsen. This notion is one which has never really been scientifically studied and clearly needs more elaboration.

If the dementia is an age-associated organic mental disorder, i.e., either PDD and/or MID, and therefore not at present treatable to cure, other types of treatment then become important. These treatments can be divided into two types: psychotherapy and pharmacotherapy; in practice usually a combination of the two is utilized. In terms of psychotherapeutic approaches to these types of dementia, three things become important: (1) The independence of the patient always should be stressed. (2) Reality testing and other treatments, such as sensory stimulation, should be utilized when possible. (3) Above all, emotional support and a sense of dignity must be maintained in the patient. It is important to stress that these dementias are progressive and will be seen at different levels of severity, from mild to severe, which will obviously affect the treatment decisions at any given point in time, necessitating a flexible and dynamic approach.

Family education, counseling, and therapy, especially during the more severe stages of these diseases, become paramount. It is important that the social isolation that an elderly patient with dementia gradually endures must be combatted both by family and professional caretakers. Also, it must be remembered that a concomitant delirium may be caused in an elderly patient with dementia secondary to any kind of stress that could exacerbate the cognitive problems. Examples of some of the stresses are: minor infections, minor pains, inappropriate medication, unexpected surprises, or even disruption of the normal routine.

The second treatment for patients with PDD or MID is thoughtful pharmacotherapy. The goal of using psychotropic medications with either delirium or dementia is to assist in controlling the signs and symptoms being exhibited (behavior which is dangerous to self or others) without adding to the already disturbed brain function by using medication which would produce excessive sedative or anticholinergic side effects. "Control" in this sense means maintaining the optimum capability of cortical function in the demented patient.

A high-potency, low-dose, nonsedating, low-anticholinergic antipsychotic agent is suggested for use in these elderly patients. It is important to point out the need to attempt to establish an effective sleep–wake cycle, since sleeplessness and nocturnal wandering is a prominent sign in these diseases. One should not, however, use sleep medications in elderly patients on a regular basis without frequent review and evaluation. The same holds true when using antianxiety agents in these patients.

Hydergine® has been tried and may have some benefit in selected patients, although its not clear whether it functions as a mild antidepressant, or in some other manner.

Precursors of acetylcholine, e.g., choline and lecithin, as well as anticholinesterases such as physostigmine, and precursors of serotonin and norepinephrine have each been tried on an experimental basis in patients with Alzheimer's with equivocal results.[75,76]

Altering the individual's immediate environment can be helpful from several perspectives. There is the matter of safety, e.g., the need to protect the patient from wandering toward a stairway, etc. There is also the matter of lowering the frustration level, such as placing different cues in the immediate environment to combat memory loss and to reduce resulting stress and disorganization. It is essential that one finds the most protective, but least restrictive, setting for care that at some point may involve a move away from home to a care facility which is equipped to deal with those with dementia.

There is the need for assistance for the family as a whole. Particularly when the patient with dementia is staying with the family, then a homemaker or other kind of aid might be sought, even on a temporary basis.

As the disease progresses, the family often experiences tremendous stress and pain at seeing unsettling changes in their loved one, and they commonly feel angry and guilty over not being able to do enough. To the extent that family members can offer emotional support to each other and perhaps seek professional consultation, they will be better prepared to help their loved one manage the illness, and in coming to know the limits of what they, as a family, can reasonably do.

This is particularly true around the time when the patient's disease has progressed to the point that the matter of placement needs to be confronted. The family must deal with the considerable anger, frustration, and guilt around which such a decision invariably occurs.

7.5. Neurologic Diseases

Among the many neurologic diseases presenting in elderly patients, two of the most common are Huntington's disease (HD) and Parkinson's disease (PD).

7.5.1. Huntington's Disease

HD, also known as Huntington's chorea, is a genetically transmitted disorder resulting in gradual degeneration of cerebral cortex and basal ganglia, especially caudate and lenticular nuclei.[77] Each child, regardless of sex, of a patient with HD has a 50–50 chance of also developing the disease since it is known to be transmitted by a single autosomal dominant gene.[78] Cognitive deterioration and classic choreiform movement disorders are the hallmarks of HD, and personality changes, such as paranoia, moodiness, irritability, hypersexuality, and also memory dysfunction, frequently occur early in the disorder. Symptoms and signs usually begin between ages 30 and 50, but may develop earlier or much later.

The onset of HD is insidious. Cognitive changes may antedate or accompany the involuntary choreic movements, which usually first appear in face, neck, and arms. Deep tendon reflexes are usually increased. The motoric dysfunction presents as jerky, irregular, and stretching movements, and contractions of the facial muscles may result in grimacing. Respiratory muscle contractions may lead to characteristic explosive speech and the gait is a dancing, shuffling one. These movements cease during sleep.

Both anterograde and retrograde memory disorders may be the only prominant sign of dysfunction early in the disease, prior to the presence of the choreiform movements.[79,80] Therefore, memory assessment is invaluable in the early diagnosis of HD.[81]

Because of a proposed cholinergic–dopaminergic imbalance in the basal ganglia, with the emphasis on cholinergic degeneration, use of strong dopamine blocking agents such as haloperidol have proven to be partially successful in treatment of the motoric component of the disease. However, the cognitive deterioration continues progressively and death occurs approximately 15 years after the diagnosis of HD is first made. Suicide in patients with HD is not uncommon.

7.5.2. Parkinson's Disease

PD is a disease of the elderly characterized by disordered movement. The classic triad of PD, i.e., tremor, rigidity, and akinesia, is well known. Other important problems are postural abnormalities, equilibrium disturbances, and autonomic dysfunction.

Early signs are slowing of movement, stooped posture, and a small-stepped gait. Subtle signs such as decreased eye blinking, lack of facial expression, or a slowness in rising from a chair may also be observed early in the course of the disease. Later, patients have bradykinesia, an essential tremor, axial rigidity, and their fine motor movements are clumsy.

The etiology of PD is unknown although there is continued interest in a variety of possible causes, including a viral etiology. There have been isolated cases of Parkinson's disease following viral infections,[82,83] but this hypothesis does not seem to account for the majority of cases of PD.[84] Additional pathogenic mechanisms have been suggested, including associations with chronic and communicating hydrocephalus, and even chronic inhalation of carbon tetrachloride, but the evidence of these associations is not strong.[85,86,87]

Although the etiology is unclear, much is known about the neurochemistry and neuropathology of PD. The substantia nigra is consistently lacking in pigmented cells, and the basal ganglia are depleted of dopamine. Even though L-dopa treatment does ameliorate the signs and symptoms of the disease, it does not slow down its progression. Interestingly, although resting rigidity responds to therapeutic agents, activated rigidity (measured during activity) does not change with therapy, even in patients who show marked clinical improvement.[88]

Lewy bodies appear to be a characteristic neuropathologic funding in PD. These intracytoplasmic inclusion bodies are found mostly in substantia nigra, but have also been reported in cerebral cortex, hypothalamus, and brain stem nuclei.[89,96] The clinical correlates of Lewy bodies are presently unknown, but these findings suggest that PD may be a more diffuse CNS disease than was previously thought.

It has become clear that abnormalities in PD are not limited to the motor system. Intellectual dysfunction appears to be quite a common finding, with dementia developing in approximately one-third of the patients with PD.[91] Dementia may affect older individuals with a more rapidly progressing, therapy-resistant disorder. There may be a direct relationship between dementia and akinetic signs, and an inverse relationship with tremor.[92] There have also been reports of patients who have a combination of PD and Alzheimer's disease.[93]

Patients with PD who are not demented also may demonstrate cognitive dysfunction, particularly in tests of concept formation, visual–spatial reasoning, and verbal memory.[94,95] The severity of these cognitive dysfunctions seems to parallel the severity of the motor signs in patients with PD.[96,97] Treatment of PD involves several pharmacologic approaches, including anticholinergic agents such as Cogentin®, dopamine precursors such as Sinemet® (L-dopa plus carbidopa, a peripheral dopa decarbosylose inhibitor), dopamine receptor antagonists such as bromocriptine, the antiviral agent Amantadine®, (thought to act by a dopaminergic rather than cholinergic mechanism), and the GABA analog baclofen.

It is thought that pharmacologic treatment masks the disease symptomatology and does not retard the underlying pathologic processes. Moreover, long-term therapy with each of the pharmacologic approaches described not only demonstrates a gradual loss of benefit, but also produces untoward side effects, including psychiatric and vasomotor complications, as well as motoric changes, including dyskinesias and hyperkinesias. Despite the increased understanding of the clinical and biochemical aspects of PD, long-term, side-effect-free therapeutic options are presently limited.

7.6. Conclusion

Two points that were made continuously throughout this chapter deserve stressing and reinforcing. One is the anatomic, physiologic, biochemical, and pharmacologic uniqueness of the elderly patient. This knowledge must be coupled with the fact that the psychosociocultural milieu in which the older person operates is also unique, when compared with that of his younger counterpart. Together, these data make it crucial for those who care for the elderly patient with neuropsychiatric signs and symptoms to look upon his patient as a rare individual in every sense of that concept.

The second point brought out is that, in the elderly patient, there are complex, varied behavioral problems. These are frequently never clear-cut, and usually have much overlapping and mixing between the straightforward "organic" and the "functional" compartments, within which we found tidy and comfortable diagnoses in the past.

With the ever-increasing numbers of elderly people who are continuing to present with neuropsychiatric problems, it behooves us to keep in mind these two points because they are interrelated. The key is the obvious fact that appropriate diagnosis must precede appropriate treatment, and, when presented with a novel clinical experience involving an elderly patient, this point must be always kept foremost in mind.

References

1. U.S. Bureau of the Census, Projections of the population of the U.S.: 1977–2050, in *Current Populations Reports*, Series P-25, No. 704, Government Printing Office, Washington.
2. Raskind, M. and Eisdorfer, C., 1978, Geriatric psychopharmacology, in: *Drug Treatment of Mental Disorders*, (L. Simpson, ed.), Raven Press, New York.
3. Kramer, M., Tauber, C., and Redick, W., 1973, Patterns of use of psychiatric facilities by the aged: Past, present and future, in: *The Psychology of Adult Development and Aging*, (C. Eisdorfer and M. Lawton, eds.), American Psychiatric Association, Washington.
4. Lowenthal, M. and Berkman, P., 1967, *Aging and Mental Disorder in San Francisco*, Jossey-Bass, San Francisco.
5. Busse, E. and Pfeiffer, E., 1969, Functional psychiatric disorders in old age, in: *Behavior and Adaptation in Late Life* (E. Busse and E. Pfeiffer, eds.), Little, Brown, Boston.
6. Stotsky, B., 1967, Allegedly nonpsychiatric patients in nursing homes, *J. Amer. Geriatr. Soc.* 15:535–544.
7. Exton-Smith, A., 1978, Neurological and mental disturbances in the elderly, *Age Ageing* Suppl:1–3.
8. Wang, H., 1977, Dementia of old age, in: *Aging and Dementia* (W. Smith and M. Kinsbourne, eds.),Spectrum, New York.
9. Engel, G., 1980, The clinical application of the biopsychosocial model, *Am. J. Psychiatry* 137:535–544.
10. Brody, H., 1980, Neuroanatomy and neuropathology of aging, in: *Handbook of Geriatric Psychiatry* (E. Busse and D. Blazer, eds.) Van Nostrand-Reinhold, New York.
11. Terry, R., 1978, Physical changes of the aging brain, in: *The Biology of Aging* (J. Behnke, C. Finch, and G. Moment, eds.), Plenum, New York.
12. Maletta, G., Use of antipsychotic medication in the elderly, in: *Annual Review of Gerontology and Geriatrics* (C. Eisdorfer, ed.), Springer, New York, in press.
13. Seltzer, B. and Sherwin, I., 1978, Organic brain syndromes: An empirical study and critical review, *Am. J. Psychiatry* 135:13–21.
14. Raskin, A. and Rae, D., 1981, Psychiatric symptoms in the elderly, *Psychopharmacol. Bull.* 17:96–99.
15. Pfeiffer, E., 1979, Handling the distressed older patient, *Geriatrics* 34:24–29.
16. American Psychiatric Association, *Diagnostic and statistical manual of mental disorders*, 3rd ed., Washington, D.C., 1980.
17. *Diagnostic and Statistical Manual of Mental Disorders*, 3rd ed., 1980, American Psychiatric Association, Washington, D.C.
18. Carstensen, L. and Fremouw, W., 1981, The demonstration of a behavioral intervention for late life paranoia, *Gerontologist* 21:329–333.
19. Manschreck, T. and Petri, M., 1978, The paranoid syndrome, *Lancet* ii:251–253.

20. Eisdorfer, C., 1980, Paranoia and schizophrenic disorders in later life, in: *Handbook of Geriatric Psychiatry* (E. Busse and D. Blazer, eds.), Van Nostrand-Reinhold, New York.
21. Murphy, E. and Brown, G., 1980, Life events, psychiatric disturbance and physical illness, *Br. J. Psychiatry* 136:326–338.
22. Shulman, K. and Post, F., 1980, Bipolar affective disorder in old age, *Br. J. Psychiatry* 136:26–32.
23. Loranger, A. and Levine, P., 1978, Age at onset of bipolar affective illness, *Arch. Gen. Psychiatry* 35:1345–1348.
24. Solomon, K., 1981, The depressed patient: Social antecedents of psychopathologic changes in the elderly, *J. Am. Geriatr. Soc.* 29:14–18.
25. Gottfries, C., 1981, Treatment of depression in the elderly. General clinical considerations, *Acta Psychiatr. Scand.* 63:401–409.
26. Salzberger, G., 1981, Anxiety and disturbed behavior in the elderly. *Am. Fam. Physician* 23:151–153.
27. Ilfeld, F., 1980, Age, stressors, and psychosomatic disorders, *Psychosomatics* 21:56–64.
28. Turner, R. and Sternberg, M., 1978, Psychosocial factors in elderly patients admitted to a psychiatric hospital, *Age Ageing* 7:171–177.
29. Bahr, H. and Cuplow, T., 1973, *Old Men Drunk and Sober,* NYU Press, New York.
30. Schuckit, M. and Pastor, P., 1979, Alcohol-related psychopathology in the aged, in: *Psychopathology of Aging,* (O. Kaplan, ed.) Academic Press, New York.
31. Rosin, A. and Glatt, M., 1971, Alcohol excess in the elderly, *Quart. J. Studies on Alcoholism* 32:53–59.
32. Maletta, G., Alcoholism in the aged, in: *American Handbook of Alcoholism* (E. Pattison and E. Kaufman, eds.), Gardner, New York, 1982.
33. Kral, V., 1978, Benign senescent forgetfulness, in: *Alzheimer's Disease: Senile Dementia and Related Disorders* (R. Katzman, R. Terry, and K. Bick, eds.), Raven Press, New York.
34. *The Aging Veteran: Present and Future Medical Needs,* Veterans Administration, Washington, D.C., 1977.
35. Blessed, G., Tomlinson, B., and Roth, M., 1968, The association between quantitative measure of dementia and of senile change in the cerebral grey matter of elderly subjects, *Bri. J. Psychiatry* 114:797–811.
36. Kay, D., 1972, Epidemiological aspects of organic brain disease in the aged, in: *Aging and the Brain* (C. Gaitz, ed.), Plenum Press, New York.
37. Hachinski, J., 1978, Cerebral blood flow differentiation of Alzheimer's Disease from multi-infarct dementia, in: *Alzheimer's Disease: Senile Dementia and Related Disorders* (R. Katzman, R. Terry, and K. Bick, eds.), Raven Press, New York.
38. Kiloh, L., 1961, Pseudo-dementia, *Acta Psychiatr. Scand.* 37:336–351.
39. Wells, C., 1979, Pseudodementia, *Am. J. Psychiatry* 136:895–900.
40. Caine, E., 1981, Pseudodementia: Current concepts and future directions, *Arch. Gen. Psychiatry,* 38:1359–1364.
41. Maletta, G., Pirozzolo, F. J., Thompson, G., and Mortimer, J., 1982, Organic mental disorders in a geriatric outpatient population, *Am. J. Psychiatry* 139:521–523.
42. Jenkyn, L., Walsh, D., Culver, C., and Reeves, A., 1977, Clinical signs in diffuse cerebral dysfunction, *J. Neurol. Neurosurg. and Psychiatry* 40:956–966.

43. Folstein, M., Folstein, S., and McHugh, P., 1975, Mini-mental state: A practical method for grading the cognitive state of patients for the clinician, *J. Psychiatr. Res.* 12:189–198.
44. Terry, R. and Davies, P., 1980, Dementia of the Alzheimers type, *Ann. Rev. Neurosci.* 3:77–95.
45. Gruenberg, E., 1978, Epidemiology of senile dementia, *Adv. Neurol.* 19:437–457.
46. Gruenberg, E., 1978, Epidemiology of senile dementia, in: *Neurological Epidemiology: Principles and Clinical Applications* (B. Schoenberg, ed.), Raven Press, New York.
47. Katzman, R., Terry, R., and Bick, K. (eds)., 1978, *Alzheimer's Disease: Senile Dementia and Related Disorders,* Raven Press, New York.
48. Cohen, D., Eisdorfer, C., and Levereng, J., 1982, Relationship of age of parents with increased incidence of Alzheimer's disease in children. *J. Amer. Geriatr. Soc.* 30:656–659.
49. Pratt, R., 1970, The genetics of Alzheimer's disease, in: *Alzheimer's Disease and Related Conditions* (G. Wolstenholme and M. O'Connor, eds.), Churchill Press, London.
50. Larsson, T., Sjögren, T., and Jacobson, G. Senile dementia: A clinical, socio-medical, and genetic study. *Acta Psychiatr. Scand.* 39(Suppl. 167):1–259, 1963.
51. Heston, L., Mastri, A., Anderson, V., and White, J., 1981, Dementia of the Alzheimer type. Clinical genetics, natural history, and associated conditions, *Arch. Gen. Psychiatry,* 38:1085–1090.
52. Theodorescu, R., 1980, Chromosome changes in women with senile dementia, *Neurol. Psychiatr.* 18:195–199.
53. Ellis, W., McCulloch, J., and Corley, C., 1974, Presenile dementia in Down's syndrome: Ultrastructural identity with Alzheimer's disease, *Neurology* 24:101–106.
54. Heston, L., 1979, Alzheimer's disease and senile dementia: Genetic relationships to Down's syndrome and hematologic cancer, in: *Congenital and Acquired Cognitive Disorders* (R. Katzman, ed.), Raven Press, New York.
55. Davies, P., 1978, Loss of choline acetyltransferase activity in normal aging and in senile dementia, *Adv. Exp. Med. Biol.* 113:251–256.
56. Perry, E., Perry, R., Blessed, G., and Tomlinson, B., 1978, Changes in brain cholinesterases in senile dementia of Alzheimer type, *Neuropathol. Appl. Neurobiol.* 4:273–277.
57. Perry, E., Gibson, P., Blessed, G., Perry, R., and Tomlinson, B., 1977, Neurotransmitter enzyme abnormalities in senile dementia. Choline acetyltransferase and glutamic acid decarboxylase activities in necropsy brain tissue, *J. Neurol. Sci.* 34:247–265.
58. Bowen, D. and Davison, A., 1980, Biochemical changes in the cholinergic system of the aging brain and in senile dementia, *Psychol. Med.* 10:315–319.
59. Crapper, D., Karlik, S., and DeBoni, U., 1978, Aluminum and other metals in senile (Alzheimer) dementia, in: *Alzheimer's Disease: Senile Dementia and Related Disorders,* (R. Katzman, R. Terry, and K. Bick, eds.), Raven Press, New York.
60. Shore, D., Millson, M., Holtz, J., Kins, S., Bridge, T., and Wyatt, R., 1980, Serum aluminum in primary degenerative dementia, *Biol. Psychiatry* 15:971–977.
61. Masters, C., Harris, J., Gajdusek, D., Gibbs, C., Bernoulli, C., and Asher, D., 1979, Creutzfeldt–Jakob disease: Patterns of worldwide occurrence and the significance of familial and sporadic clustering, *Ann. Neurol.* 5:177–188.
62. Gibbs, C. and Gajdusek, D., 1978, Subacute spongiform virus encephalopathies: The

transmissible virus dementias, in: *Alzheimer's Disease: Senile Dementia and Related Disorders,* (R. Katzman, R. Terry, and K. Bick, eds.) Raven Press, New York.

63. Masters, C., Gajdusek, D., and Gibbs, C., 1981, The familial occurrence of Creutzfeldt-Jakob disease and Alzheimer's disease, *Brain* 104:535–558.

64. Kay, M., 1976, Aging and the decline of immune responsiveness, in: *Basic and Clinical Immunology* (H. Fudenberg, D. Stites, J. Caldwell, and J. Wells, eds.), Lange, Los Altos, California.

65. Alzheimer, A., 1907, Uber eine Eigenartige Erkrankung der Hirnrinde, *Allg. Z. Psychiat.* 64:146–148.

66. Alzheimer, A., 1911, Uber eigenartige, Krankheitsfalle des Spateran Alters, *Z. Ges. Neurol. Psychiat.* 4:356–385.

67. Herzos, A. and Kemper, T., 1980, Amygdaloid changes in aging and dementia, *Arch. Neurol.* 37:625–629.

68. Farmer, P., Peck, A., and Terry, R., 1976, Correlation among numbers of neuritic plaques, neurofibrillary tangles, and the severity of senile dementia, *J. Neuropath.* 35:367–371.

69. Boller, F., Mizutani, T., Roessman, U., and Gambetti, P., 1980, Parkinson disease, dementia, and Alzheimer's disease: Clinicopathological correlations, *Ann. Neurol.* 7:329–335.

70. Yamaguichi, F., Meyer, J., Yamamoto, M., Sakai, F., and Shaw, T., 1980, Noninvasive regional cerebral blood flow measurements in dementia, *Arch. Neurol.* 37:410–418.

71. Kazniak, A., Garron, D., and Fox, J., 1979, Differential effects of age and cerebral atrophy upon span of immediate recall and paired-associate learning in older patients suspected of dementia, *Cortex* 15:285–295.

72. Wilkinson, A. and Davies, I., 1978, The influence of age and dementia of the neurone population of the mammillary bodies, *Age Aging* 7:151–160.

73. Mancardi, G., Perdelli, F., Rivano, C., Leonardi, A., and Bugiani, O., 1980, Thickening of the basement membrane of cortical capillaries in Alzheimer's disease, *Acta. Neuropathol.* 49:79–83.

74. Ball, M. and Lo, P., 1977, Granulovacuolar degeneration in the aging brain and in dementia, *J. Neuropathol. Exp. Neurol.* 36:474–487.

75. Caine, K. and Mohs, R., 1982, Enhancement of memory processes in Alzheimer's disease with multiple-dose intravenous physostigmine, *Am. J. Psychiatry* 139:1421–1424.

76. Davis, K. and Mohs, R., 1982, Enhancement of memory processes in Alzheimer's Disease with multiple-dose intravenous physostigmines, *Am. J. Psychiatry* 139:1421–1424.

77. Bruyn, G., Bots, G., and Dom, R., 1979, Huntington's chorea: Current neuropathological status, in: *Advances in Neurology* (T. Chase, N. Wexler, and A. Barbeau, eds.), Raven Press, New York.

78. Sjogren, T., 1935, Genetical investigations of Huntington's chorea in a Swedish peasant population, *Z. Mensche. Vereb. U. Konstit.* 19:131–135.

79. Albert, M., 1981, Geriatric neuropsychology, *J. Consul. Clin. Psych.* 49:835–850.

80. Wexler, N., 1979, Perceptual-motor, cognitive, emotional characteristics of persons at risk for Huntington's disease, in: *Advances in Neurology* (T. Chase, N. Wexler, and A. Barbeau, eds.), Raven Press, New York.

81. Albert, M., Butters, N., and Brandt, J., 1981, The development of remote memory loss in patients with Huntington's disease, *J. Clin. Neuropsychol.* 3:1–12.

82. Schultz, D., Barthal, J., and Garrett, G., 1977, Western equine encephalitis with rapid onset of Parkinsonism, *Neurology* 27:1095–1096.

83. Miyaski, K. and Fujita, T., 1977, Parkinsonism following encephalitis of unknown etiology, *J. Neuropath. Exp. Neurol.* 36:1–8.

84. Moore, G., 1977, Influenza and Parkinson's disease, *Pub. Health Rep.* 92:70–80.

85. Tohgi, H., Tomonaga, M., and Inoue, K., 1978, Parkinsonism and dementia with acoustic neurinomas, *J. Neurol.* 217:271–279.

86. Botez, M., Bertrand, G., and Leveille, J., 1977, Parkinsonism-dementia complex, hydrocephalus and Paget's disease, *Can. J. Neurol. Sci.* 4:139–142.

87. Melamed, E. and Lavy, S., 1977, Parkinsonism associated with chronic inhalation of carbon tetrachloride, *Lancet* i:1015.

88. Webster, D. and Mortimer, J., 1977, Failure of L-dopa to relieve activated rigidity in Parkinson's disease, *Adv. Exp. Med. Biol.* 90:297–313.

89. Ikeda, K., Ikeda, S., and Yoshimura, T., 1977, Idiopathic Parkinsonism with Lewy-type inclusions in cerebral cortex, *Acta. Neuropathal.* 39:173–175.

90. Langston, J. and Farno, L., 1978, The hypothalamus in Parkinson's disease, *Ann. Neurol.* 3:129–133.

91. Lieberman, A., Dziatolowski, M., Kupersmith, M., Serby, M., Goodgold, A., Korein, J., and Goldstein, M., 1979, Dementia in Parkinson disease, *Ann. Neurol.* 6:355–359.

92. Mortimer, J. A., Pirozzolo, F. J., Hansch, E. C., and Webster, D. D., 1982, Relationship of motor symptoms to intellectual deficits in Parkinson disease, *Neurology* 32:133–137.

93. Hakim, A. and Mathieson, G., 1979, Dementia in Parkinson Disease: A neuropathologic study, *Neurology* 29:1209–1214.

94. Matthews, C. and Haaland, K., 1979, The effect of symptom duration and cognitive and motor performance in Parkinsonism, *Neurology* 29:951–956.

95. Pirozzolo, F. J., Hansch, E. C., Mortimer, J. A., Webster, D. D., and Kuskowski, M. A., 1982, Dementia in Parkinson disease: A neuropsychological analysis, *Brain Cognit.* 1:71–83.

Bibliography

Adolfsson, R., Gottfries, C., Oreland, L., Wibers, A., and Winblad, B., 1980, Increased activity of brain and platelet monoamine oxidase in dementia of Alzheimer type, *Life Sci.* 27:1029–1034.

Anderson, J. and Hubbard, B., 1981, Age-related changes in Alzheimer's disease, *Lancet* 1:1261.

Andrews, G., Tennant, C., Hewson, D., and Schonell, M., 1978, The relation of social factors to physical and psychiatric illness, *Am. J. Epidemiol.* 108:27–35.

Ball, M. and Vis, C., 1978, Relationship of granulovacuolar degeneration in hippocampal neurones to aging and to dementia in normal-pressure hydrocephalics, *J. Gerontol.* 33:815–824.

Ban, T., 1979, Pharmacological treatment of psychosomatic manifestations in geropsychiatric patients, *Act. Nerv. Super.* 21:116–121.

Basavaraju, N., Silverstone, F., Libow, L., and Paraskevas, K., 1981, Primitive reflexes and perceptual sensory tests in the elderly: Their usefulness in dementia, *J. Chronic Dis.* 34:367–377.

Bell, M. and Ball, M. Morphometric comparison of hippocampal microvasculature in aging and demented people: Diameters and densities, *Acta Neuropathol.* 53:299–318.

Branchey, M., Lee, J., Amin, R., and Simpson, G., 1978, High- and low-potency neuroleptics in elderly psychiatric patients, *JAMA* 239:1860–1862.

Brink, T., Janakes, C., and Martinez, N., 1981, Geriatric hypochrondriasis: Situational factors, *J. Am. Geriatr. Soc.* 29:37–39.

Brinkman, S., Sarwar, M., Levin, H., and Morris, H., 1981, Quantitative indexes of computed tomography in dementia and normal aging, *Radiology* 138:89–92.

Buell, S. and Coleman, P., 1979, Dendritic growth in the aged human brain and failure of growth in senile dementia, *Science* 206:854–856.

Buell, S. and Coleman, P., 1981, Quantitative evidence for selective dendritic growth in normal human aging but not in senile dementia, *Brain Res.* 214:23–41.

Busse, E. and Wang, H., 1974, The multiple factors contributing to dementia in old age, in: *Normal Aging 2* (E. Palmore, ed.) Durham, Duke University Press.

Cheah, K., Baldridge, J., and Beard, O., 1979, Geriatric evaluation unit of a medical service: Role of a geropsychiatrist, *J. Gerontol.* 34:41–45.

Cheah, K. and Beard, O., 1980, Psychiatric findings in the population of a geriatric evaluation unit: Implications, *J. Am. Geriatr. Soc.* 28:153–156.

Comfort, A., 1979, The myth of senility: Diagnosing nonspecific major illness in the elderly, *Postgrad. Med.* 65:130–142.

Comfort, A., 1981, Geriatric psychiatry: Mental symptoms in old people, *Ala. J. Med. Sci.* 18:177–183.

Corsellis, J. and Brierley, J., 1959, Observations on the pathology of insidious dementia following head injury, *J. Ment. Sci.* 105:714–720.

Goldstein, G., 1980, Psychological dysfunction in the elderly: Discussion, *Proc. Annu. Meet. Am. Psychopathol. Assoc.* 69:137–144.

Goodin, D., Squires, K., and Starr, A., 1978, Long latency event-related components of the auditory evoked potential in dementia, *Brain* 101:635–648.

Granacher, R., 1981, The neurologic examination in geriatric psychiatry, *Psychosomatics* 22:485–499.

Hirano, A., Dembitzer, H., Kurland, L., and Zimmerman, H., 1968 The fine structure of some intraganglionic alterations: Neurofibrillary tangles, granulovacuolar bodies and "rod-like" structures as seen in Guam amyotrophic lateral sclerosis and Parkinsonism-dementia complex, *J. Neuropath. Exp. Neurol.* 27:167–182.

Hubbard, B. and Anderson, J., 1981, Age, senile dementia and ventricular enlargement, *J. Neurol. Neurosurg. Psychiatry* 44:631–635.

Hubbard, B. and Anderson, J., 1981, A quantitative study of cerebral atrophy in old age and senile dementia, *J. Neurol. Sci.* 50;135–145.

Hughes, C. and Gado, M., Computed tomography and aging of the brain, *Radiology* 139:391–396.

Jacoby, R. and Levy, R., 1980, Computed tomography in the elderly. 2. Senile dementia: Diagnosis and functional impairment, *Br. J. Psychiatry* 136:256–269.

Jarvik, L., Ruth, V., and Matsuyama, S., 1980, Organic brain syndrome and aging: A six-year follow-up of surviving twins, *Arch. Gen. Psychiatry* 37:280–286.

Kaszniak, A., Garron, D., Fox, J., Bergen, D., and Huckman, M., 1979, Cerebral atrophy, EEG slowing, age, education, and cognitive functioning in suspected dementia, *Neurology* 29:1273–1279.

Katzman, R., 1976, The prevalence and malignancy of Alzheimer disease, *Arch. Neurol.* 33:217–222.

Katzman, R., 1981, Early detection of senile dementia, *Hosp. Pract.* 16:61–76.

Kral, V., 1980, Psychosocial problems of the aged: A shared medical responsibility, *J. Am. Geriatr. Soc.* 28:68–70.

Liston, E., 1979, Clinical findings in presenile dementia: A report of 50 cases, *J. Nerv. Ment. Dis.* 167:337–342.

Mann, D. and Sinclair, K., 1978, The quantitative assessment of lipofuscin pigment, cytoplasmic RNA and nucleolar volume in senile dementia, *Neuropathol. Appl. Neurobiol.* 4:129–135.

McConnachie, R., 1978, The clinical assessment of brain failure in the elderly, *Pharmacology* 16:27–35.

McMordie, W. and Blom, S., 1979, Life review therapy: Psychotherapy for the elderly, *Perspect. Psychiatr. Care* 17:162–166.

Murkofsky, C., Conte, H., Plutchik, R., and Karasu, T., 1978, Clinical utility of a rapid diagnostic test series for elderly psychiatric outpatients, *J. Am. Geriatr. Soc.* 26:22–26.

Paulson, G., 1977, The neurological examination in dementia, in: *Dementia* (C. Wells, ed.), Philadelphia, F. A. Davis.

Peck, A., Wolloch, L., and Rodstein, M., 1978, Mortality of the aged with chronic brain syndrome: Further observations in a five-year study, *J. Am. Geriatr. Soc.* 26:170–176.

Perry, E., 1980, The cholinergic system in old age and Alzheimer's disease, *Age Aging* 9:1–8.

Perry, R., Blessed, G., Perry, E., and Tomlinson, B., 1980, Histochemical observations on cholinesterase activities in the brains of elderly normal and demented (Alzheimer-type) patients, *Age Aging* 9:9–16.

Pfeiffer, E., 1979, Psychiatric problems in elderly patients, *Geriatrics* 34:23.

Pfeffer, R., Kurosaki, T., Harrah, C., Chance, J., Bates, D., Detels, R., Filos, S., and Butzke, C., 1981, A survey diagnostic tool for senile dementia. *Am. J. Epidemiol.* 114:515–527.

Phillips, M., 1979, Theoretical aspects of psychometric testing in the elderly, *Age Aging* 8:294–298.

Reisberg, B., Ferris, S., and Gershon, S., 1980, Pharmacotherapy of senile dementia, *Proc. Annu. Meet. Am. Psychopathol. Assoc.* 69:233–264.

Schneck, M., Reisberg, B., and Ferris, S., 1982, An overview of current concepts of Alzheimer's disease, *Am. J. Psychiatry* 139:165–173.

Schuckit, M., Miller, P., and Berman, J., 1980, The three year course of psychiatric problems in a geriatric population, *J. Clin. Psychiatry* 41:27–32.

Shraberg, D., 1980, An overview of neuropsychiatric disturbances in the elderly, *J. Am. Geriatr. Soc.* 28:422–425.

Spar, J., Ford, C., and Liston, E., 1979, Bipolar affective disorder in aged patients, *J. Clin. Psychiatry* 40:504–507.

Stoudemire, A. and Thompson, T., 1981, Recognizing and treating dementia. *Geriatrics* 36:112–120.

Sylph, J., Ross, H. and Kedward, H., 1977, Social disability in chronic psychiatric patients, *Am. J. Psychiatry.* 134:1391–1394.

Task force sponsored by the National Institute of Aging, 1980, Senility reconsidered: Treatment possibilities for mental impairment in the elderly, *JAMA* 244:259–263.

Tomlinson, B., The pathology of dementia, 1977, in: *Dementia* (C. Wells, ed.), Philadelphia, Davis.

Uemura, E. and Hartmann, H., 1978, RNA content and volume of nerve cell bodies in human brain. I. Prefrontal cortex in aging normal and demented patients, *J. Neuropathol. Exp. Neurol.* 37:487–496.

Vitaliano, P., Peck, A., Johnson, D., Prinz, P., and Eisdorfer, C., 1981 Dementia and other competing risks for mortality in the institutionalized aged, *J. Am. Geriatr. Soc.* 29:513–519.

Walker, J. Helping elderly patients deal with emotional problems. *Geriatrics* 36:137–138, 1981.

Wang, H., 1977, Dementia in old age, *Contemp. Neurol. Ser.* 15:15–26.

Wells, C. and Buchanan, D., 1977, The clinical use of psychological testing in evaluation for dementia, in: *Dementia* (C. Wells, ed.), Philadelphia, F. A. Davis.

White, P., Hiley, C., Goodhardt, M., Carrasco, L., Keet, J., Williams, I. and Bowen, D., 1977, Neocortical cholinergic neurons in elderly people, *Lancet* 1:688–671.

Wilson, W., Musella, L., and Short, M., 1977, The electroencephalogram in dementia. *Contemp. Neurol. Ser.* 15:205–221.

Wisniewski, K., Howe, J., Williams, D., and Wisniewski, H., 1978, Precocious aging and dementia in patients with Down's syndrome, *Biol. Psychiatry* 13:619–627.

Nutritional Problems in the Elderly

Cornelius J. Foley and Rein Tideiksaar

8.1. Statement of Purpose

The intent of this chapter is to provide insights to the difficulties inherent in assessing the nutritional status of the elderly. It advocates caution in the interpretation of current age-related nutrition data. The confusing overlap of age with disease is discussed to highlight these difficulties of interpretation. Approaches to assessing estimates of nutritional status and the current nutritional recommendations in the elderly are presented. Finally, geriatric information is provided on areas of broad clinical concern such as nutritional history taking, the hazards of the kitchen, and the interactions of drugs with nutrients. The summary details future research imperatives.

This chapter is not intended to be comprehensive—rather it provides an overview of issues regarded by the authors to be of geriatric interest. A number of recent texts on nutrition in old age are referenced for more detailed review.[1-7]

CORNELIUS J. FOLEY • Jewish Institute for Geriatric Care, New Hyde Park, New York 11042; School of Medicine, State University of New York at Stony Brook, Stony Brook, New York 11794; and Long Island Jewish and Hillside Medical Center, New Hyde Park, New York 11040. REIN TIDEIKSAAR • Department of Geriatrics and Adult Development, Mt. Sinai School of Medicine, New York, New York 10029.

8.2. Introduction

In the continuum of aging, there clearly exists a state produced only by "normal aging" in which disease has had no influence. There is, however, great difficulty in identifying this conceptually "healthy" state in which there exists neither overt nor occult disease. In fact, as a cohort ages, there is a progressive variability in biological efficiency among its members. Thus, at a chronological age of 75, one person may appear physiologically or psychologically to be 90 years old, while another presents and performs as a 60-year-old. This variability is caused by the disparate influences of time, disease, environment, and genetic profile on the individual aging process. In contrast, a group at maturity shows little intergroup deviation from its mean value for biological efficiency.

There is a wide range of "normal" aging changes that interface with the pathologies of late life. This results in a significant overlap in the spectrum of "healthy old age" with that of "sick old age." It is an imperative that research clearly demarcate those changes that divide aging changes considered "normal" from those caused by disease. With respect to nutrition, it is unfortunate that such demarcation points are not clearly defined. Neither is there agreement on the measurements that might be used to establish cut-off points between adequate nutrition and malnutrition.

Limitations of Nutritional Indicators in the Aged

Nutritional indicators must be accurate and have their validity established on representative populations. In addition, it is the precision and reliability with which such indicators can be measured that determines the accuracy and value of nutritional research. To assure such accuracy, an array of extraneous factors must be controlled. In the case of research with the elderly, complicating factors include age, the frequency of disease and disabilities, multiple medications, and underlying genetic or heredity factors. For example, in calculating body water, its significant, but normal, change with age can be further confounded by dehydration or edema resulting from disease or social factors. These and other factors can, for instance, critically impair the value of body weight as an indicator of an individual's energy status.

Nutritional measurements, appropriate in clinical settings, may become technologically inappropriate because of their complexity, expense, or degree of invasiveness when applied to large populations.

Clinical correlates of the nutritional indicators used in large surveys have not, in many instances, been well established. This is especially true for older populations. To illustrate, a drop in serum albumin does not generally occur early in states of protein deficiency; rather, it declines significantly only in advanced or severe deficiency. Interpreting such a fact with respect to an elderly patient is difficult, since there is a gradual decline in serum albumin[8] that normally accompanies advancing age. Thus, in an older patient, a serum albumin, below the standard range for adults, is compatible with either normality or protein malnutrition. The relevance of an abnormal nutritional indicator in an aged patient is also questionable. For example, an altered hematocrit, which etiologically might be multifactorial and which might include nutritional factors in its genesis, may have few or arbitrary clinical consequences.

In summary, the validity and reliability of indicators of malnutrition (undernutrition or overnutrition) in the elderly are questionable since their interpretation may frequently be little more than guesswork. In addition, when nutritional indicators are abnormal, they may have no clinical significance.

8.3. Aging Influences on Nutritional Data Interpretation

8.3.1. Metabolic Change

Basal metabolic rate (BMR) declines rapidly from infancy to age 20, with a further but gradual decline to age 75. Whether this latter slow decline in BMR reflects a real decrease in metabolic activity or a decline in cell mass is debatable. Cellular mass and body musculature slowly decline after age 30; muscle mass is partially replaced by fat and connective tissue.[9-10] The decline in lean body mass is reflected in a 15 to 20% decrease in exchangeable potassium per kilogram from age 20 to 75.[11] (This exchangeable body potassium is viewed as an indicator of lean body mass.) The decline of BMR with advancing age parallels that of exchangeable potassium. Thus, energy requirements, as a reflection of BMR, appear proportional to lean body mass at all ages.[12] This underscores the difficulty in evaluating age-related changes and highlights different interpretations that are possible when standards of measurement are compared or changed.

8.3.2. Physical Activity

There is a mild reduction in physical activity from age 20 to retirement when additional variable declines occur. Further advances in age do not appear to significantly influence energy expenditure unless there are additional factors, such as cardiovascular or pulmonary illnesses, degenerative arthropathies, or stroke. For the elderly involved in moderately strenuous exercise, significantly more energy output is required than in the young. This occurs because of decreased neuromuscular coordination and consequently increased muscular inefficiency which occurs with age and which results in wasted energy. This potential for greater energy loss is balanced by a reduction in extraneous movements and less indulgence in exercise. Overall, the decrease in energy requirement coupled to the decrease in demand of reduced lean body mass results in decreasing caloric requirements with advancing age.

Table I. Age-Related Changes in Body Composition and Function[59-60]

	Increase	Decrease
Lean body mass[a]		*
Body fat[b]	*	
Total body weight	*	
Total body water		*
Kidney weight		*
Liver weight		*
Cellular enzymes		*
Cardiac output		*
Renal blood flow		*
Skeletal muscle		*
Bone density[b]		*
Cellular immunity (T- and B-cell function)		*
Basal metabolism		*
Nutrient intake by cells		*
Glucose metabolism		*
Lipid metabolism		*
Protein synthesis[61]		*

[a]Greater in men.
[b]Greater in women.

Other specific age-related changes occur in body composition and function which influence the interpretation of actual nutritional status and nutritional requirements. These changes are detailed in Table I. The extent of change in many of the parameters listed is debated and is the focus of continuing research.

In addition to the physiological and metabolic parameters discussed in Table I, an additional array of biopsychosocial changes occur with normal aging. They can significantly influence the evaluation of older persons. Of these multiple factors, those considered to influence the nutritional aspects of health are listed in Table II.

Table II lists the normal physiological, psychological, and/or social accompaniments of aging in relation to their potential effects on function. The clinical outcomes which might accrue are then related to simple measures intended to limit potentially adverse functional or nutritional consequences.

8.4. Nutritional Assessment in the Elderly

Approaches to the nutritional assessment of the older patient include: (1) dietary history, (2) clinical evaluation, and (3) laboratory tests.

Table II. Biopsychosocial Changes to Consider in the Nutritional Care of the Elderly

Physiologic changes that accompany aging	Potential functional outcome	Probable clinical outcome	Recommended action to prevent nutritional difficulty
Eye			
Degenerative changes in muscles of accommodation	Pupils become smaller	Impaired visual acuity; decreased socialization while dining	Increase lighting in dining room and kitchen Refer to ophthalmologist to rule out reversible decline in vision
Degenerative changes[66] in vitreous, retina, choroid	Decreased color vision; decreased night vision	Susceptibility to accidents in the kitchen	Geriproof kitchen[a] Activity of Daily Living (ADL) training
Degeneration of intrinsic/extrinsic ocular muscles	Impaired upward gaze	Susceptibility toward tripping and falling in the kitchen	Geriproof kitchen[a] ADL training
Sclerosis of lens	Cataract, decreased peripheral vision	Impaired peripheral vision; susceptibility to accidents in the kitchen	Geriproof kitchen[a] ADL training
Central Nervous System			
Cerebral atrophy, senile plaques, neurofibrillary tangles	Parkinson's disease; supranuclear palsy	Confusion, and decreased ADL; possible diminished response and perception; memory loss leading to poor nutritional compliance	Memory aids to indicate when to go shopping, need to purchase specific foods, quality and frequency of meals
Decreased sensory function	Decreased reaction to pain, touch, heat, and cold	Decreased perception leading to accidental injury	Geriproof kitchen[a] ADL training
Impaired proprioception	Diminished mechanisms controlling balance	Increased susceptibility to falls in the kitchen	Geriproof kitchen[a] ADL training
Musculoskeletal System			
Decreased number and bulk of muscle fibers	Decrease in lean body mass	Decreased muscular strength leading to impairment in handling heavy kitchen pots and pans; decreased mobility	Use lightweight aluminum pots Geriproof kitchen[a] ADL training
Density of bone decreases	Osteoporosis	Increased risk of fractures	May respond to calcium diet
Loss of resilience in joints	Joint narrowing; bony sclerosis	Arthritis leading to impairment of using kitchen utensils, accidents in the kitchen	Analgesics and anti-inflammatory medication, heating pads, exercise, geriproof kitchen
Skin			
Thinning of epithelial and subcutaneous layers	Tissue and vascular fragility	Increased susceptibility to abrasions, bruises, burns in the kitchen	Geriproof kitchen[a]

(cont.)

Table II. (continued)

Physiologic changes that accompany aging	Potential functional outcome	Probable clinical outcome	Recommended action to prevent nutritional difficulty
Ear			
Degeneration of organ[67-68] of corti	Less of high-frequency tones	Decreased hearing leading to decreased socialization while dining	Audiologic evaluation Provide patient with working hearing aid
Nose			
Atrophy of olfactory mechanism[69]	Impaired sense of smell	Increased susceptibility to gas poisoning; decreased appreciation of foods	Geriproof kitchen[a] Suggest the use of herbs and spices
Mouth			
Resorption of gums and bony tissue surrounding teeth	Loss of teeth; impaired biting force	Preference for softer foods; increased incidence of malfunctioning dentures	Refer to gerodontist for oral evaluation
Decreased salivary flow	Dry mouth	Poor oral hygiene; increased incidence of gingivitis; impaired food bolus formation	Artificial saliva Avoid drugs that cause dry mouth, i.e., anticholinergics
Loss of tastebuds for sweet and salt[70-71]	Increased salt and sugar consumption	Diet high in sugar and salt	Monitor diet compliance in patients with high blood pressure, diabetes, and cardiac heart disease
Gastrointestinal			
Decrease in esophageal smooth muscle; lower esophageal sphincter dysfunction	Decreased esophageal mobility	Difficulty swallowing high-bulk foods, hiatus hernia	Serve foods in small quantities and provide water with meals
Decreased intestinal blood flow; decreased liver size[72-73]	Impaired intestinal absorption and liver metabolism	Malnutrition potential— probably subclinical	High nutrient content, relative to calories, in the diet
Decreased contractile function of intestinal smooth muscle[74]	Decreased intestinal motility	Constipation	High-fiber diet, exercise, fluids
Decrease in HCl secretion; decrease in number of absorbing cells	Achlorhydria; defective absorption of nutrients (Ca^{2+} and iron)	Pernicious anemia; iron deficiency anemia; osteoporosis	Vitamin B_{12} therapy; iron fortified foods with vitamin C; calcium diets may be beneficial
Decreased gallbladder motility	Gallstones	Gastrointestinal upsets; fatty food intolerance	Low-fat and high-fiber diet; possibly surgery for gallstones
Renal			
Decrease in nephrons; renal atherosclerosis in conjunction with decreased cardiac output	Decreased ability to dilute and concentrate urine; renal blood flow is diminished	Renal insufficiency; increased potential for dehydration	Provide fluids and encourage their intake

Table II. (*continued*)

Physiologic changes that accompany aging	Potential functional outcome	Probable clinical outcome	Recommended action to prevent nutritional difficulty
Endocrine			
Pancreatic beta cells or their function, or insulin end-organ responsiveness, may be diminished	Progressive glucose intolerance with advancing age	Special criteria for defining and treating diabetes mellitus; susceptibility to hypoglycemia if treating with insulin or long-acting oral hypoglycemic drugs	Caution in establishing diagnosis of diabetes; monitor serum glucose levels; observe for signs or symptoms of diabetes; cautious drug treatment
Psychological Changes			
Role changes[76–77]	Retirement; loss of productivity; increased leisure time	Depression; decreased nutritional intake; decreased finances	Psychosocial counseling Economic history Social history
Loss[78]	Multiple physical, mental, financial, and social loss	Depression; isolation; decreased nutrient intake	Psychological counseling Economic history Social history History of dining practices, facilities, and companionship Physical examination

[a]See Table X.

8.4.1. Dietary History

8.4.1.1. Nutritional Interview and History-Taking in the Elderly

Since the elderly often underreport illness, the clinician must maintain a high index of suspicion for potentially reversible diseases. In addition, many of the clinical indicators of disease in the young are diminished, absent, or altered in the elderly. Symptoms must therefore be carefully evaluated, since they may relate to potentially reversible conditions. It would be an error to dismiss findings or information on the basis of presumed normal aging changes without considering pathological states. Such clinical judgments can be difficult since the patient may have multiple overlapping and nonspecific complaints. Thus, it is necessary to place symptoms in rank order, recognizing that an apparently minor symptom may have major diagnostic or therapeutic significance for an older patient. Such difficulties reflect the challenge of geriatric medicine.

Multiple sensory deficits accompany aging and may limit history-taking. To overcome such difficulties and to facilitate communication, it is essential that the patient wear appropriate eyeglasses and/or a hearing aid; the patient must be allowed to lip read; the examiner must speak slowly and place proper light on his own face; and, in addition, extraneous background noises must be eliminated. To comprehend the edentulous patient's speech, the interviewer should ensure, if possible, that the patient wear correctly fitting dentures.

A patient's memory, orientation, or emotional state may significantly affect the reliability of a history. Early recognition of confusion or memory deficits will avoid a protracted and inaccurate interview. In this context, even subtle changes in mentation can be identified with simple, rapidly administered mental status tests.[13,14] In those patients who are mentally impaired, the history should be confirmed or supplemented by other sources such as relatives, previously involved health professionals, or hospital records.

8.4.1.2. Geriatric Nutritional History

An adequate nutritional history is rarely taken in any patient and is often performed poorly due to a lack of nutritional knowledge or training in nutritional assessment. This history must review not only the direct influence of disease, medication, and diet on nutritional status, but also the more indirect influences, such as finances, transportation, and ability to prepare meals.

Table III provides insights to the clinical relevance of the geriatric nutritional history. It identifies a broad range of factors influencing nutritional health in old age.[15–21]

8.4.1.3. Major Tools of Dietary History

The major tools of dietary history include: (1) dietary recall (24 hr), (2) food intake record, (3) dietary history.

8.4.1.3a. Twenty-Four-Hour Dietary Recall. One limitation of a 24-hr recall is that it may not represent the usual pattern of food intake. Variables such

Table III.   A Suggested Geriatric Nutrition History

Questions to consider	Clinical significance
(1) How many total meals are eaten per day? Per week? How many of these meals are hot?	(1) These questions provide information as to the quantity of diet. The number of hot meals correlates positively with nutritional content.
(2) What is the content of the meals? Special diets? Fad diets? Religious prohibitions?	(2) Assesses quality of diet, types of snacks consumed, and amount of fiber in diet, and also helps identify a patient on a special medical diet. Also, assesses the cost and nutritional value of special diets.

Table III. (*continued*)

Questions to consider	Clinical significance
(3) Who prepares the meals?	(3) The presence of a spouse or relative in helping to prepare meals can positively affect the diet.
(4) How and where is food stored?	(4) Availability of a refrigerator or freezer to store perishables.
(5) What cooking facilities are available?	(5) Whether a person has a kitchen or uses hot plate for cooking may influence dietary choices.
(6) Where are foods purchased? What is the distance to the store? Is transportation available? Who does the marketing?	(6) Whether food is purchased at a small grocery store or large supermarket will affect price. This is also dependent on type of transportation available.
(7) How much money is spent on food? What percentage of the income is this?	(7) The elderly are often restricted in their choice of food by lack of income.
(8) What is the level of physical activity?	(8) One's level of activity determines calorie requirements.
(9) What is the patient's dental status? Do dentures fit?	(9) The enjoyment and quality of food is dependent on one's oral hygiene.
(10) Does the patient have visual problems?	(10) Ocular problems may limit the preparation of meals.
(11) Do physical limitations affect cooking ability?	(11) Arthritis, tremors, or paralysis limit the utilization of cooking and eating utensils.
(12) Does the patient live alone?	(12) The level of socialization will affect the enjoyment of foods.
(13) What is the patient's emotional state?	(13) Depression will negatively affect nutritional status.
(14) What medications is the patient taking?	(14) There are many drugs which will negatively affect one's nutrition.
(15) Is there excessive alcohol consumption?	(15) Alcoholism is often related to nutritional deficiencies.
(16) Does the patient have anorexia, increased appetite, or weight change? Are these recent or long-standing complaints?	(16) These may indicate depression, medication side effects, or system illness (diabetes mellitus, hyperthroidism, etc.).
(17) Are flatulence, diarrhea, constipation, or difficulty in swallowing problems?	(17) These indicate gastrointestinal problems that may affect appetite.

as weekends, holidays, travel, paydays, receipt of food stamps, or illness can affect food intake. Furthermore, estimates of portion size may be inaccurate since the elderly can have perceptual difficulty in relating their usual food intake to the unusual measuring containers used in nutritional studies. With such difficulties, the accuracy of dietary recall is probably greater for those elderly subjects whose dietary habits have little variation.

8.4.1.3b. Food Record. Three- or seven-day time periods are usually selected. As in the case of dietary recall, the accuracy of a food record increases if the spouse, relative, or friends provide confirmation or additional information. The elderly may have significant problems in writing or recording their food intakes. Conditions such as arthritis, tremor, Parkinson's disease, stroke, benign senile memory loss, and presbyopia may limit usefulness of a food record. The value of such records is further questioned since a subject, completing a food record, may alter their usual intake pattern toward that of perceived normality because of involvement in a study.

8.4.1.3c. Dietary History. The dietary history focuses on food patterns and habits for periods of time up to 1 year. This approach provides information on the quality of the diet and can focus on specific nutrients, such as salt, fat, or sugar.

The nutrient content of a subject's average or usual food intake (obtained by history) can be determined from food composition tables. The amount of ingested nutrient actually absorbed can be calculated by allowing for factors that interfere with absorption.[22–23] Thus, an individual's total nutrient intake can be calculated and compared to standard norms. This approach provides a measure or indicator of an individual's nutritional status without recourse to physical examination or laboratory studies. With this methodology, difficulties arise in calculating the fraction of nutrients absorbed in elderly subjects, since age, disease, and drug prescription can significantly influence gastrointestinal function. In addition, "standard norms" similar to those accepted for young and middle-aged populations have not been firmly established for the aged.

Dietary history must therefore be combined with clinical examination, and when malnutrition is suspected, with laboratory studies.

8.4.2. Clinical Evaluation

8.4.2.1. Introduction

There are many classical descriptions of the physical findings related to malnutrition. Some descriptions relate to the specific findings of an isolated nutritional deficiency while others portray the picture of a more generalized malnutritive state. As discussed, many of the normal changes of aging may mimic clinical findings described as pathognomic of malnutritive states in adults. Competent geriatric assessments are necessary, for example, in interpreting ecchymoses in late life, which are almost invariably of the senile type and unrelated to vitamin C deficiency. Similarly, cheilosis and angular stomatitis, which can be caused by ribo-flavin, iron, or pyridoxine deficiency, are probably related to local causes in the elderly, such as lack of teeth, loose-fitting dentures, or drooling of saliva found in the conditions of stroke with facial involvement or Parkinsonism. Periodontal disease is relatively frequent in the aged and can present a clinical picture of spongy gums with marginal bleeding and hemorrhagic interdentate papillae similar to that found in vitamin C deficiency.

In the aged, clinically overt malnutrition is rarely due to a primary deficit in nutritional intake. It is more likely to be associated with a malignancy, frequently of the gastrointestinal (GI) tract, or with one of the chronic debilitating illnesses common to the elderly. In contrast, subclinical malnutrition[24] (by definition, undetectable on simple clinical examination) is probably frequent in certain at-risk older populations. These subgroups include: (1) those with mental disturbances or gross central nervous system disease; (2) those who are institutionalized; or (3) those who suffer from poverty. During subclinical malnutritive states, a patient may manifest depleted nutritional reserves by problems which might be described as "failure to thrive." Typical examples in the aged are the contribution of this state to postoperative confusion, delayed recovery times of homeostatic function, slow wound healing, and increased susceptibility to infection.[25]

8.4.2.2. Anthropometric Indicators of Nutritional Status

Anthropometric variables[26] provide estimates of body composition that, when standardized, provides an indicator of nutritional status. These variables may not correlate well with formal indicators of nutritional status such as hematological or biochemical parameters. There are two areas of anthropometric measurement of relevance, namely those of weight and skin-fold thickness.

8.4.2.2a. Weight Measures. Weight, which is easily obtained, is a measure of all the constituents of the body.[29] Since it is all-encompassing, it does not reflect any of the alterations or changes in the relative proportions of body constitutents which accompany aging—specifically the increase in fat and decline of other tissues such as muscle. Variables such as food or fluid intake, constipation, or diseases producing edema may further reduce its value. Note that it is insufficient to obtain weight values by interview since patients are frequently inaccurate.[27]

Andres[28] has reviewed the literature that suggested that obesity was related to reduced life expectancy and its corollary that those who were thin should live longest. He suggests that the weight-for-height tables define as undesirable those aged who are 10 to 25% overweight, but whom he suggests, when appropriate corrections are made for the lean body mass/body fat ratio change with age, may be a group with long survival. His interpretation may be skewed by the presence of unrecognized disease producing the decreased weight of those who are thin; or that the thin may have lifestyles with high levels of stress; or habits such as smoking or excessive alcohol concumption, which may be life-limiting.

8.4.2.2b. Weight/Stature. Actual height must be measured to determine the value of this ratio[2] accurately. The statures claimed by adults when interviewed are approximately 2 cm greater on average than that found on measurement. When performed accurately, this measure provides moderate correlation with percent body fat and a high degree of correlation with total body fat in the elderly. In both instances, however, the degree of correlation is less than in the middle-aged.

8.4.2.2c. Relative Weight. As in the case of weight/stature,[2] height must be measured in the estimation of relative weight.[29] Height decreases by 3 cm during an average life span, secondary to the postural changes of kyphosis or kyphoscoliosis and of intervertebral disk shrinkage or vertebral fractures. Inaccuracies in this estimating of height are significant in that a 3-cm inaccuracy results in a 2-kg change in the median reference value for weight when it is calculated from standard tables.[30]

Because of the potential inaccuracies in the estimation of height, other closely related measures are used, for example, recumbent length; this measure includes many of the inaccuracies of height estimates. Arm span may also be difficult to estimate in the elderly subject with postural changes. Thus, measures such as total arm length or alternatively ulnar length have been used and standardized tables are being developed.

8.4.2.2d. Triceps/Subscapular Skin-Fold Thickness. The accuracy of skin-fold thickness has been questioned in the elderly since age-related changes in the skin are variable and result in altered skin compressability. Two measurements of skin-fold are necessary (one on the trunk, the other on an extremity), since there are differentials in the aging changes of skin in various areas of the body.

8.4.2.2e. Upper Arm Circumference. There are progressive muscular changes associated with aging, specifically an increase in fibrous tissue, muscle fiber dropout, and an increase in intramuscular fat. There is significant variability in the extent of muscular mass decline and correlation of studies in the elderly are lacking. This is unfortunate since upper arm circumference is a good measure of total body fat in edematous patients in cases in which weight might be misleading.

8.4.2.2f. Anthropometrics: Summary. Total body fat is strongly correlated with upper arm circumference and with weight/stature[2] to a high degree; percent body fat is highly correlated with triceps skin-fold thickness. It is important to recognize that these measures do not actually measure nutritional status, but rather provide an indicator of such status. When compared with standardized norms, these measures provide a percentile nutritional rank for a studied individual. The inaccuracies involved in such projections are in the order of 3 to 5%.

Techniques used to validate the simpler anthropometric definitions include estimates of lean body mass estimates with total body ^{40}K measurements, estimates of total body water through neutron activation, fat-soluble gas inhalation to estimate total body fat, electrical conductivity to provide a measure of lean body mass, and finally, hydrostatic weight to provide a measure of total body composition. Other approaches are used but all must be placed in perspective. For example, the value of lean body mass must be questioned since the extensive changes in muscle that occur with normal aging have not been accurately determined or standardized.

8.4.2.3. Clinical Evaluation: Summary

The clinical or physical examination may reveal findings referable to nutritional deficiencies. Table IV provides pointers to possible clinical presentations of nutritional deficiencies that can occur in the aged. However, before ascribing any physical findings elicited on examination to nutritional inadequacies, the clinician should consider whether the findings are consistent with normal aging or with an underlying disease state.

Table IV provides rhetorical questions for the clinician to ask; for example, whether the patient has poor night vision or not. If the response is tentatively "yes," the table on its horizontal axis indicates possible related nutritional deficiency states. In this instance, vitamin A deficiency might be considered if night vision were poor. In addition, on this horizontal axis other physical findings are listed that might be found in association with that specific deficiency. In the case of vitamin A deficiency, an associated finding of protophobia is listed. The chart also lists physical findings that aid in distinguishing deficiency states which produce similar symptoms. For example, it lists the differential physical findings in iron and folic acid deficiencies, since either deficiency might be considered when the symptom of a sore tongue is obtained by history.

If the response to the rhetorical question is "no," proceed vertically down the table to the next question, namely, to ask "Do your gums bleed easily?" Again, the response will cue to progressing horizontally or vertically.

If followed, this format will identify most isolated or combined nutritional deficiencies.

8.4.3. Biochemical and Laboratory Evaluations of Nutritional Status

A number of laboratory studies exist for the evaluation of nutritional status. Some measures are taken randomly; others must be performed within specific time frames relative to nutrient intakes. A measure of body nutrient stores can be established by providing a standardized intake of a nutrient and determining its effect on serum or tissue concentrations, or by measuring its subsequent rate of excretion.

Studies frequently performed include:

(1) Hemoglobin and hematocrit
(2) White cell count with differential

Table IV. Pointers to Nutritional Deficiencies in the Aged

History		Nutritional disorders to consider	Physical signs
Do you have poor night vision? Dry eyes? Dry skin?	yes →	Vitamin A deficiency	**Eyes**—photophobia; decreased lacrimation; corneal ulceration; loss of light reflex; Bitots spot (white spots under bulbar conjunctivas)
↓ no			**Gums**—gingivitis **Skin**—dry skin; follicular hyperkeratosis (gooseflesh skin)
Do your gums bleed easily? Do small hemorrhages occur easily?	yes →	Vitamin C deficiency	**Gums**—gingival hypertrophy **Skin**—petechiae; purpura **Muscular**—intramuscular hematomas
no ↓ Is your tongue sore?	yes →	Iron deficiency . . . . . ↓ no	**Eyes**—pale conjunctivae **Tongue**—atrophic, smooth, sore papillae **Skin**—pallor **Nails**—spoon-shaped koilonychia **Vulva**—vulvovaginitis
no		Folic acid deficiency	**Eyes**—pale conjunctivae **Mouth**—stomatitis **Tongue**—glossitis **Skin**—pallor
	yes →	Riboflavin deficiency	**Eyes**—angular blepharitis **Nose**—nasolabial exfoliation **Lips**—cheilosis, inflammation of the mucous membranes **Gums**—gingivitis **Mouth**—angular stomatitis **Tongue**—atrophic lingual papillae
↓ Do you become overexcited easily?	yes →	Magnesium deficiency . . . . ↓ no	**CNS**—tremor, convulsions, behavioral disturbances
no ↓		Niacin deficiency . . .	**Gums**—gingivitis **Tongue**—raw, atrophic lingual papillae; fissures

Table IV. (*continued*)

History	Nutritional disorders to consider	Physical signs
		Skin—increased pigmentation, thick skin, atrophic in intertriginous areas; dermatitis **CNS**—dementia **GI**—diarrhea

Do you have:
  Trouble tasting?
  Burning lips?
  Tingling, numbness of hands or feet?
  Difficulty walking? → yes
	Thiamine deficiency	**Muscular**—calf muscle tenderness and weakness
		CNS—hyporeflexia; foot and wrist drop; hyperesthesia; paresthesia

no ↓		
Are you apathetic or tired? → yes	Protein deficiency . .	**Hair**—dry, brittle **Skin**—pitting, edema **Muscular**—wasting, loss of subcutaneous fat **Liver**—hepatomegaly **GI**—diarrhea
no ↓		
Do you have low back pain? → yes	Calcium deficiency . no ↓	**Skeletal**—osteoporosis/ osteomalacia; fracture
no ↓	Fluoride deficiency .	**Teeth**—caries
Do you have frequent diarrhea? → yes	Lactose deficiency . .	Low weight
no ↓		
Do you have trouble walking? → yes	Vitamin B$_{12}$ deficiency	**Eyes**—optic neuritis **CNS**—dementia **GI**—anorexia, diarrhea
no ↓		
Are you dizzy, depressed, or suffering from headaches? → yes	Hypoglycemia	Tachycardia, sweating, fainting

(4) Total protein and serum albumin
(5) Serum iron and total iron-binding capacity
(6) Serum calcium and phosphorus
(7) Fat and water-soluble vitamins (those easily measured)
(8) Skin tests of delayed hypersensitivity

Studies performed less frequently include:

(1) Fat and water soluble vitamins (those not readily measurable)
(2) Trace elements
(3) Various proteins such as transferrin, thyroxine binding prealbumin and retinol-binding protein; and various amino-acids

8.5. Nutritional Surveys

8.5.1. Introduction

In epidemiological studies, the aim is to establish a range of "normal" values or to compare the research values to accepted norms. Attempts to establish such norms for the nutritional status of groups in the population, including the aged, have been based on two approaches. One is to survey major population groups,

Table V. Recommended Daily Dietary Allowances (Revised 1980) [a]

	Men older than 51 years	Women older than 51 years
Weight (kg)	70	55
Weight (cm)	178	163
Protein (g)	56	44
Calcium (mg)	800	800
Phosphorus (mg)	800	800
Magnesium (mg)	350	300
Iron (mg)	10	10
Zinc (mg)	15	15
Iodine (μg)	150	150
Vitamin A (μg retinol equivalents)	1000	800
Vitamin D (μg)	5	5
Vitamin E (mg α-tocopherol equivalents)	10	8
Vitamin C (mg)	60	60
Thiamine (mg)	1.2	1.0
Riboflavin (mg)	1.4	1.2
Niacin (mg niacin equivalents)	16	13
Vitamin B_6 (mg)	2.2	2.0
Folacin (μg)	400	400
Vitamin B_{12} (μg)	3.0	3.0
Energy needs (kcal)		
Age 51–75	2400	1800
Age 76 +	2050	1600

[a]Reprinted with permission from: Committee on Dietary Allowances of the Food and Nutrition Board of the National Academy of Sciences/Nutrition Research Council.

the other is to survey small representative groups in great detail and to extrapolate, if possible, to the larger population. Based on such surveys, the Committee on Dietary Allowances of the Food and Nutrition Board within the National Academy of Sciences/National Research Council (NAS/NRC) has established Recommended Dietary Allowances (RDAs). The current allowances, revised in 1980, are presented in Table V.[31]

RDAs are defined, on the basis of available scientific knowledge, as levels of essential nutrient intake considered to be adequate in meeting the nutritional needs of practically all healthy persons. RDAs are not the requirements of a particular individual, rather they are recommendations for population groups. RDAs tend to overestimate the average requirements of an individual subject, thus some surveys have used two-thirds of RDAs as their standard.

Although the RDAs appear comprehensive, they are but a consensus of informed opinions on nutritional needs. In addition, it is important to note that the RDAs are "recommended" allowances that are constantly being revised and updated. Thus, it is difficult to make comparisons between nutritional studies that have standards based on the RDAs of different years; on a percentage of RDAs (rather than on 100% of RDAs); or on their own standards.

8.5.2. Major Nutritional Surveys

8.5.2.1. Introduction

The following major nutritional surveys have assisted in the establishment of nutritional data and standards for the United States populations and are outlined in Table VI.[32–38]

(1) The U.S. Department of Agriculture's (USDA) Household Food Consumption Surveys (HFCS) have been conducted at intervals (now approximately once per decade) since 1935. The most recent is the 1977–78 National Household Food Consumption Survey referred to as the Nationwide Food Consumption Survey (NFCS).
(2) The Department of Health, Education and Welfare, now of Health and Human Services, through the National Center of Health Statistics has conducted two Health and Nutrition Examination Surveys (HANES I and II).[35]
(3) The National Ten State Nutritional Survey was completed by the U.S. Department of Health, Education and Welfare's Center for Disease Control (HEW—CDC) at the request of Congress.[36]

8.5.2.2. Details

The HANES and USDA are both ongoing studies. Each has a different focus: namely on nutritional status in the HANES studies and on dietary intake

Table VI. Major Nutritional Surveys

	Time constraints for survey	Population sample	Methodologies	Caveats
USDA HFCS 1965–1966 and NFCS 1977–1978	Adequate	Representative of all U.S. households, including the aged	(1) Primary food preparer gave 7-day food consumption data (2) Others in household gave 24-hr food recall plus an additional 2-day food record (3) Data on all food consumed both in and out of the home (4) Source of food supply (5) Expenditures for food and housing	(1) Primarily a diet survey (2) No biochemical measures (3) Only reported heights and weights recorded (4) Food supplements not studied (5) The aged only provided 24-hr food recall
HANES I HANES II	Adequate	(1) Representative of population groups from age 1 to 74 (2) Selected at-risk subgroups: poor, preschoolers, and the 65- to 74-year-old age group	(1) 24-hr food recall for intake and a food frequency recall for dietary pattern (2) Anthropometric measures (3) Laboratory studies: hematological and biochemical (4) Extensive medical history and physical exam	(1) Dietary intake information limited (2) Those greater than 74 not included
National or Ten State Nutrition Survey—1967	Severe constraints	Unrepresentative: Evaluated those ten states with highest expected malnutrition; included inner-city, poor, migrants, and hispanic groups	(1) 24-hr food recall and household food consumption patterns (2) Food sources and expenditures (3) Anthropometric measures (4) Laboratory studies (5) Medical history and physical examination	(1) A skewed population; extrapolation not possible to general population or to the aged

in the USDA studies. Unfortunately, the persons included in one study are not included in the other. Thus, there are major inadequacies in relating actual dietary intakes and social situation to observed nutritional status and biochemical or laboratory indices of nutritional adequacy. The USDA in their HFCS do not relate dietary intake to nutritional status, which was not measured, and the dietary intake evaluations of the HANES studies are inadequate in comparison to their comprehensive medical and laboratory studies. Those over 74 years of age are not surveyed, as reflected in the absence of RDAs for the aged. Additional difficulties are that it takes many years for survey data to become available and that surveys are not sufficiently frequent to detect trends.

It is hoped that the two population bases might be incorporated and, with common standards, the HANES and USDA surveys would provide more comprehensive data on the nutritional status of the population.

Note that there are no RDAs for specific nutrients for those over 65 years of age, but the 1980 RDAs do make a recommendation for total caloric intake for those over 75 years of age.

8.5.2.3. Summary

The elderly appear to maintain approximately the same ratio of protein, fat, and carbohydrate in their diets to that of younger groups, namely, protein: 13–30%; carbohydrate: 50–55%; and fat: 30–35%.

Caloric requirements of the aged, however, appear significantly different to those of younger adults. For elderly men aged 51 to 75, the requirements are 2400 kcal, and for those over 76, 2050 kcal. For the older woman, the recommendations are 1800 kcal at age 51 to 75 and 1600 kcal for women over age 76. In contrast, the recommended caloric intakes in 19- to 20-year-old men and women are 2900 and 2100 kcal, respectively.

These large surveys suggest that some 35% of elderly subjects have caloric or energy intakes less than the RDA. Even if 50% of the RDA were taken as a norm, some 50% of white women and 60 to 95% of elderly black women would have intakes less than this reduced standard. Surveys note a decrease in caloric intake with advancing age of 24% in men and 17% in women as they age from 70 to 87.

Mean protein intake is adequate except for low-income black women. However, although the mean or average intake is acceptable, approximately 35% of all subjects have protein intakes significantly below the RDA.

Calcium appears to be one of the nutrients most frequently lacking in the diets of the elderly, with women having a lower, and proportionately a greater inadequacy in, intake than men. For example, in the Ten State survey, approximately 30% of elderly women living in high-income states and 50% of those living in low-income states fell below the standards of that survey, which was 400 mg of calcium (50% of the current RDA for calcium). The diets of 30 to 50% of elderly men and 70 to 100% of elderly women have less than the current 10-mg RDA for iron. The lower the income and the older the person, the more the diet appears to be deficient in iron. Vitamin A appears to be adequate in the diet although only 67% of the elderly appear to have diets which provide 100% of vitamin A's RDA. Those subjects over 75 years, especially women, have lower intakes of vitamin A. Vitamin C was found to be adequate in the subjects of the major surveys, although the level for low-income black women fell below the 45-mg RDA. In general, the intake of niacin has been found to be adequate and that of thiamin and riboflavin is probably adequate. Intake of Vitamin B_6 appears to be below the 1980 RDA for those 65 and older. In addition, there appears to be a decline in magnesium intake below RDA levels for those 65 and older.

In summary, total caloric intake, iron, calcium, magnesium, and Vitamin B_6, and perhaps Vitamin B_{12} in elderly women, appear deficient in the diets of elderly Americans.

8.5.3. Detailed, but Limited, Nutritional Surveys

8.5.3.1. Introduction

A significant number of limited nutritional surveys[39-43] have been performed in recent years.[39-43] These studies, in addition to the healthy elderly, have studied ill and institutionalized groups. They have, in general, attempted to focus on either a specific subgroup of older persons or on a limited or specific perspective of nutritional status. Surveys have, for example, attempted: (1) to accurately correlate dietary intake with biochemical and anthropometric indices of nutritional status; (2) to determine the incidence of, not only clinical, but subclinical malnutrition; (3) to determine the level of nutrient intake in those suffering from disease; (4) to determine the response of these diseases to replacement therapy; and (5) to assess specifically the effects of nutrient supplementation on biochemical parameters of nutrition.

8.5.3.2. Details of Surveys

An Oregon study in 1980, of 100 elderly men and women, determined that vitamin A, thiamine, and calcium were the nutrients most likely to be deficient.[44] Forty-one percent of the group had low serum protein concentrations. Biochemical values were abnormal in only 10% of subjects. Abnormal values were not significantly correlated with dietary nutrients, except for hemoglobin with dietary iron and vitamin C with its dietary intake. Dietary and serum folate values were in the lower limits of normal. Twenty-seven of the subjects took nutrient supplements. These supplements were generally inappropriate because of excessive intake. A subsegment of 20 patients residing in a retirement community, which provided one large meal daily, consumed less food than those who were completely independent. Significantly, there were no biochemical discrepancies between these two last mentioned groups.

A 1981 report[45] detailed the difficulties of interpreting data from national cohort studies. It reviewed data on the consumption of alcoholic beverages. By including additional "side information," it revealed that the previously predicted patterns were likely to be incorrect. It suggested that inadequate allowances had been made for the differential effects of aging on the various cohorts.

In 1980, a Swedish group studied[46] vitamin D deficiency by measuring serum concentrations of 25-OH-D in a group of 47 elderly patients of advanced age living in welfare institutions. They compared the welfare group with matched control groups living in their own homes. There were no differences between the groups for ionized calcium, alkaline phosphatese, parathyroid hormone, inorganic phosphate, or magnesium. Thus, the relevance of the reduction in 25-OH-D is difficult to determine. Speculatively, it might be related to decreased physical activity, reduced exposure to sunlight, and perhaps smaller dietary vitamin D intake in welfare homes.

A Wisconsin program[47] in 1980 sampled 372 households in an urban Midwest county. It reported that meat was the only food consumed with appropriate frequency by all age groups. The elderly consumed less milk, but increased amounts of fruit and vegetables and more cereals and breads than younger groups. The elderly skipped fewer meals, but ate less frequently on the average.

A 1979 New Jersey study[48] of 327 elderly patients of mean age 87 residing in nursing homes, and 146 patients with a mean age of 77 residing at home were compared with a group of 204 healthy volunteers aged 20 to 50. Levels of vitamins A, B_6, B_{12}, C, E, folate, biotin, pantothenate, riboflavin, thiamine, the carotenes, and nicotinate were measured. Deficiencies identified in order of decreasing severity in the institutionalized group were vitamin B_6, nicotinate, vitamin B_{12}, folate, thiamine, and vitamin C. In the noninstitutionalized group deficiencies were noted for vitamin B_{12}, thiamine, vitamin C, vitamin B_6, nicotinate, and folate. Overall, vitamin B_6, nicotinate, and vitamin B_{12} were the most common deficits. It was noted that vitamin supplementation reduced the prevalance of folate and vitamin B_{12} deficits.

This New Jersey group[48] studied an additional 228 ambulatory nursing home patients, of whom 30% showed vitamin deficits despite oral supplementation. Three months after a single intramuscular injection of the deficient vitamins, a rise to acceptable levels was found in 90 to 100% of this group. The intramuscular route apparently overcame oral absorption difficulties.

In 1979, a study in Belfast, Ireland,[49] reviewed 196 geriatric patients in hospitals, residential accommodations, sheltered dwellings, and of a home-residing group. The study compared the various groups with respect to the presence or absence of vitamin supplementation. Subclinical nutritional deficiency was apparently highly prevalent. Deficiencies included vitamin D, 47%; vitamin B_6, 42.3%; vitamin C, 29.2%; thiamine, 13.8%; and riboflavin, 7.1%. A biochemical deficit was detected in 91.3% of the nonvitamin supplemented group compared to 64.3% in the supplemented group. Oral multivitamins appeared to increase blood levels of riboflavin and vitamin C to normal levels in all patients, but failed in the case of thiamine and vitamin B_6 in 3% and 20% of subjects, respectively.

A 1980 study in Cardiff, Wales,[50] demonstrated that although serum folate rose rapidly, the levels of serum iron, total iron-binding capacities, and vitamin B_{12} were not influenced by food intake. Serum iron and total iron-binding capacity were, however, influenced by the time of day; their levels dropped significantly from 8:00 a.m. to 8:00 p.m.

Roth in 1975[51] demonstrated that corticosteroid hormone receptors diminished significantly in aging rats, although Sugarman and Munro in 1980[52] demonstrated that aged cultured cells had a decrease of up to 40% in zinc uptake. These data, coupled to the apparent diminished response to vitamin supplementation in the elderly, might suggest an age-related decline in cellular nutrient uptake.

8.5.3.3. Summary

The data from these more detailed studies indicate that little is as yet known about the specifics of nutrition in the elderly, that a multiplicity of factors complicate nutritional assessment in the aged, and that further research is clearly necessary.

These studies indicate (1) that significant nutritional deficits may exist without associated biochemical correlates; (2) that in those cases in which biochemical abnormalities are found, they are not necessarily associated with obvious deficits in nutrient intake; (3) that nutritional supplements, if taken, may not correct biochemical deficits, although the intramuscular route for supplementation may be superior to the oral one; and (4) that if supplements are taken, they are perhaps frequently inappropriate. In addition, factors such as the standardization of food intake and the time of day or of the year may be critical in nutrition studies. Finally, data from ongoing cellular nutritional research may demand a review of clinical data.

8.6. Nutrient Recommendations for Older Americans

A concensus of opinion on dietary recommendations for the elderly[53-55] as developed by Winick of the Institute of Human Nutrition is presented in Table VII. A number of general principles that underlie these recommendations are important: The elderly have, on average, a progressive decline in exercise (and a proportional decrease in energy expenditure) which, when linked to the decrease in their basal metabolic rate, suggests the need to progressively reduce caloric intake. Nutrient requirements, however, remain constant with advancing age, thus

Table VII.   Nutrient Recommendation for the Elderly[a]

Nutrient	Men	Women
Calories	2300/day	2000/day
Protein	56 g/day	45 g/day
Fat	25–30% of total daily calories (64–76 g/day)	25–30% of total daily calories (55–66 g/day)
Carbohydrates	55–60% of total daily calories (310–345 g/day)	55–60% of total daily calories (275–300 g/day)
Fiber (dietary)	Increase to approximately 10 g	Increase to approximately 10 g
Vitamins	Increase B_{12} to greater than 3 μg	Increase B_{12} to greater than 3 μg
Calcium	1000 mg/day	1000 mg/day
Phosphorus	Reduce	Reduce
Iron	18–40 mg/day	18–40 mg/day

[a] Developed by Winick for Institute of Human Nutrition.

Protein recommendations are similar to those of younger adults. Red meats can be replaced by fish, poultry, low-fat dairy products, and combinations of vegetables and grains. This reduces the intake of saturated fats and increases calcium intake.

Calcium intake should approximate 1000 mg/day (higher than current RDA) especially in women. This will aid in preventing postmenopausal osteoporosis. In addition, since calcium maintains an inverse relationship to phosphorus, carbonated soft drinks and meats, which have high levels of phosphorus, should be reduced. This reduction in dietary phosphorus will result in higher total body calcium and perhaps delay or reduce the rate of development of osteoporosis. Exercise has a further beneficial effect.

Iron supplementation is important in the elderly since its intake appears to be borderline. Iron is available from a variety of sources including lean meats, vegetables, and enriched or fortified food products.

It is difficult to make any specific recommendations on vitamin supplementation since the clinical benefits that might accrue are equivocal. In the case of vitamin B_{12}, the recommendation for its level of intake is most pertinent in those patients suspected of intrinsic factor deficits. Many nutritional experts have suggested that appropriate multivitamin supplementation in the aged is without serious side effects, and perhaps beneficial. Certainly multivitamins are less expensive than attempting to provide all required nutrients in the diets of the elderly, especially since the recommendations include a reduction in the caloric content of the diets. Balanced against this recommendation must be the apparent excessive intake, to toxic levels, by some older patients when advised to take nutrient supplements.

8.7. Drug–Diet Interactions in the Aged

The elderly consume 25% of all prescription drugs and an even greater percentage of over-the-counter medication.[56–58] In fact, the average patient, with multiple chronic diseases, probably takes as many as 7 to 8 different medications daily. Thus, the possibility of incurring a drug–drug or drug–diet interaction is great.

Table VIII provides a listing of potential drug–diet interactions in the elderly with suggested approaches to the preventive management of such interactions.

Table IX lists medications, or drug groups, whose actions or effects may influence the levels of specific nutrients. There is inadequate information on nutrient–drug effects, on the susceptability of individuals to them, or on their appropriate management if they should occur. For example, vitamin D supple-

Table VIII.   Potential Drug–Diet Interactions in the Aged

Drug–drug group	Diet	Potential effect of interaction	Preventive recommendation
Acetaminophen	High carbohydrate	Decreased absorption of acetaminophen	Avoid high-carbohydrate meals
Anticoagulants	Foods rich in vitamin K	Decreased anticoagulant effect	Limit or keep constant intake of vitamin K foods (citrus fruits, eggs, fish, leafy green vegetables)
Digoxin	Milk	Decreased absorption of digoxin	Avoid taking digoxin with milk; milk may be taken 2 hr after digoxin dose
Erythromycin	Acidic fruit juices, carbonated drinks	Decreased absorption of erythromycin	Give erythromycin 1 hr before or 3 hr after meals
Iron	Milk	Decreased absorption of iron	Avoid taking iron with milk
Levodopa	Foods rich in vitamin B_6	Decreased effect of levodopa	Avoid foods with vitamin B_6; use Sinemet® (this drug does not interact with vitamin B_6)
Lithium	Insufficient salt and water intake	Lithium toxicity	Monitor lithium blood levels; ensure adequate salt and water intake (especially if patient is taking diuretics)
MAO inhibitors	Aged cheese, beer, wine, chocolate, avocado, herring	High blood pressure	Avoid tyramine-containing foods
Penicillin	Acidic fruit juices	Decreased absorption of penicillin	Take penicillin with water 1 hr before or 2 hr after meals
Tetracycline	Milk and other dairy products	Decreased absorption of tetracycline	Take medication 1 hr before or after meals
Tolbutamine	Alcohol	Nausea, vomiting, photosensitivity	Avoid alcoholic beverages

Table IX. Drug–Nutrient Interactions

Drug-drug group	Nutrients influenced by drug action	Preventive recommendations
Antacids with phosphorus	Phosphorus	Monitor serum phosphorus levels Use antacids which do not interfere with absorption of phosphorus
Aspirin	Vitamin C	Prescribe vitamin C
Colchicine	Potassium	Monitor serum potassium Add potassium supplements Use potassium-sparing diuretics Increase dietary potassium
Digoxin	Potassium Thiamine	Monitor potassium levels Prescribe vitamin B
Diuretic	Potassium	Monitor serum potassium Add potassium supplements Use potassium-sparing diuretics Increase dietary potassium
Hydralazine	Vitamin B_6	Monitor B_6 levels
Isoniazid	Vitamin B_6[80]	Prescribe vitamin B_6 with isoniazid
L-dopa	Potassium Vitamin B_6	Monitor serum potassium Avoid B_6 supplements
Mineral oil	Vitamins A, D, K	Prescribe multivitamins
Neomycin	Potassium	Monitor serum potassium Add potassium supplements Use potassium-sparing diuretics Increase dietary potassium
Oral hypoglycemics	Vitamin B_{12}	Monitor vitamin B_{12} levels
Phenobarbital	Folic acid	Monitor folic acid levels
Phenytoin	Vitamin D Calcium	Prescribe vitamin D Increase dietary calcium
Potassium chloride	Vitamin B_{12}	Monitor vitamin B_{12} levels
Prednisone	Calcium	Calcium diets may be beneficial
Warfarin	Vitamin K	Keep diet constant Provide list of foods which contain vitamin K

ments might modify the therapeutic effects of phenyton, but reduce its potential to cause osteomalacia. On the other hand, the significant effect of vitamin K in reducing the therapeutic efficacy of anticoagulants is well appreciated.

Tables VIII and IX are intended to increase the clinician's index of suspicion for potential interactions between drugs and diet. The tables are simplified and are not intended to be comprehensive, and do not provide details of the many mechanisms proposed for diet-drug effects or interactions. The references[56–58] provide comprehensive information on drugs and diet.

Table X.   Geriproofing the Kitchen

Potential problems	Preventive recommendation
Excessive reaching, bending, and standing on chairs or stepladders in the kitchen increases the risk of accidental falling.	Place all shelves at eye level, or put all commonly used foods at counter level. Place refrigeration on 18-inch platform or store all foods in the refrigerator at waist level.
Kitchen chairs without armrests, or seats that are either too high or low, increase the risk of accidental falling. Chairs without high backs allow the head to fall backward, increasing the risk for vertebral basilar ischemic attacks.	Provide kitchen chairs that have high backs and armrests. Seat height should be no higher or lower than 18 inches to allow the older person to easily get on and off the chair.
Sense of smell decreases as a result of age-related decrease in olfactory nerve endings that can lead to nondetection of kitchen fires and smoke or gas inhalation.	Provide smoke detectors in the kitchen. Use electric stoves (the danger with gas stoves comes when an unlighted gas stove can lead to gas intoxication). Provide a kitchen fire extinguisher. Keep baking soda available in the kitchen to put out fires.
The risk of accidental falling increases with wet or slippery kitchen floors.	Provide water-absorbing mats around sink. Use nonskid floor wax. Clean up spills immediately. Use shoes that are nonskid.
Dim lighting in the kitchen can lead to accidental injuries. Accidental injury is increased with kitchen appliances that do not clearly indicate the "On" or "Off" position.	Provide adequate illumination in the kitchen, especially around cooking and cutting areas. Provide that the "Off" position is clearly marked on all kitchen appliances, especially the stove. Red fingernail polish can be used to mark the "Off" position.
Accidental falling from chairs or ladders which are unsteady.	Use stepladders which are of sturdy quality. Caution against using kitchen chairs to stand on.
Accidental injury from kitchen equipment knives which are left about the counter top.	Provide that special equipment such as knives and other dangerous devices are kept in clearly marked storage spaces.
Accidental injury is increased with age-related decrease in mobility and strength.	Wear garments of nonflammable material. Avoid clothing with long sleeves that can get caught on appliances. Avoid plastic aprons. Use pot holder mittens which cover the forearms.

8.8. The Kitchen: A Geriatric Health Hazard

The home environment in which the elderly prepares food, namely the kitchen, should be of concern to the health professional. More accidents occur in the home than anywhere else. In addition to the bedroom and bathroom, the kitchen is a high-risk area for accidental injury. Since environmental factors play a significant role in the nutritional management of an older person, knowledge of the possible etiologies for kitchen accidents and their prevention is important. Major problems that may lead to accidental injury in the kitchen and suggested preventive recommendation are presented in Table X. Insights of this nature allow for preventive geriatrics.

Table XI. Nutritional Research Imperatives

Establish the prevalence of nutritional deficiencies in old age.
Determine the appropriateness of extrapolation from young to old subjects of the parameters that measure nutritional deficiency.
Delineation of normal old age from diseased states.
Delineation of clinical data which define malnutritive states in old age.
Establishment of parameters which determine the adequate treatment of malnutritive states.
Determine the influences of nutrition on the normally occurring changes which accompany advancing age.
Determine the specific parameters of absorption, distribution, metabolism, and excretion of nutrients with age.
Establishment of specific RDAs for the elderly which provide reference norms for the age groups 65–74, 75–84, and 85+.
Extension of epidemiological data and clinical correlates of age, dietary intake, nutritional status, and health.
Determination of the influences of specific diseases and drug therapies on nutritional status, for example, the effect of anticonvulsants on bone, of chronic cardiac failure, and of dental disease on nutritional status.
Determination of the associations of nutrition with specific diseases such as vitamin K and calcium on osteoporosis.
Establish the effects of dietary manipulation on organ function such as water and fiber on intestinal mobility and absorption of zinc on taste or wound healing.
Determine the influence of food coloring or flavor enhancement on levels of intake.[84]
Determine the functional outcomes resulting from nutrient additives in the diets of older persons.
Establish the influence of dietary manipulation on the aging immune system.
Determine the influence of practical and tolerable dietary restrictions on longevity.
Determine whether the nutritional approach to disease prevention influences general nutritional status.
Determine the influence of environment (i.e., social systems, safety, mass media, and transportation) on nutrition.[85]
Delineate the nutritional differences between free living and institutionalized elderly groups.

8.9. Final Summary and Nutritional Research Imperative for the Elderly

Future updates on nutrition in contemporary geriatrics will focus on developments in nutritional research applicable or specific to the elderly. These, and the topics discussed in this chapter, are summarized in Table XI, which lists current areas of concern and interest. In addition, updates will detail the relationship of disease in old age to nutrition and the nutritional approaches to the management of the disabilities and diseases associated with advanced age.

References

1. Nsu, J. M. and Davis, R. L. (eds.), 1981, *Handbook of Geriatric Nutrition,* Moyes Publications, New Jersey.
2. Natow, A. B. and Heslin, J., 1980, *Geriatric Nutrition,* CBI Publishing Company, Inc., Boston.
3. Albanese, A. A., 1980, *Nutrition for the Elderly,* Alan R. Liss, Inc., New York.
4. Posner, B. M., 1979, *Nutrition and the Elderly,* Lexington Books, Lexington.
5. Web, R. B., 1978, *Nutrition and the Later Years,* The Ethel Percy Andrus Gerontology Center, University of Southern California Press, California.
6. Winick, M. (ed.), 1976, *Nutrition and Aging,* John Wiley and Sons, New York.
7. Rockstein, M. and Sussman, M. L. (eds.), 1976, *Nutrition, Longevity and Aging,* Academic Press, New York.
8. Greenblatt, D. J., 1979, Reduced serum albumin concentration in the elderly: A report from the Boston collaborative drug surveillance programme, *J. Am. Geriatr. Soc.* 27:20-23.
9. Tzanoff, S. P. and Norris, A. H., 1977, Effect of muscle mass decrease on age related BMR changes, *J. Appl. Physiol.* 43:1001-1006.
10. Tzankoff, S. P. and Norris, A. H., 1978, Longitudinal changes in basal metabolism in man, *J. Appl. Physiol.* 45:536-539.
11. Forbes, G. B. and Reina J. C., 1980, Adult lean body mass declines with age: Some longitudinal observations, *Metabolism* 19:653-663.
12. McGandy, R. B., Barrows, C. H., Spanias, A., Meridith, A., Stone, J. L., and Norris, A. H., 1966, Nutrient intakes and energy expenditure in men of different ages, *J. Gerontol.* 21:581-587.
13. Kahn, R. L., Goldfarb, A. I., Pollack, M., and Peck, A., 1960, Brief objective measures for the determination of mental status in the aged, *Am. J. Psychiatry* 117:326-328.
14. Libow, L. S., 1977, Senile dementia and pseudosenility: Clinical diagnosis, in: *Cognitive and Emotional Disturbance in the Elderly* (C. Eisdorfer and R. O. Friedel, eds.), Yearbook Medical Publishers, Inc., Chicago.
15. Sherwood, S., 1973, Sociology of food and eating: Implications for action for the elderly, *Am. J. Clin. Nutr.* 26:1108-1110.

16. Busse, E. W., 1978, Eating in late life: Physiologic and psychologic factors, *N.Y. State J. Med.* 80:1496–1497.
17. Busse, E. W., 1978, How mind, body and environment influence nutrition in the elderly, *Postgrad. Med.* 63:118–122; 125.
18. Moore, H. B., 1957, The meaning of food, *Am. J. Clin. Nutr.* 5:77–82.
19. Krehl, W. A., 1974, The influence of nutritional environment on aging, *Geriatrics* 29:65–76.
20. Lyons, J. S. and Tralson, M. F., 1956, Food practices of older people living at home, *J. Gerontol.* 11:66–72.
21. Sherwood, S., 1970, Gerontology and the sociology of food and eating, *Aging Human Develop.* 1:61–165.
22. Adams, K., 1975, Nutritive value of American foods, *Agriculture Handbook No. 456,* Washington, D.C.
23. Southgate, D. A. T. and Durnin, J. V. G. A., 1970, Caloric conversion factors: An experimental reassessment of the factors used in the calculation of the energy value of human diets, *Br. J. Nutr.* 24:517–535.
24. Exton-Smith, A. N., 1968, The problem of subclinical malnutrition in the elderly, in: *Vitamins in the Elderly* (A. N. Exton-Smith and D. L. Scott, eds.), Wright and Sons, Ltd., Briston, pp. 12–18.
25. Gambert, S. R. and Guansing, A. R., 1980, Protein-calorie malnutrition in the elderly, *J. Am. Geriatr. Soc.* 28:272–275.
26. Vir, S. C. and Love, A. H. G., 1980, Anthropometric measurements in the elderly, *Gerontology* 26:1–8.
27. Master, A. M., Lasser, R. B., and Beckman, G., 1959, Analysis of weight and height of apparently healthy populations, ages 65 to 94 years, *Proc. Soc. Exp. Biol. Med.* 102:367–370.
28. Andres, R., 1981, Influence of obesity on longevity in the aged, in: *Aging: A Challenge to Science and Society,* Volume 1-Biology (D. Danson, N. W. Shock, and M. Marois, eds.), Oxford University Press, New York, pp. 196–203.
29. Dyer, A. R., Stamler, J., Berkson, D. M., and Lindberg, H. A., 1975, Relationship of relative weight and body mass index to 14-year mortality in the Chicago People Gas Co. Study, *J. Chronic Dis.* 28:109–123.
30. Master, A. M., Lasser, R. P., and Beckman, G., 1960, Tables of average weight and height of Americans aged 65–94 years, *JAMA,* 172:658–662.
31. Food and Nutrition Board, Committee on Dietary Allowances, H. N. Munro, Chairman, 1980, *Recommended Dietary Allowances,* Ninth Revised Edition. National Research Council, National Academy of Sciences, Washington, D.C.
32. Food and Nutrient Intakes of Individuals in One Day in the United States, Spring 1977, *Nationwide Food Consumption Survey 1977–1978,* Sept. 1980, Preliminary Report No. 2, U.S. Department of Agriculture, Science and Education Administration, Washington, D.C.
33. Household Food Consumption Survey, 1965–66, November 11, 1972, *Food and Nutrient Intake of Individuals in the United States–Spring 1965,* U.S. Dept. of Agriculture, Agriculture Research Service Report, Washington, D.C.
34. Consumer and Food Economics Research Division, Agricultural Research Service: Food and nutrient intake of individuals in the United States, Spring 1965, *USDA*

Household Food Consumption Survey, 1965–66, Dept. No. 11, 1972, U.S. Government Printing Office, Washington, D.C.

35. Anthropometric and clinical findings, preliminary findings of the first Health and Nutrition Examination Survey (HANES) U.S. 1971–1972. DHEW Publication No. (HRA) 75-1229, 1975, U.S. Government Printing Office, Washington, D.C.

36. Department of Health, Education and Welfare, Health Service and Mental Health Administration, Center for Disease Control. *Ten States Nutrition Survey, 1968–70,* 1972, DHEW Publication No. (HSM) 72-8130-34, Atlanta.

37. U.S. Department of Agriculture, 1972, *Household Food Consumption Survey, 1965–66.* Report No. 17, U.S. Government Office, Washington, D.C.

38. Department of Health and Social Security, 1972, A nutrition survey of the elderly. Reported by the panel on nutrition of the elderly, *Reports on Health and Social Subjects* No. 3, Her Majesty's Stationary Office, London, pp. 28–29.

39. O'Hanlon, P. and Kohrs, M. B., 1978, Dietary studies of older Americans, *Am. J. Clin. Nutr.* 31:1257–1269.

40. Beauchene, R. E. and Davis, T. A., 1979, The nutritional status of the aged in the U.S.A., *Age* 2:23–28.

41. Brown, P. T., Bergan, J. G., Parsons, E. P., and Krol, L., 1977, Dietary status of elderly people, *J. Am. Diet. Assoc.* 71:41–45.

42. Department of Health and Social Security, 1972, A nutrition survey of the elderly. Reported by the panel on nutrition of the elderly. *Reports on Health and Social Subjects* No. 3, Her Majesty's Stationery Office, London.

43. Grotkowski, M. L. and Sims, L. S., 1978, Nutritional knowledge, attitudes, and dietary practices of the elderly, *J. Am. Diet. Assoc.* 72:499–506.

44. Yearick, E. S., Wang, M. S. L., and Pisias, S. J., 1980, Nutritional status of the elderly: Dietary and biochemical findings, *J. Gerontol.* 35(5):663–671.

45. Glenn, N. D., 1981, Age, birth, cohorts, and drinking: An illustration of the hazards of inferring effects from cohort data, *J. Gerontol.* 36(3):362–369.

46. Toss, G., Almqvist, S., Larsson, L., and Zettergvist, H., 1980, Vitamin D deficiency in welfare institutions for the aged, *Acta Med. Scand.* 208:87–89.

47. Slesinger, D. P., McDivitt, M., and O'Donnell, F. M., 1980, Food patterns in an urban population: Age and sociodemographic correlates, *J. Gerontol.* 35(3):432–441.

48. Baker, H., Frank, O., Thind, I. S., Jaslow, S. P., and Louria, D. B., 1979, Vitamin profiles in elderly persons living at home or in nursing homes, versus profile in healthy young subjects, *J. Am. Geriatr. Soc.* 27(10):444–450.

49. Vir, S. C. and Love, A. H. G., 1979, Nutritional status of institutionalized and non-institutionalized aged in Belfast, Northern Ireland, *Am. J. Clin. Nutr.* 32(9):1934–1947.

50. Pathy, M. S. and Newcombe, R. G., 1980, Temporal variation of serum levels of vitamin B12, folate, iron and total iron-binding capacity, *Gerontology* 26(1):34–42.

51. Roth, G. S., 1975, Age related changes in glucocorticoid binding by rat splenic leukocytes: Possible cause of altered adaptive responsiveness, *Fed. Proc.* 34:183–185.

52. Sugarman, B. and Munro, H. N., 1980, Altered accumulations of zinc by aging human fibroblasts in culture, *Life Sci.* 26:915–920.

53. Nutrition for the elderly, 1979, *Nutr. Health* 1.

54. Todhunter, E. N. and Darby, W. J., 1978, Guidelines for maintaining adequate nutrition in old age, *Geriatrics* 33(6):49–56.

55. Select Committee on Nutrition and Human Needs, United States Senate, 1977, *Dietary Goals for the United States,* 2nd. ed., U.S. Government Printing Office, Washington, D.C.

56. Roe, D. A., 1971, Drug induced deficiency of B vitamins, *N.Y. State J. Med.* 71: 2770–2777.

57. Roe, D. A., 1976, *Drug-Induced Nutritional Deficiencies,* AVI Publishing, Westport, CT.

58. Weg, R. B., 1973, Drug interaction with the changing physiology of the aged: Practice and potential, in: *Drugs and the Elderly* (R. David, ed.), Andrus Gerontology Center, Los Angeles, pp. 71–91.

59. Shock, N. W., 1981, Indices of functional age, in: *Aging: A Challenge to Science and Society,* Volume 1 (D. Dansen, N. W. Shock, and M. Marois, eds.), Oxford University Press, New York, pp. 270–286.

60. Towbin, J. D., 1981, Physiological indices of aging, in: *Aging: A Challenge to Science and Society,* Volume 1 (D. Dansen, N. W. Shock, and M. Marois, eds.), Oxford University Press, New York, pp. 286–295.

61. Uauy, R., Winterer, J. C., Bilmazes, C., Haverberg, L. N., Scrimshaw, N. S., Munro, H. N., and Young, V. R., 1978, The changing pattern of whole body protein metabolism in ageing humans, *J. Gerontol.* 33:663–671.

62. Masoro, E. J. (ed.), 1981, *CRC Handbook of Physiology in Aging,* CRS Press, Inc., Florida.

63. Finch, C. E. and Hayflick, L., (eds.), 1977, *Handbook of the Biology of Aging,* Van Nostrand-Reinhold Co., New York.

64. Libow, L. S., 1974, Interaction of medical, biologic and behavioral factors on aging adaptation and survival. An 11-year longitudinal study, *Geriatrics* 29:75–88.

65. Bernard, A., 1977, Sociological factors in nutrition for the elderly, in: *The Later Years* (R. Kalish, ed.), Brooks/Cole, Monterey.

66. Birren, J. E., Bick, M. W., and Fox, C., 1948, Age changes in the light threshold of the dark-adapted eye, *J. Gerontol.* 3:267–271.

67. Gaitz, C. and Warshaw, H., 1964, Obstacles encountered in correcting hearing loss in the elderly, *Geriatrics* 19:83–86.

68. Rupp, R., 1970, Understanding the problems of presbycucis, *Geriatrics* 25:100–110.

69. Schiffman, S., 1977, Food recognition by the elderly, *J. Gerontol.* 32:586–592.

70. Cohen, T. and Gitman, L., 1959, Oral complaints and taste perception in the aged, *J. Gerontol.* 14:294–298.

71. Grzegorczyk, P. B., Jones, S. W., and Mistretta, C. M., 1979, Age related differences in salt-taste acuity, *J. Gerontol.* 34:834–846.

72. Guth, P. H., 1968, Physiologic alteration in small bowel function with age: The absorption of D-xylose. *Am. J. Digest. Dis.* 13:565–571.

73. Webster, S. G. P. and Leeming, J. T., 1975, Assessment of small bowel function in the elderly using a modified xylose tolerance test, *Gut* 16:109–113.

74. Strode, J. E., 1968, The large intestine as a geriatric problem, *Geriatrics* 23(7):102–112.

75. Eastwood, M. A., 1975, The role of vegetable dietary fibre in human nutrition, *Med. Hyp.* 1:46–53.

76. Weinberg, J., 1972, Psychologic implications of the nutritional needs of the elderly, *J. Am. Diet. Assoc.* 60:293–296.

77. Blumenthal, M. D., 1980, Depressive illness in old age: Getting behind the mask, *Geriatrics* 35:34–48.
78. Williams, L. M., 1978, A concept of loneliness in the elderly, *J. Am. Geriatr. Soc.* 26:183–187.
79. Kruse, H. D., Sydenstricker, V. P., Sebrell, W. H., and Cleekley, H. M., 1940, Ocular manifestations of ariboflavinosis, *Public Health Rep.* 55:157–169.
80. Biehl, J. P. and Wilter, R. W., 1954, Effect of isoniazid on vitamin B6 metabolism: Its possible significance in producing isoniazid neuritis, *Proc. Soc. Exp. Biol. Med.* 85:389–392.
81. Barrows, C. H. and Kokkonen, G. C., 1977, Relationship between nutrition and aging, in: *Advances in Nutritional Research,* Volume 1 (H. Draper ed.), Plenum Press, New York, pp. 253–298.
82. Watkin, D. M., 1978, Logical bases for action in nutrition and aging, *J. Am. Geriatr. Soc.* 26:193–202.
83. National Institute on Aging, 1979, *Nutrition and Aging,* U.S. GPO, Washington, D.C.
84. White, P. and Mondeika, T. D., 1980, Foods fads and faddism, in: *Modern Nutrition in Health and Disease* (R. S. Goodhart and M. E. Shills, eds.), 6th ed., Lea and Febiger, Philadelphia, pp. 456–462.
85. Clancy, K. L., 1975, Preliminary observations on media use and food habits of elderly, *Gerontologist* 15:529–532.
86. Administration on Aging, U.S. Department of Health, Education and Welfare, 1980, *Longitudinal Evaluation of the National Nutrition Program for the Elderly. Report of First-Wave Findings by Kirschner Associates, Inc. and Opinion Research Corporation,* DHEW Publication No. (OHDS) 80-20249. U.S. Government Printing Office, Washington, D.C.
87. Watkin, D. M., 1977, Aging, nutrition and the continuum of health care. *Ann. N.Y. Acad. Sci.* 300:200–297.
88. Watkin, D. M., 1979, Nutrition, health and aging, in: *Nutrition and the World Food Problem* (M. Recheigl, Jr., ed.), S. Karger, Basel, pp. 20–62.
89. U.S. Department of Agriculture and U.S. Department of Health, Education and Welfare, 1980, *Nutrition and Your Health: Dietary Guidelines for Americans,* U.S. Government Printing Office, Washington, D.C.

Preventive Medicine for the Elderly

Ronald D. Adelman, Michele G. Greene, and Michael M. Stewart

9.1. Introduction

This chapter will explore the importance of prevention as a health care issue for the elderly. This subject has a special impact because of the increasing number of elderly who are living much longer today. In the past, diseases that occurred in the aged were often considered to be natural consequences of the aging process and so prevention was infrequently considered. In fact, disease prevention and an understanding of the impact of diet, exercise, drug use, and environment for people of all ages has received more emphasis only in recent years.

Since we are committed to increasing life span, efforts should be made to ensure a high quality of life for as long as one lives. Differential diagnosis, which can discern what ailments are a function of aging and what are really disease processes, is crucial for maintaining wellness.

There are now many useful preventive interventions for older adults. Primary preventive tactics for the elderly refer to those measures that may avert the

RONALD D. ADELMAN and MICHELE G. GREENE • Division of General Medicine, Department of Medicine, College of Physicians and Surgeons, Columbia University, New York, New York 10032.   MICHAEL M. STEWART • Division of General Medicine, Department of Medicine, College of Physicians and Surgeons, Columbia University, New York, New York 10032; and The Rockefeller Foundation, New York, New York 10036.

occurrence of disease. Health promotion, rather than disease prevention, is the focus. For example, it is clear that carefully prescribed exercise programs can promote improved physiologic function. Similarly, minimizing adverse drug reactions through understanding of normal pharmacokinetic changes in the aged can be a useful primary preventive measure. Also, a physician's awareness of the potential for alcoholism in the aged can result in increased early detection and prevention. Secondary prevention involves the detection and early treatment of disease. It is important for the physician to be aware of screening procedures that are beneficial for all elderly patients as well as those case-finding strategies that are relevant to individuals at high risk. Perhaps tertiary preventive intervention is the most important consideration in preventive medicine for the geriatric patient. Tertiary preventive strategies are concerned with limiting further complications of disease, restricting disabilities, and delaying death. Because so many older adults have chronic illness, physicians should direct their energy into preserving as much remaining function as possible.

The health provider–patient relationship plays a major role in disease prevention especially for the increasingly dependent and isolated aging patient. A good relationship can have a great impact on patient compliance, satisfaction, and health status.[1] Therefore, primary care practitioners should be aware of their attitudes regarding their elderly patients. The manner in which the health provider copes with his/her own mortality—fearfully, avoidantly, realistically—may account for the manner in which the aging patient is treated.

9.2. Primary Prevention

9.2.1. Anticipatory Guidance for the Elderly Patient

Although the concept of anticipatory guidance was originally developed as an approach for understanding developmental changes in the pediatric age group, it may have merit in a geriatric practice as well.

Anticipatory guidance involves preparation of elderly individuals and their families for the common physiologic, psychologic, and social changes that usually accompany the aging process. When patients and their families understand and are prepared for the changes that are probable and possible as a patient ages, they may be better able to cope with those changes and then be prepared to identify aberrations from the norm. The health provider can assist patients and their families in anticipating major life events and their sequelae, in recognizing the early signs and symptoms of disease, and in identifying when professional help may be necessary. The time spent educating the geriatric patient and his/her family early on will, in the long run, save the practitioner time. Although knowledge about the normal aging process is not as yet well defined, whatever information primary care physicians can share with patients and their families will be of assistance.

9.2.2. Nutrition in the Elderly

Nutritional assessment is an important and often overlooked aspect of health promotion. The value of appropriate nutritional practice clearly has an immense impact on health maintenance for all age groups, including the elderly (see Chapter 8).

At this point in time, the dietary requirements for people over 65 have not been explicitly established. Present recommendations are extrapolated from the dietary requirements mandated for younger individuals. There is a clear need for further research concerning the specific dietary requirements of elderly individuals.

Nutritional evaluation, promotion, and education is important for the geriatric patient who is particularly vulnerable to inadequate nutrition for a variety of economic, physiologic, social, and psychologic factors.[2]

Economic factors play a major role in determining a patient's overall nutritional status. The majority of the elderly are on fixed incomes, and approximately one-quarter of our nation's older adults live at or below the poverty level.[3] Somers points out that the average income for the elderly decreases as they age.[4] The cost of foods high in protein, such as meat and fish, may inhibit elderly persons from purchasing these items. Instead the elderly may select the cheaper, more filling, or more easily prepared foods which are usually high in carbohydrates and which may contribute to an unbalanced diet. Limited mobility and reduced exercise tolerance in the elderly may prevent comparative food shopping which earlier in life may have enabled purchasing food at the most competitive prices. The disabled elderly patient often shops out of necessity at local, high-cost markets. Physical limitation may also necessitate "interval shopping," whereby a homebound patient is entirely dependent on a relative or friend to assist with shopping. Often assistance is available only once monthly, leading to a diet deficient in fresh fruits and vegetables. In addition, economic factors such as limited cooking facilities (e.g., a furnished room only equipped with a hot plate) often determine dietary practice.

Physiologic factors, such as decreased senses of smell and taste, may significantly decrease interest in food.[5] Diminished salivary function may make swallowing more difficult. Decreased physical exercise may also play a role in decreased appetite stimulation. Physical immobility and poor vision may influence the patient's ability to prepare food. Edentulous patients and those with ill-fitting dentures may have mechanical difficulties with food consumption leading indirectly to specific deficiency states.

The primary care physician should be aware that certain drugs may lead to nutritional deficiencies as well as potential pharmacologic interactions with adverse effects. Although anorexia may be the heralding symptom of a variety of disorders, an anorexic patient being treated with drugs such as digitalis should be evaluated for possible drug-related toxicity. Potassium intake must be closely monitored when patients are taking digitalis in conjunction with diuretics or L-dopa since a hypokalemic environment further increases the likelihood of digitalis toxicity.[6] Anorexia due to drug toxicity must also be considered in the depressed, hypertensive patient being treated with reserpine. Isoniazid, L-dopa, and hydralazine, all commonly used medications, can lead to vitamin B_6 deficiency.[7] In addition to causing hypokalemia, chronic use of diuretics may also induce a magnesium deficiency. Antacids containing aluminum inhibit the gastrointestinal absorption of fluoride and phosphorus and promote calcium excretion.[7] Laxative abuse is an important cause of diarrhea in the geriatric population potentially leading to weight loss and fluid and electrolyte disturbances. In addition, many laxatives contain mineral oil that, when used chronically, can deplete patients of the fat-soluble vitamins A, D, E, and K.[8] Patients on long-term anticonvulsant therapy with phenobarbital or Dilantin® may become depleted of vitamin D and folate.[7]

Deficiency in calcium, either through inadequate dietary intake or due to decreased absorption, may additionally predispose the elderly person to the development of osteoporosis. Other factors that appear to be significant in the development of metabolic bone disease include one's level of physical activity, postmenopausal status, diminished estrogen levels, and a decreased intake or absorption of vitamin D (see Chapter 6).

A deficiency of iron is common in the elderly. This most likely results from either poor dietary intake, blood loss, or decreased parietal cell function leading to improper conversion of dietary iron, ferric, to absorbable iron, ferrous. Diets deficient in meat, vegetables, and eggs lack proper iron.

Constipation is a major problem requiring a nutritional evaluation and assessment. Constipation may result when a diet lacks sufficient bulk and inadequate fluid intake to stimulate peristaltic activity. Dietary fiber supplements can often relieve the problem. Bran is a readily available and cheap source of crude fiber. It is important to note, however, that commercially purchased bran is processed with sugar. Increased dietary fiber content may be obtained from fruits and vegetables. High-fiber diets may also be useful in diverticulosis as well as diabetes, since fiber appears to promote a more gradual absorption of carbohydrate.

Obesity has been associated with the development of diabetes, arthritis, gout, hypertension, coronary heart disease, and decreased rehabilitation potential. A decreased metabolic rate coupled with a decreased activity level place some elderly at risk for weight gain, especially if dietary intake is not proportionately decreased. With obesity there is often a pattern of decreased mobility, placing the already obese elder at further risk for weight gain and subsequent loss of independent function. Whenever dietary changes are indicated, it is usually best to advise gradual changes, since the elderly may have fixed dietary practices and may be resistant to major changes. Reducing caloric intake with or without increased caloric expenditure by exercise is the only way to lose weight; no instant method is available. Ultimately, the patient's motivation to lose weight is crucial for success.

Although psychological factors have a great impact on the eating pattern of all age groups, some factors are perhaps more specific and pronounced in the elderly. Loneliness is a common complaint of many elderly; often the impetus to cook and prepare food is lost when a patient lives alone, after years of cooking for, or eating with, family members or a partner. Depression with resultant anorexia may be commonly seen.[8] Homebound patients may benefit from the "Meals on Wheels" program and ambulatory elderly may find eating at their senior citizen center, within a social context, beneficial.

9.2.3. Exercise for the Elderly

It is important that the clinician appreciate the benefits of an exercise program designed for the elderly. The failure of many physicians to do so may stem from uncertainty as to the need for continued exercise in the geriatric age group and a concern about the risk involved in exercise at an older age. Health professionals also often underestimate the abilities of elderly patients, believing that their capacity for physical activity is intrinsically limited. Many of the misconceptions concerning the suitability of the exercise prescription in the elderly patient result from educational inadequacies. Doctors are often not taught a systematic approach to ordering such prescriptions. Although it is true that certain patients with specific medical problems, regardless of age, are ill-advised to participate in an exercise regimen, this high-risk group would be limited to patients with congestive heart failure, acute myocardial infarction, angina, recent embolism, severe aortic stenosis, and various other readily identified conditions.[2] For the most part, exercise for the elderly provides appreciable benefits including increased endurance, improved coordination, enhanced body image, and an improved sense of well-being.[2,9] Exercise regimens need to be individually tailored to each patient, in response to differing physiologic needs, tolerances, and individual activity preferences.

Clearly, physical conditioning helps to preserve independent functioning, the basic goal in preventive geriatric care. Physiologic data measured in conditioned elders document benefits to exercise, including significant increases in pulmonary vital capacity, oxygen uptake, and stroke volume.[10,11] Other important secondary effects resulting from exercise include further opportunities for socialization, improved psychological well-being, and weight control. Fewer sleep disturbances, less constipation, and perhaps decreased advancement of coronary artery disease have also been suggested as possible benefits from regular exercise. Improved coordination may decrease the incidence of falls in this age group.

Prior to initiating an exercise program, the elderly patient should have a thorough physical examination and complete review of systems. Although the American College of Sports Medicine recommends a stress test prior to beginning exercise, the test is quite expensive and many elderly patients may not be able to afford it.[2] To ascertain the safety of an elderly patient's participation in an exercise program, a resting electrocardiogram and observation of the patient's response to exercise is suggested especially when endurance training other than walking is considered.[11] Prior to initiating an exercise program, the physician should question the patient as to what activities are most appealing. The exercise should be prescribed to the individual's tastes. Sports or activities that promote isometric activities are not recommended for the elderly since this form of exercise will place an unwise amount of stress on the cardiovascular system. Isotonic exercise, whereby multiple muscle groups are engaged, is preferred. Probably most important is the need for careful graduation in intensity and duration of exercise, as monitored by heart rate.

Before prescribing an exercise program, the physician should consider several factors:

(1) In the beginning, the elderly patient may be discouraged by an increased amount of muscle and joint soreness. This is to be expected and the patient should probably start with a more gradual regimen and understand that a conditioned effect takes time, extended effort, patience, and committment.

(2) Patients should avoid eating substantial amounts of food for approximately 2 hr before and 1 hr after exercise.[12]

(3) Elderly patients often have less ability to adapt to temperature extremes. Elderly exercising in warm climates should be careful to guard against dehydration. Elderly exercising in cold climates should protect against hypothermia by wearing proper clothing (i.e., multiple layers of absorbent, preferably cotton, materials). The intensity of exercise should be decreased with climatic extremes.

(4) All exercise sessions should be preceded with a gradual warm-up period and terminated with a full cool-down period.

(5) Care should be taken not to take excessively hot showers or baths, since sometimes this can be deleterious to cardiac function.

(6) When ill, patients should refrain from exercising. Exercise may potentiate dehydration possibly already present due to elevated body temperature and increased sweating.[12]

(7) Patients should know when to stop exercising—unusual discomfort, shortness of breath, chest pain, or palpitations require immediate exercise termination and medical consultation.

(8) Often the elderly have impaired vision. Older adults who exercise should do so in well-lighted, flat-surfaced areas where the risk of falling is reduced. Elderly with impaired hearing should exercise in nontrafficked areas to minimize dangers resulting from the diminished hearing.

Physical activity can minimize the loss of physical function that may accompany aging as well as confer a protective effect on the heart. Most importantly, however, by maintaining good physical function, the goal of preserving independence is further advanced.

9.2.4. Smoking and the Elderly

Although some health practitioners condone smoking among their elderly patients, thinking it is one of their "few small pleasures," smoking does have a detrimental effect upon older individuals and hastens many of nature's otherwise normal aging processes. In addition, elderly patients, especially those with a long smoking history, are at increased risk for lung cancer and chronic obstructive pulmonary disease. Moreover, cigarette smoking in the elderly is associated with increased lower respiratory tract infections and peripheral vascular and cardiovascular disease. The reduction or complete elimination of smoking is likely to affect the severity, complications, and in some instances, the incidence of these conditions.[13] Therefore, primary care practitioners should routinely obtain a smoking history from their patients as part of a regular workup and advise them of the hazards of smoking.

9.2.5. Promoting the Safe Use of Drugs in the Elderly

To one degree or another, aging effects all pharmacokinetic parameters including absorption, distribution, metabolism, and excretion. Normal physiologic consequences of aging have profound influences on drug therapy in the elderly in terms of adequacy of treatment and potential for toxicity.

Drug absorption in the elderly may be altered due to several factors. The secretion of hydrochloric acid by the stomach's parietal cells diminishes with age, influencing the rate of absorption of many drugs due to altered solubility characteristics.[14,15] There is a reduction in splanchnic blood flow, a decrease in gastrointestinal peristaltic activity, and a reduction in surface area for absorption, all contributing to a changed absorptive capacity with age.[14]

Several important physiologic alterations occur with age which affect the distribution of drugs. The composition of the body changes with age; the percentage of lean body mass is significantly reduced; there may be a marked decrease in the percentage of body water; and there is a proportionately increased percentage of body fat as compared to total body weight.[16,17] Increased adipose tissue may produce an increased reservoir of lipid soluble drugs allowing for an increased duration of action and potential for toxicity.[17] Also the amount of plasma albumin may be decreased, a factor which has great influence on how much and how long the drug will be active for those drugs that are highly protein bound. In addition to a decrease in albumin, there may also be a change in protein-binding ability.[17]

Most drugs are metabolized in the liver. With age, the process by which drugs are converted into forms that allow for excretion may be affected by a decrease in liver mass, hepatic flow, and possibly diminished hepatic enzyme activity.[17]

Excretory changes with age can be partially explained by the decrease in renal mass, the end result of a gradual loss of nephrons through the course of a lifetime. Both cardiac output and renal blood flow attenuate with age such that renal plasma flow decreases by 50% from age 20 to 90. Tubular mass and glomerular filtration rate also decline with age.[14] Age-related decline in renal reserve make the elderly more vulnerable to further impairments of renal function precipitated by conditions such as dehydration and congestive heart failure. It is important for the practitioner caring for the elderly to remember that due to reduced muscle mass and creatinine formation, creatinine may be in the normal range despite a significantly reduced creatinine clearance. Therefore, to adequately assess renal function, a creatinine clearance is a necessity. Additional research is needed to further delineate how aging alters drug usage.

In addition to the physiologic factors described above, many social factors place elderly patients at high risk for adverse drug reactions. Elderly patients are particularly vulnerable because of the large quantities of prescription and nonprescription drugs they consume. Although comprising about 11% of the nation's population, the elderly use about 25% of prescribed drugs.[16] With the multiple chronic and often serious diseases that may accompany old age, the elderly may take many different drugs. The necessity to take many different drugs at different times of the day and at different dosages may often lead to patient noncompliance with resultant ineffective or adverse drug reactions.

Other factors, which might be called environmental, also contribute to the problems patients may have in following a drug regimen. Bad weather, housing barriers (such as multiple flights of stairs to an apartment), and fear of crime may prevent elderly patients from getting to the pharmacy to purchase their needed medication. The child-resistant medication caps may also make it difficult for patients with painful arthritis to comply.

Concurrent health problems may also limit an elderly individual's ability to comply with a prescribed regimen. For instance, poor vision, hearing, or memory may prevent the patient from completely understanding the physician's often long and complicated instructions.

Finally, the excessive costs of drugs may be a major problem for the elderly patient. Medicare and many other insurance plans do not pay for medications, and patients on fixed or negligible incomes may not be able to afford their prescribed or over-the-counter drugs.

There are steps, however, that the primary care physician may take to help elderly patients help themselves. The relatively simple interventions recommended below should assist in preventing those adverse drug reactions that are caused by some of the previously described social factors:

(1) Patients should be given *written* instructions which simply and graphi-

cally describe the drug regimen. Drug companies, nurses, patient educators, and other health care groups concerned with the drug compliance of the elderly patient have developed a variety of innovative techniques, including day-by-day drug dispensers, to simplify the medication-taking process.

(2) Written instructions should avoid generalities such as "take as needed" or "as directed." Additionally, specific directions about the time of day, dosage, and the relationship to food, over-the-counter drugs, alcohol, and smoking should be explicit. Common side effects of the medications should be explained.

(3) Instructions should take individual patient problems into account. For instance, if a patient has poor vision, large print should be employed.

(4) The prescribing physician should review the instructions with the patient verbally. Patients should be asked to repeat the physician's directions.

(5) At the initial office visit and regularly thereafter, the physician should take a drug history. Special attention should be given to the social and economic barriers that may influence patient compliance. Most geriatricians find it useful to request that patients bring in all their prescriptions and over-the-counter drugs at the time of visit.

Although each of the suggested interventions takes time, it is time well spent. Ultimately, these recommendations may prevent adverse drug reactions. The primary care practitioner, as patient educator, can play a vital role in the prevention of adverse drug reactions and the assurance of patient compliance.

9.2.6. Mental Health of the Elderly

The life cycle approach, advocated by Butler and Lewis,[18] provides a sensible conceptual framework for understanding the mental status of the elderly. The social relationships and experiences of individuals throughout their lives influence attitudes and adjustment in the later stages of life. Aging, when considered within this framework, should be a time of continued emotional growth and development and should not be viewed as a period of decline. The mental health of the elderly may be affected by a wide variety of physical, psychological, and social factors, many of which may be beneficially altered through appropriate primary, secondary, and tertiary preventive interventions.

The elderly individual is often confronted by many new life situations. The loss of a spouse with resulting social isolation may leave an elderly individual overwhelmed by depression. Living alone, perhaps for the first time, can be a frightening experience for many elderly. Grieving over the loss of a loved one and the realization of one's own mortality often requires new coping and adaptation skills on the part of the elderly individual. Those who live alone and are recently bereaved are at high risk not only for depression, but also for suicide.

Retirement, loss of a regular income, and greatly increased leisure time may also prove to be life crises for the elderly. The elderly individual is often confused about the meaning of his/her daily existence, fearful about the management of routine expenses, and bewildered by the lack of regular activities.

The depression that often accompanies these new and stressful life changes must be given serious consideration by both the individual's family and health care provider. The suicide rate among individuals 65 and over is considerably higher than it is for younger age groups (23/100,000 vs. 12/100,000 population).[19] This is especially true for elderly men, who have a greatly increased risk of suicide. Additionally, the elderly rarely fail at suicide, i.e., the proportion of successful to unsuccessful suicide attempts is greater for the elderly. Kopell suggests that "suicide attempts among elderly are more likely to be motivated by the genuine desire to die than by a desire for sympathy and attention, and therefore suicide constitutes a significant hazard."[19]

The stresses and major life changes that accompany old age often lead to alcoholism among the elderly (see 9.2.7).

There are many primary and secondary preventive measures that can be employed to help the elderly cope with these life crises. Education and preparation are good primary preventive strategies. For instance, preparation for retirement and education about budgeting and the financial assistance available to the elderly (i.e., SSI and Medicare) may help the individual cope and adjust at this most difficult time. Patients may also be helped by being directed to appropriate social supports and services in the community. Additionally, because the elderly may be isolated and withdrawn, outreach services may be particularly helpful.[18,20] Services which provide health, social service, housing and other information and referral can help the elderly to lead an independent existence. Family members should be alerted to the particular needs of the elderly at this time.

Secondary prevention involves evaluation and treatment activities. Complete psychological and sociocultural assessments should include a review of the personal and family history, mental status, social supports, financial status, work experience, and housing and transportation needs. Screening for depression, alcoholism, drug use, and abuse by family members is also indicated. Early recognition and treatment of these conditions are of great benefit to the elderly. Screening activities should also focus on ruling out organic brain syndrome, particularly due to "reversible" causes.[18] The practitioner should be aware that physical disease or particularly stressful life crises may precipitate an acute confusional state. Butler and Lewis warn: "One consequence of failure to identify the syndrome is that older people are often considered chronic patients and are sent to long-term institutional care facilities or nursing homes when active hospital care and return to the community would be the appropriate course of treatment."[18]

The difficulties in distinguishing treatable functional disorders from organic disorders are also well-known. There are many new diagnostic evaluation tools being developed that can help the clinician with this most difficult assessment. The early diagnosis and treatment of depression among the elderly can reduce further complications. Geropsychiatrists are good resources for helping to manage clinically depressed patients.

Gaitz and Varner provide a realistic perspective for the practitioner who deals with the mental health of the elderly. They argue that the focus must be on "altering, modifying and delaying, rather than curing, totally reversing, or completely preventing." Moreover, even with the best possible quality of medical and health care "some patients may improve only minimally and some patients will deteriorate. If one has reason to believe that deterioration is the natural history of a process—and this is the fate of many conditions associated with aging—therapists may take some satisfaction with efforts, primary and secondary, that delay decline."[21]

Finally, tertiary preventive tactics in managing the mental health of the elderly include appropriate rehabilitation services and counseling. It is estimated that presently 1.1 million persons in the United States have some form of dementia.[22] Services for patients and their families are now available to help with the difficult tasks of coping and adjusting to chronic irreversible changes in cognitive function. Support groups, such as the Alzheimer's Disease and Related Disorders Association provide practical advice, education, information, and referrals for both patients and their families.

9.2.7. Alcoholism in the Elderly

The number of elderly who are alcoholics is generally underestimated due to difficulties inherent in its identification in this age group.[23] Underreporting occurs because many older adults live in isolation, are retired, and often do not readily admit to alcohol abuse. There are two types of alcoholics generally identified in the geriatric age group; those who have been habitual drinkers and have survived to old age, and those elderly with the onset of alcoholism in old age.[23] Elderly widowers are at particular risk for alcoholism—the incidence of alcoholism in this population is the highest for all age groups.[18]

Alcohol abuse implies an impairment of an individual's health and ability to function in society. Loss of judgment, disorientation, the tendency to have more accidents, and poor nutrition are associated with alcoholism and serve to aggravate symptoms of age and chronic illness. One of the problems in the detection of alcoholism in the elderly is that symptoms of the disease can be mistaken for the ravages of age. It is therefore important to consider the possibility of alcohol abuse in the elderly person who may be malnourished and suffering from multiple falls, physical deterioration, and/or dementia.[23]

As habitual drinkers age, there is a tendency toward a decrease in alcohol consumption.[23] Social drinking also usually decreases with age due to financial limitations and changing social habits after retirement which may diminish opportunities for social drinking. The reasons for the onset of alcoholism in old age usually relate to loneliness, bereavement, depression, chronic disease, or loss of status after retirement.[24] Younger alcoholic individuals are often motivated to obtain treatment either from fear of job loss or family pressure.[25] However, often the elderly adult is retired, alone, and without external pressures to seek treatment. It is important to identify those elderly patients who may have alcohol-related problems or whose life situation may make them potentially vulnerable to alcohol abuse. Patients with confusion, weakness, sleep disturbances, gastritis, or those who have experienced loss of a close relative, in particular widowers, deserve special attention.[25] Detection of alcohol abuse can be difficult especially in this age group either because the health provider is too embarrassed to assess the patient's true alcohol status or is reluctant to designate a patient as alcoholic. Although this may result from a lack of training in evaluating alcohol abuse, more important it may result from the lack of awareness of the possibilities for therapeutic intervention.

Treatment of the elderly alcoholic can clearly be beneficial. Zimberg noted an excellent response in the nonhabitual elderly alcoholic to therapy consisting of antidepressant medication and socialization programs.[26] He also found that habitual elderly alcoholics readily responded to the same therapy as well, despite his prior belief that they would be resistant to treatment. A treatment approach which specifically focuses on the social and psychologic elements of aging may also be helpful.[24] Zimberg's results provide some optimism for positive treatment outcome in both groups of elderly alcoholics.

Alcoholics Anonymous can also be extremely useful for the older alcoholic, especially when a specific geriatric group is formed. The potential for beneficial treatment underlines the usefulness of case detection of alcohol abuse in the elderly patient.

9.2.8. Environmental Geriatrics

Environmental geriatrics refers to those environmental conditions that pose a particular hazard for older patients. Although individuals at all ages are susceptible or at risk for these conditions, elderly individuals are particularly vulnerable to hypothermia, hyperthermia, falls, and architectural barriers which prevent independent living. All of these conditions are amenable to preventive interventions.

Prolonged exposure to cold may induce hypothermia. Many elderly patients live on fixed incomes and thus reside in suboptimal housing, often with nonfunctioning boilers or insufficient heat. During winter months under these conditions, elderly individuals are particularly susceptible to hypothermia. The health provider can help the geriatric patient by making appropriate referrals to social service and community resources to assist the elderly in altering their living environment. A heightened awareness for the differential possibility of hypothermia may help diagnose this condition at an early stage. Signs and symptoms of hypothermia such as dysarthria, decreased coordination, and ataxia may be interpreted as changes consistent with aging. Shivering may or may not be present and is usually absent if body temperature falls below 32°C, at which time delirium and stupor may set in.[27] Certain drugs such as phenothiazines may interfere with temperature regulation; an elderly person's ability to detect changes in environmental temperature and respond accordingly may be altered, leading to hypothermia.

Heat stroke in the elderly can be anticipated and therefore prevented. Elderly patients as a group are more susceptible to environmental temperature extremes and in particular have a decreased capacity to deal with temperature elevations due to decreased thermoregulatory sensitivity and a diminished ability to sweat. Usually heat stroke occurs in summer months after a period of days when the ambient temperature is greater than 38°C. It is important for the practitioner to realize that a patient need not be overexposed; heat stroke can as easily occur in a patient never venturing outside his/her apartment. The practitioner should also be aware that the morbidity and mortality related to a succession of hot days may occur several days after the time of maximum temperature elevations.[28]

There is a particular subset in the elderly population who have been shown to have increased susceptibility to hyperthermia. The foremost factor which predisposes to heat stroke is cardiovascular disease.[29] In particular, patients with congestive heart failure and those patients on diuretic therapy have an increased susceptibility to hyperthermia. Anticholinergic medications pharmacologically inhibit sweating and place patients at increased risk for the development of heat stroke.[29] Geriatric patients who are bedridden or with dementia are also at increased risk due either to the lack of physical capacity or mental awareness to remove excess clothing. In addition, fluid consumption may not be appropriately increased. Elderly patients who are obese or alcoholic, or have an infection causing fever are all at higher risk for hyperthermia.

In one study during the 1980 heat wave in Memphis, it was concluded that poor, elderly, and black inner-city residents were disproportionately affected with increased morbidity and mortality associated with heat stroke.[28] The authors hypothesized that lack of air-conditioning and inadequate ventilation were responsible for the dramatically increased susceptibility and mortality of the elderly. The authors also noted that the inner-city elderly living in high-crime areas were particularly reluctant to open windows to promote adequate ventilation for fear of intrusion. Additionally, some of the elderly poor actually did have access to fans and air-conditioning, but did not use them because of concerns about expensive electric bills.

To assist in prevention of hyperthermia, elderly patients, their families, and homemakers should be made aware of the phenomenon. Patients who are at increased risk should be made especially aware of the possibility of hyperthermia and the setting in which it is likely to occur. Those patients with poorly ventilated apartments, especially those inhabiting apartments on higher floors, should be made aware of the need for special surveillance of body temperature and the need to promote cooling. Patients should decrease the amount and intensity of physical activity during extremely hot weather and increase their fluid consumption accordingly. Light clothing should be worn. Patients should also be instructed to use air-conditioners or fans, if available. Their utilization, especially during periods of prolonged temperature elevation, can be life-saving and therefore well worth the extra utility costs. Those who are able to mobilize themselves and do not have access to air-conditioning in the home should seek out air-conditioned environments for relief (e.g., senior citizens' centers). It is advisable to encourage sponging, bathing, or showering with cool water to lower body temperature, if necessary.

Much of an individual's life is spent at home and the environmental conditions found there can make a major difference in health status. Although home visits are usually not made by the primary care physician, home visits by a visiting nurse service or other health professionals for patients at risk (e.g., patients with a past history of home accidents, poor vision, decreased muscular control, postural instability, and osteoporosis) can be arranged. Assessment of the hazards in the physical environment can be made and the patient and the primary care physician advised accordingly. In the case of falls, the health provider's primary preventive task involves patient and family education. Patients should be warned to avoid throw rugs, loose mats, trailing wires, and waxed floors. Worn-out carpets and uneven floors or stairs are also hazards. All areas in the home, as well as the hallway, should be well lighted. Handrails on stairs and grabrails by the toilet and bathtub will assist the patient.

The secondary effects of many drugs may cause drowsiness or loss of concentration, and elderly patients must be warned about these possibilities.

One author has suggested on-the-floor alarm systems with a pull-cord to assist elderly patients once they have fallen.[30] Other similar innovations need to be developed. Once most of these hazards are removed from the environment and the patient is aware of some common pitfalls (e.g., walking in the dark, attempting ambulation on ice), there is also the possibility of prescribing some physical activity for the elderly; exercise, even if only walking, improves coordination and may help to prevent potential accidents.

Accidents in the aged may be the first manifestation of the onset of an underlying disease process. Secondary preventive tactics should, for example, focus on detection of alcoholism, neurological disease, and possible hypoglycemia. Moreover, the health provider should be prepared to manage the psychological ramifications of falling (including secondary fear and anxiety) which may further impede mobility and normal functioning.

The ability of the elderly to live and function independently can be severely hampered by architectural barriers at home. Innovative architectural planning is a part of environmental geriatrics. The health provider can assist in making plans for a living space which will facilitate the creation of safe, independent accommodations. Of special concern is the disabled elderly patient who lives in the community. For example, wider door spaces; ramps instead of stairs; more accessible work spaces, telephones, kitchen countertops, and appliances; and handbars by the bathtub and toilet will be a great help to the disabled elderly patient. Often, these simple architectural changes make the difference between independent living and institutionalization.

9.2.9. Geriatric Dentistry

Dental health impacts greatly on one's general health, with implications both for the patient's nutritional status and psychosocial functioning (e.g., impaired self-image in the edentulous patient may result in isolation), among other factors.

Although regular dental evaluation is required, elderly patients on fixed incomes are often unable to afford routine dental follow-up visits. Medicare coverage does not reimburse for dental expenses. Even those elderly with private insurance often have only limited dental care coverage. Since elderly patients generally have much more frequent contact with their physician than with their dentist, the primary care practitioner who is interested in providing comprehensive care must assume a larger role in dental evaluation.

The extent of dental problems in the elderly population is enormous. More than 50% of people at 65 years of age are edentulous, and many require dentures but are unable to obtain them.[5,31] Patients wearing dentures require routine reevaluation, but frequently elderly patients seek dental attention only when encountering severe problems.

Chewing difficulties in the elderly may stem from several interacting forces including diminished sensation, impaired motor function, and the phenomenon of bone resorption occurring with age.[31] Increased bone resorption can change the adequacy of denture fit and adversely affect the ability to masticate. With decreased ability to chew, food preferences progressively change towards a diet consisting of soft foods. This change in dietary choice directly relates to the integrity of prosthetic fit and may profoundly compromise nutritional adequacy.

Drugs may also affect the patient's dental health. For example, drugs that reduce salivary flow through their anticholinergic side effects place the patient at high risk for developing caries and may create an uncomfortable, sometimes painful, oral environment.

The primary care practitioner should make a thorough observation of the oral cavity without dentures. The incidence of oral tumors increases with age and the practitioner should carefully examine for any obvious pathology. The dentures should be evaluated for cracks or other deficiencies. The patient should also be asked directly about denture-related problems and general dental concerns. Good dental hygiene requires removal and daily cleaning of dentures and all patients should be instructed about proper care. When the denture wearer is disabled or unable to perform dental maintenance activities independently, some assistance may be required.

9.3. Secondary Prevention

9.3.1. Introduction

As defined by the Canadian Task Force report, secondary prevention "interrupts or minimizes the progress of a disease or irreversible damage from a disease by early detection and treatment."[32] Secondary prevention involves case-finding and screening strategies to promote disease detection in asymptomatic individuals. Unfortunately, at this juncture, techniques in secondary prevention are still in their infancy. Much research is currently in progress and further studies must be done to validate current practice and guide future preventive intervention. Since certain diseases in the elderly may present atypically or with a greater prevalence, there is a need to evaluate and refine existing secondary prevention screening specifically for elderly individuals.[2]

At the present time, three major studies[32,33,34] have developed rationales for periodic health maintenance of patients over 65 years of age. The Canadian Task Force[32] is the most comprehensive and widely accepted. Currently, only a handful of secondary preventive measures have "good evidence" to support inclusion in a periodic health examination.[32,35] This indicates that ample evidence is provided "to support the recommendation that the condition be specifically considered in a periodic health exam."[32] Assessment must be based on a careful review of the existing data, risks and benefits, and cost and acceptability to the patient.[32] Although the health provider has few validated screening tests available, he/she should be atuned to discretionary inclusion of those unvalidated interventions which are relevant for individual patients. Clinical judgment must guide the practitioner when measurement validity is absent. The need for more research is painstakingly evident.[36]

9.3.2. Assessment of Psychosocial and Physical Function

Most agree that periodic screening should be done every 2 years between the ages of 65 and 74, and on an annual basis thereafter. Although only fair evidence is cited, some authors feel screening in this sphere should be accepted on faith alone. Screening may have practical clinical implications and may dictate beneficial interventions as well.

In an assessment of psychosocial function of the elderly, the health provider may inquire about the following: social support structures, family relationships (including parent abuse), recent losses, financial pressures, housing/environmental status, alcohol use, medication use/abuse, affective wellness, and sleeping patterns. Lack of update or awareness on a wide variety of issues may prevent comprehensive geriatric care.

An assessment of physical function especially relevant for older adults includes the following: (1) activities of daily living (adequacy of performance); (2)

environmental limitations (is the patient still able to negotiate the four story walk-up?); (3) mobility; (4) dizziness or other abnormal neurological symptoms or signs; (5) changes in vision or hearing; (6) chest pain or other cardiovascular complaints; (7) ability to chew, denture fit, appetite, weight loss, change in bowel habits, blood in rectum, melena; (8) dysuria, hesitancy, polyuria, impotence, incontinence; (9) vaginal bleeding; (10) status of feet; (11) claudication; (12) mental status; (13) dyspnea; and (14) nutritional adequacy.

Recommendations for physical examination procedures and laboratory tests to be used as secondary preventive strategies are shown in Table I.

9.4. Tertiary Prevention

9.4.1. General Rehabilitation for the Geriatric Patient

An understanding of the concepts of rehabilitation medicine and the ability to implement these principles is essential for providing comprehensive geriatric care, both in the inpatient and the ambulatory care settings. The principles of rehabilitation usually are not well developed in the general practitioner's armamentarium of skills; this may be linked to the almost total omission of this branch of medicine in medical school training. The multidisciplinary approach inherent in the practice of rehabilitation medicine is prototypic of what primary care geriatric medicine emcompasses, namely input from many different fields in a team effort, with the goal of offering much more to the patient than any one physician would be able to provide individually.[37] Traditionally, the physician has been trained to function as an individual with little or no input from other health professionals. In both geriatric and rehabilitation medicine, the health care team approach is essential for the provision of optimal and coordinated care.

A rehabilitative medicine approach is applicable both to the elderly patient recovering from a stroke and to the elderly patient who is temporarily ill with a resultant weakness. Acute illness may require substantial rehabilitative efforts to restore function to the level antecedent the illness.

The goals of rehabilitative practice in the elderly are quite different from the expectations for rehabilitative intervention in the young. In the young patient, the goal is usually to attain full prior-to-illness function with the expectation of return to employment. Of course, the hope exists for return to optimal functional status in the elderly patient as well; however, the main aspiration is to maintain independent functioning.

Special problems may arise in the rehabilitation process in an elderly patient that can significantly affect outcome.[37] Stumbling blocks to effective rehabilitation outcome include the level of intellectual and perceptual awareness of the patient, the extent of multi-organ system involvement which can restrict rehabilitative intervention (e.g., the degree of cardiac dysfunction may limit the level of ambu-

Table I.   Physical Examination and Laboratory Tests in Secondary Prevention

	Recommendation
1. Skin	Assess for basal cell and squamous cell carcinomas on a discretionary basis.
2. Breasts	Good evidence exists for a full exam and annual mammogram in women 50–59 years of age. The American Cancer Society recommends yearly mammograms for women over age 65.
3. Cardiovascular	Good evidence exists for checking blood pressure specifically at least every 2 years; measurements should be taken at every visit made for other reasons. ECG is discretionary, but may be an extremely useful baseline for future reference.
4. Pulmonary	There is no evidence for the validity of chest X ray as a screen. PPD testing has good evidence for inclusion in high-risk individuals. Even though prophylactic measures are limited because of potential INH toxicity in this age group, reactivation of TB is primarily a disease of the elderly and knowledge of PPD reactivity is useful.
5. Gastrointestinal	Mouth: There is good evidence to include an examination for dental caries on an annual basis and a dental X ray, if indicated. Although there is an increased incidence of oral cancer with increasing age, an exam for oral cancer is not yet a valid screen. Colon and rectum: Only fair evidence exists for inclusion of a stool guaiac on an annual basis. Rectal examination is discretionary.
6. Endocrine	Thyroid function testing is discretionary; but occult thyroid disease in the elderly should be considered.
7. Genitourinary	Discretionary assessment of prostate size and character. Use of urine cytology is discretionary in high-risk patients. No good evidence for inclusion of urinalysis in the asymptomatic individual. Discretionary use of VDRL is recommended.
8. Gynecologic	Discretionary use of Pap smear in high-risk groups, i.e., women over 59 years, is recommended.
9. Neurologic	None of the following procedures is validated, but they can be included on a discretionary basis: assessment of coordination, ability to walk, muscular strength; full assessment of vision and hearing; assessment of mental status (if evidence of dementia, look for reversible component).
10. Immunizations	There is good evidence for giving a pneumovax every 5 years. There is good evidence for giving a flu vaccine every year in patients without an egg allergy. There is good evidence for giving a diphtheria/tetanus vaccine with a booster injection of toxoid every 10 years with diphtheria vaccination optional. This should be given only to patients in good health.

lation), and the motivation of the participating patient. This last factor probably has the most profound effect on outcome. A patient's rehabilitative potential must be thoroughly assessed prior to accepting a patient for extensive rehabilitation.[38]

The initial assessment of a candidate for rehabilitation must include an evaluation of functional capacity and psychological readiness for therapeutic intervention. When functional evaluation is complete, the type and extent of disability can be determined. Disabilities range in severity from: (1) temporary loss of function with expectation of complete return of function (e.g., resolved weakness after pneumonia) to (2) a permanent impairment where the loss of function remains, but function can be promoted by rehabilitative measures (e.g., use of an artificial limb after amputation) to (3) a progressive type of disability where the loss of function occurs over time with little opportunity for functional restoration (e.g., slowly dymelinating neurological disorder).[39] The particular disability and the stage at which the impairment is being evaluated will determine the rehabilitative approach and outcome.

The ability of the primary care practitioner to perform a functional assessment can be extraordinarily important in prevention for the geriatric patient. Gresham[37] addresses the need for close collaboration between the primary care practitioner and the physiatrist. A primary care practitioner should perform frequent functional assessments so that diminished function can be recognized early on and appropriate rehabilitative intervention implemented prior to significant loss of function. To enable the generalist to recognize a change in functional capacity, Gresham endorses the Barthel index[37,40] as an effective evaluative instrument providing an objective systematic index of physical function. This approach to assessment is far superior to the narrative accounts generally found in medical charts.

9.4.1.1. Preventive Aspects of Rehabilitation

9.4.1.1a. Prevention of Contractures. Primary care physicians must be particularly careful to guard against contractures. The preventive approach entails careful positioning of patients and passive range of motion exercising in paralyzed extremities. The placement of a footboard is also essential to prevent footdrop.[41]

9.4.1.1b. Prevention of Respiratory Complications. Prolonged periods of immobilization may lead to congestion at the lung bases and an increased susceptibility to pulmonary infection and other complications. To prevent such developments, the physician should request regular deep-breathing exercises which allow for adequate basilar aeration. Regular coughing and frequent change of position is also beneficial.

9.4.1.1c. Prevention of Decubitus Ulcers. Although there is a great need for early mobilization in the elderly, a balance must be reached between the longer time often required for healing in the elderly and the active initiation of rehabilitative activities. Once again, careful positioning and daily care can help prevent decubiti.

9.4.1.2. Potential Problems with Rehabilitating the Elderly

The health practitioner should be aware of several pitfalls in rehabilitating the elderly patient.[38,42] The geriatric patient often has decreased sensory awareness. If heat is used as a treatment modality, there must be an awareness of the potential for burning patients without their knowledge (this can also occur with ultrasound). There also should be an awareness that immersion into a hot tub may place increased stress on the cardiovascular system potentially leading to hypotension and syncope. One must be aware that heat applied to a patient with metal implants can radiate excessively and harm adjacent tissue. Another potential hazard involves the application of heat in the presence of occlusive peripheral vascular disease. If one is referring a patient with a pacemaker to rehabilitation, the physiatrist must be notified as shortwave and microwave heating devices may cause significant problems. Passive range of movement exercise must be done cautiously to avoid trauma or bleeding in or around the joint. The risk of damaging a joint is further increased by the frequent presence of impaired sensation.[38]

Rehabilitation medicine must also address the need for environment to facilitate optimal functioning. Minor changes in the environmental architecture can clearly maximize independent function. Architectural barriers to function are described elsewhere in this chapter (see 9.2.8.).

9.4.2. Cardiac Rehabilitation

For the postmyocardial infarction, patient appropriate rehabilitation can decrease disability and help restore function. Wenger[43] describes in detail the rehabilitation responsibilities necessary in caring for the coronary patient. Tasks involved include: initial functional assessment, prescription for appropriate interventions to increase functioning, monitoring of interventions, and continuing re-evaluation.[43]

After myocardial infarctions uncomplicated by congestive heart failure, ectopy, hypotension, or recurrent chest pain, all patients are candidates for early ambulation. In the not-too-distant past, prolonged bedrest was prescribed for all coronary patients. However, it is now clear that early ambulation has many positive features including the prevention of deconditioning that occurs with extended bedrest, muscle disuse, and a decreased incidence of thrombotic complications, and a significant psychological effect with decreased feelings of anxiety, depression, and helplessness.[43] In addition, no increase of complications secondary to the initiation of early ambulatory activity has been reported.

While still in the coronary care unit, the patient with an uncomplicated myocardial infarction should be allowed to participate in various self-care activities. The patient should begin feeding himself, using the bedside commode, sitting in bed with feet dangling, and gradually advance to sitting in a chair. In order to maintain muscular tone and joint flexibility, low-level arm and leg exercise should be started early. Limited activity such as sitting in a chair several times daily may prevent the development of orthostatic symptoms expected to occur after prolonged bedrest.[43] These self-care activities may offer important psychological support to patients suffering from this emotionally traumatic experience. Patients must realize that independent functioning is still possible.

After leaving the coronary care unit, the goal of in-hospital rehabilitation is to reach an activity level that approximates the level required for the performance of normal activities within the home. Under the careful monitoring of the cardiac rehabilitation therapist, patients should continue with self-care activities and progressively add arm, leg, and trunk exercises. With supervision, the level of activity can be gradually increased. Patients who will have steps to negotiate at home should receive special instruction, with gradual increase in duration and intensity. Prior to discharge, activity plans should be extensively discussed with patients and their families. Patient education and family education are a major component of the rehabilitation process. A discussion of risk factors associated with coronary heart disease should be addressed (i.e., smoking and obesity). The drugs prescribed to the patient should be discussed in detail—the purpose of the medication and possible side effects should be included. For example, a patient discharged with a prescription for nitroglycerin should realize that a severe headache may develop after taking this medication. A discussion outlining the reasons behind initial activity restrictions and an estimate of when progressive activities may be undertaken is useful. It is also important that patients involved in an exercise regimen be able to evaluate their response to a given exercise by taking their pulse and restricting it to below that previously prescribed. Chest pain, palpitations, shortness of breath, and a heart rate greater than that prescribed by the physician are important warning signs for the patient. Should any of these occur, the patient should be instructed to notify his/her physician immediately.

Once the immediate hospitalization period is over and daily activity level requirements are met without difficulty, cardiac rehabilitation in the form of exercise training is of benefit. It must be made quite clear that although exercise training may produce favorable psychological benefits, enable earlier return to work, improve oxygen uptake, and improve myocardial function by reducing oxygen requirements for a given work load, exercise training probably does not increase coronary collaterals or affect recurrence rate and survival.[44] Once at home, patients should continue with the regimen instituted in the hospital and gradually increase distance and intensity of walking as prescribed. Generally, patients who can walk 3 to 3½ miles comfortably will be able to easily perform the tasks of most sedentary work.[43] After myocardial infarction, low-level stress testing is often prognostically important. Later, a full exercise test may be helpful in evaluating the response and safety of a particular exercise prescription. Sexual activity can be resumed when other features of daily living are well integrated into the patient's life. Patients should be encouraged to participate as tolerated in activities such as jogging, swimming, running, walking and bicycling which exercise the large muscle groups. The desired objective is to "train," whereby there is a reduction in myocardial oxygen demand for a given amount of submaximal work, systolic blood pressure, and heart rate.[43,44] Training programs for coronary patients can reduce the threshold for anginal symptoms and may result in a markedly improved oxygen uptake by as much as 20%. In addition, patients participating in a training program tend to develop an improved sense of self-esteem and frequently a strong motivation to reduce other coronary risk factors as well.[44]

9.4.3. Pulmonary Rehabilitation

Since chronic obstructive pulmonary disease (COPD) is prominent in the geriatric population and the level of morbidity is profound, tertiary prevention is an important part of primary care (see Chapter 2). The limiting symptoms of COPD often manifest in the fifth and sixth decades of life.[45] The development of increased physical limitations such as breathlessness on exertion and at rest and the increased numbers of hospitalizations that may be required may have significant emotional implications for the patient. There is a high prevalence of depression and anxiety in COPD patients.[46]

The goals of pulmonary rehabilitation are very similar to those outlined for cardiac rehabilitation. Tertiary preventive goals include maximizing function and making the patient as comfortable as possible within the confines of the underlying disease process. Patients should be able to: (1) recognize signs of decompensation and be aware of how to proceed when there is a change in medical status; (2) understand the goals and techniques of pulmonary hygiene and its individualized application; and (3) participate, if feasible, in a pulmonary rehabilitation program with the goal of augmenting exercise capacity and general endurance. Implicit in all of the above measures is a high degree of patient motivation.

The importance of early treatment of infection is often emphasized in patients with chronic pulmonary diseases. Although it is difficult to prove that early antibiotic intervention lessens morbidity, most practitioners find that there is an advantage to such intervention in many cases. Patients should be clearly informed of symptoms and signs which may signal decompensation of respiratory status. McDonald and Hudson[45] succinctly outline the most salient of these features: (1) change in sputum color or character; (2) increased shortness of breath; (3) weight gain; (4) increased edema; (5) drowsiness; and (6) confusion or other behavioral changes. Reliable patients who have been taught to recognize symptoms consistent with acute bacterial bronchitis may be directed to initiate antibiotic therapy independently. The physician should be informed when antibiotic therapy is initiated.

All patients with COPD should be informed that smoking is hazardous and especially so once one has contracted severe pulmonary problems. The patient must realize that discontinuing the smoking habit is highly relevant to tertiary prevention. Smoke as well as other environmental pollutants act as irritants and enhance sputum production and ultimately may compromise respiratory reserve. Effective bronchial hygiene and the termination of smoking can help in the maintenance of a stable respiratory status.[47] Use of bronchodilators, chest percussion, and postural drainage along with proper coughing techniques may all aid in the preservation of respiratory function. Secretions tend to collect during the night; appropriate pulmonary toilet prior to retiring and upon rising may be beneficial. Family members or homemakers can be instructed in percussive techniques.

It should be remembered that some patients with COPD have unexpected reversibility of obstruction with the use of bronchodilator therapy. Many authors agree that every COPD patient deserves a trial of bronchodilators.[45-47] The role of steroid therapy is more controversial, however. A trial of steroids may be useful in patients showing only limited response to bronchodilator therapy or in those with severe restrictions in activities of daily living.[48] Hudson stresses the need for objective data via spirometry to measure the physiologic response to steroids during a trial period before steroid therapy is given on a chronic basis.[48]

The importance of physical fitness cannot be emphasized enough in patients with COPD. Although patients who undergo endurance training may not necessarily have objectively improved pulmonary function tests, the benefits of such training, i.e., improved endurance, better sleep, and improved energy conservation, are impressive.[48] Patients seem to feel better after exercise training. Their improved psychologic status and heightened performance of the activities of daily living add substantially to their quality of life. Even if the patient does not participate in a full program of pulmonary rehabilitation, all patients should learn to incorporate the technique of pursed-lip breathing. This technique allows for an extended expiratory phase and is helpful in alleviating the anxiety induced by increased dyspnea.[48]

Sedatives and antidepressants must be prescribed with caution to chronic pulmonary patients. These medications can further depress respiratory function and produce serious changes in mental status and other unhealthy side effects.

Patient and family education play an important role in pulmonary rehabilitation. The negative psychological sequelae of COPD can be reduced with support from the patient's family. Additionally, sympathetic attention by the primary care practitioner can also be of benefit.

9.5. Summary

The number of elderly is increasing at a rapid rate. Although the population as a whole will double in the next 35 years, the population over age 65 will double in only 30 years, and those over the age of 75 will increase at an even faster rate. With socioeconomic advances, more and more people are living to the mean maximum life span of the human species, i.e., 100 to 110 years. This phenomenon has been referred to as the "rectangularization" of society. Despite this apparent increase in longevity, the finite maximum life-span of 100 to 110 years has not changed. In fact, computer specialists tell us that even if medical advancements lead to the conquering of cancer, heart disease, and stroke, mankind's mean maximum life span will still not change; only more people will live to this finite point. It is essential, therefore, that the health care provider work to improve one's quality of life for as long as one lives.

Prevention can play a major role in minimizing some of the normal processes of aging which eventually lead to degenerative disorders. One does not have to be a geriatrician to realize that it is normal for joint cartilage to undergo changes with age; excess body weight may lead to a more rapid decline in normal joint function. Although certain aspects of preventive health (in this case, weight loss) will not prevent the normal processes of aging, preventive health care can play a major role in the maintenance of optimal functioning and independence. This may lead to improved quality of life and the prevention of premature physiological aging.

In addition, practicing good preventive health care can minimize the effects of harmful environmental factors, that due to prolonged length of exposure as one ages or changes in biological defense with age, may lead to significant health risks.

By approaching the elderly person holistically, with attention to psychosocial as well as physiological needs, an optimal quality of life can be best maintained. The health provider should be familiar with aspects of primary, secondary, and tertiary prevention and seek to include these in his/her clinical practice.

References

1. Greene, M. G., 1981, *The Physician-Patient Relationship in Three Medical Primary Care Settings,* Unpublished doctoral dissertation, Columbia University, New York, pp. 50–56.
2. Johnson, J. J. and Pawlson, L. G., 1981, Health maintenance, in: *Eldercare* (M. O'Hara-Devereaux, L. H. Andrus, and C. D. Scott, eds.), Grune and Stratton, Inc., New York, pp. 293–306.
3. Barberis, M., 1981, America's elderly: Policy implications, *Pop. Bull.* 35:2–13.
4. Somers, A. R., 1980, Demographics can help guide health policy, *Hospitals* 54:67–82.
5. Elkowitz, E. B., 1981, Gastrointestinal and related disorders, in: *Geriatric Medicine for the Primary Care Practitioner* (E. B. Elkowitz, ed.), Springer Publishing Company, New York, pp. 98–110.
6. Sherman, F. T. and Libow, L. S., 1981, Pharmacology and medication, in: *The Core of Geriatric Medicine* (L. S. Libow and F. T. Sherman, eds.), C. V. Mosby Company, St. Louis, pp. 92–126.
7. Foley, C. J., Libow, L. S., and Sherman, F. T., 1981, Clinical aspects of nutrition, in: *The Core of Geriatric Medicine* (L. S. Libow and F. T. Sherman, eds.), C. V. Mosby Company, St. Louis, pp. 280–304.

8. Moolten, S. E., 1981, Nutrition in the elderly, in: *The Geriatric Imperative* (A. R. Somers and D. R. Fabian, eds.), Appleton-Century-Crofts, New York, pp. 205–217.

9. Naughton, J., 1982, Physical activity and aging, *Prim. Care* 9:231–238.

10. deVries, H. A., 1977, Physiology of physical conditioning for the elderly, in: *Guide to Fitness After Fifty* (R. Harris, L. J. Frankel, and S. Harris, eds.), Plenum Press, New York, pp. 47–52.

11. deVries, H. A., 1979, Tips on prescribing exercise regimens for your older patient, *Geriatrics* 34:75–81.

12. Hellerstein, H. K., and Franklin, B. A., 1978, Exercise-testing and prescription, in: *Rehabilitation of the Coronary Patient* (N. K. Wenger, and H. K. Hellerstein, eds.), John Wiley and Sons, New York, pp. 149–202.

13. Glick, S. M., 1976, Preventive medicine in geriatrics, *Med. Clin. N. Am.* 60:1325–1332.

14. Poe, W. D. and Holloway, D. A., 1980, How drugs work, in: *Drugs and the Aged* (W. D. Poe and D. A. Holloway, eds.), McGraw-Hill Book Company, New York, pp. 14–24.

15. Ward, M. and Blatman, M., 1979, Drug therapy in the elderly, *Am. Fam. Prac.* 19:143–152.

16. Hollister, L. E., 1981, Prescribing drugs for the elderly patient, in: *Management of Common Problems in Geriatric Medicine* (F. G. Ebaugh, Jr., ed.), Addison-Wesley Publishing Company, California, pp. 82–102.

17. Vestal, R. E., 1978, Drug use in the elderly: A review of problems and special considerations, *Drugs* 16:358–382.

18. Butler, R. and Lewis, M., 1977, *Aging and Mental Health,* C. V. Mosby Company, St. Louis.

19. Kopell, B. S., 1981, The management of depression in the elderly patient, in: *Management of Common Problems in Geriatric Medicine* (F. G. Ebaugh, Jr., ed.), Addison-Wesley Publishing Company, California, pp. 118–138.

20. Gurian, B., 1982, Mental health outreach and consultation services for the elderly, *Hosp. Commun. Psych.* 33:142–147.

21. Gaitz, C. M. and Varner, R. V., 1980, Preventive aspects of mental illness in late life, in: *Handbook of Mental Health and Aging* (J. Birren and B. Sloane, eds.), Prentice-Hall, Inc., New Jersey, pp. 959–970.

22. Information Exchange, 1982, *Service Center for Aging Information,* InterAmerica Research Associates, Inc., Virginia, pp. 1–6.

23. Rosin, A. J. and Glatt, M. M. 1971, Alcohol excess in the elderly, *Q. J. Stud. Alcohol* 32:53–59.

24. Zimberg, S., 1978, Diagnosis and treatment of the elderly alcoholic, *Alcoholism: Clin. Exp. Res.* 2:27–29.

25. Pattee, J. J., 1982, Uncovering the elderly "hidden" alcoholic, *Geriatrics* 37:145–146.

26. Zimberg, S., 1974, The elderly alcoholic, *Gerontologist* 14:221–224.

27. Kurtz, K. J., 1982, Hypothermia in the elderly: The cold facts, *Geriatrics* 37:85–93.

28. Applegate, W. B., and Runyan, J. W. Jr., Brasfield, L., Williams, M. L., Konigsberg, C., and Fouche, C., 1981, Analysis of the 1980 heat wave in Memphis, *J. Am. Geriat. Soc.* 29:337–342.

29. Wheeler, M., 1976, Heat stroke in the elderly, *Med. Clin. N. Am.* 60:1289–1296.
30. Overstall, P. W., 1978, Falls in the elderly: Epidemiology, aetiology and management, in: *Recent Advances in Geriatric Medicine* (B. Isaacs, ed.), Churchill Livingstone, New York, pp. 61–72.
31. Chauncey, H. H. and House, J. D., 1978, Dental Problems, in: *The Geriatric Patient* (W. Reichel, ed.), H. P. Publishing Company, New York, pp. 166–171.
32. Spitzer, W. O., 1979, Report of the task force on the periodic health examination, *Can. Med. Assoc. J.* 121:1193–1254.
33. Frame, P. S., and Carlson, S. J., 1975, A critical review of periodic health screening using specific screening criteria, *J. Fam. Prac.* 2:29–36, 123–129, 189–194, 283–289.
34. Breslow, L., and Somers, A. R., 1977, The life-time health-monitoring program: A practice approach to preventive medicine. *N. Eng. J. Med.* 296:601–608.
35. Sackett, D. L., 1982, Preventive geriatric medicine, *Prim. Care* 9:3–6.
36. Charap, M. H., 1981, The periodic health examination: Genesis of a myth, *Ann. Int. Med.* 95:733–735.
37. Gresham, G. E., 1982, Rehabilitation of the geriatric patient: Stroke rehabilitation, the rehabilitation team, and the usefulness of functional assessment, *Prim. Care* 9:239–247.
38. Hunt, T. E., 1978, Rehabilitation of the elderly, in: *The Geriatric Patient* (W. Reichel, ed.), H. P. Publishing Company, Inc., New York, pp. 172–180.
39. Birchenall, J. and Streight, M., 1973, Restorative nursing, in: *Care of the Older Adult* (J. Birchenall and M. Streight, eds.), J. B. Lippincott Company, New York, pp. 62–79.
40. Granger, C. V. Albrecht, G. L., and Hamilton, B. B., 1979, Outcome of comprehensive medical rehabilitation: Measurement by PULSES profile and the Barthel index, *Arch. Phys. Med. Rehab.* 60:145–154.
41. Vallarino R. and Sherman, F. T., 1981, Stroke, fractured hip, amputation, pressure sores and incontinence: Principles of rehabilitation treatment, in *The Core of Geriatric Medicine* (L. S. Libow and F. T. Sherman, eds.), C. V. Mosby Company, St. Louis, pp. 127–168.
42. Tobis, J. S., 1979, Rehabilitation of the geriatric patient, in: *Clinical Geriatrics* (I. Rossman, ed.), J. B. Lippincott, New York, pp. 502–515.
43. Wenger, N., 1981, Rehabilitation of the coronary patient: Scope of the problem and responsibility of the primary care physician, *Cardiovasc. Rev. Rep.* 12:1249–1261.
44. Rechnitzer, P. A., 1982, Specific benefits of postcoronary exercise programs, *Geriatrics* 37:47–51.
45. McDonald, G. J. and Hudson, L. D., 1982, Important aspects of pulmonary rehabilitation, *Geriatrics* 37:127–134.
46. Dudley, D. L., Glaser, E. M., Jorgenson, B. N., and Logan, D. L., 1980, Psychosocial concomitants to rehabilitation in chronic obstructive pulmonary disease, *Chest* 77:413–420, 544–551, 677–684.
47. Reichel, J., 1978, Pulmonary problems in the elderly, in: *Clinical Aspects of Aging* (W. Reichel, ed.), Williams and Wilkins, Maryland, pp. 85–89.
48. Hudson, L. D., and Pierson, D., 1981, Comprehensive respiratory care for patients with chronic obstructive pulmonary disease, *Med. Clin. N. Am.* 65:629–643.

Index